WEEDON'S
SKIN PATHOLOGY
ESSENTIALS

RONALD B. JOHNSTON MD

Colonel, USAF
Chief of Dermatology
Eglin AFB, Florida, USA
and
Affiliate Assistant Professor
Department of Dermatology and Cutaneous Surgery
University of South Florida College of Medicine
Tampa, Florida, USA

For additional online content visit expertconsult.com

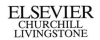

ELSEVIER
CHURCHILL
LIVINGSTONE

CHURCHILL LIVINGSTONE an imprint of Elsevier Limited

Notices

Knowledge and best practice in this field are constantly changing. As new research and experience broaden our understanding, changes in research methods, professional practices, or medical treatment may become necessary.

Practitioners and researchers must always rely on their own experience and knowledge in evaluating and using any information, methods, compounds, or experiments described herein. In using such information or methods they should be mindful of their own safety and the safety of others, including parties for whom they have a professional responsibility.

With respect to any drug or pharmaceutical products identified, readers are advised to check the most current information provided (i) on procedures featured or (ii) by the manufacturer of each product to be administered, to verify the recommended dose or formula, the method and duration of administration, and contraindications. It is the responsibility of practitioners, relying on their own experience and knowledge of their patients, to make diagnoses, to determine dosages and the best treatment for each individual patient, and to take all appropriate safety precautions.

To the fullest extent of the law, neither the Publisher nor the authors, contributors, or editors, assume any liability for any injury and/or damage to persons or property as a matter of products liability, negligence or otherwise, or from any use or operation of any methods, products, instructions, or ideas contained in the material herein.

Churchill Livingstone

ISBN: 978-0-7020-3574-6

Printed in Spain

Last digit is the print number: 9 8 7 6 5 4 3 2 1

WEEDON'S
SKIN PATHOLOGY
ESSENTIALS

For Elsevier
Commissioning Editor: *Michael Houston*
Development Editor: *Louise Cook*
Project Manager: *Elouise Ball*
Design: *Kirsteen Wright*
Illustration Manager: *Merlyn Harvey*
Marketing Manager (UK/USA): *Gaynor Jones/Tracie Pasker*

Contents

v

Preface

During my career as a fighter pilot and then a pilot-physician, checklists were an integral part of procedures and flying. Similarly, this book was created as a study guide, review book, rapid reference and microscope "wingman". *Weedon's Skin Pathology Essentials* indicates the classic features, both clinically and histologically, including numerous photographs of each side-by-side. Additionally, genetic defects, classic treatments, commonly associated disorders and "memory joggers" were included to assist in remembering the vast amount of information.

As a result, this book describes the more common location and appearance, and not every variation or possibility is described. Thus, to complement this book, it is designed for use in conjunction with the primary reference *Weedon's Skin Pathology*. Enjoy my dermatologist's "checklist"!

Ronald "R.J." Johnston

"Check six"

F-15C Pilot-Physician/Dermatologist

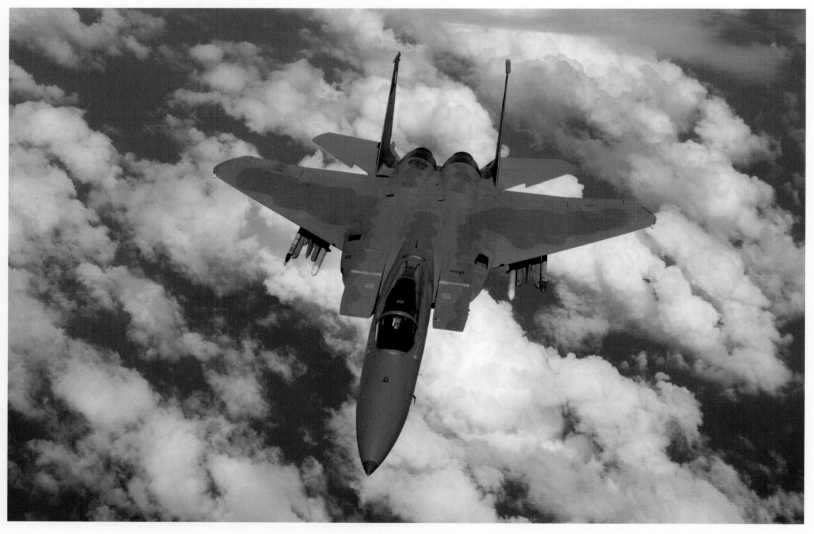

Photo of the author preparing to air-to-air refuel off a tanker.

Dedication

A special thank you to my wife, Christy, and our son, Gage, for all your support
and encouragement during this endeavour.

Love,

R.J.

(Dad)

Acknowledgments

Special thanks to the following individuals and organizations for their support and/or use of images and pathology slides (alphabetical order):

- Brooke Taylor Baldwin, MD, Dermatologist, Tampa, FL
- Carlos Canton, DermPath Diagnostics, Miami, FL
- Ann A. Church, MD, Departments of Dermatopathology and Dermatology, University of Florida, Gainesville, FL
- Christopher P. Crotty, MD, Orlando, FL
- Department of Dermatopathology, University of Florida, Gainesville, FL
- Department of Dermatology and Cutaneous Surgery, University of South Florida, Tampa, FL
- L. Frank Glass, MD, University of South Florida, Tampa, FL
- Ricardo J. Gonzalez, MD, Sarcoma and Cutaneous Department, H. Lee Moffitt Cancer Center and Research Institute, Tampa, FL
- John N. Greene, MD, Division of Infectious Diseases and Tropical Medicine, H. Lee Moffitt Cancer Center and Research Institute, Tampa, FL
- Ronald Johnston, Colonel (Ret.), USAF, Destin, FL
- Tim McCardle, MD, H. Lee Moffitt Cancer Center and Research Institute, Tampa, FL
- J.D. Morgan, MD, Capt. (Ret.), USMSN, private practice, Lake Wales, FL
- Michael Morgan, MD, Professor Pathology USFCOM, Clinical Professor Dermatology UFCOM, MSUCOM, Managing Director, Bay Area Dermatology, Tampa, FL
- Jonathan Newberry, MD, Capt., USAF, Department of Pathology, Eglin AFB, FL
- Carlos H. Nousari, MD, Institute for Immunofluorescence, Pompano Beach, FL (DIF, salt-split, scalded skin H & E and clinical PNP images provided courtesy of Dr Nousari)
- David A. Riggs, Col (ret), D.O., AAFP, USAFP, 96th Medical Group, Eglin AFB, FL
- Lubomir Sokol, MD, PhD, Department of Malignant Hematology, Moffitt Cancer Center and Research Institute, Tampa, FL
- Donald R. Stranahan, MD, Easton Dermatology Associates, Easton, MB
- Isabel C. Valencia, MD, Dermpath Diagnostics, Tampa, FL
- Vladimir Vincek, MD, PhD, Director of Dermatopathology, University of Florida, Gainesville, FL

Further reading

Weedon, D. *Weedon's Skin Pathology*, 3rd edition. 2009.

Bolognia, JL, Jorizzo, JL, Rapini, RP. *Dermatology*, 2nd edition. 2008.

McKee, PH, Calonje, E, Granter, SR. *Pathology of the Skin*, 3rd edition. 2005.

Spitz, JL. *Genodermatoses: A Clinical Guide to Genetic Skin Disorders*, 2nd edition. 2005.

The Basics

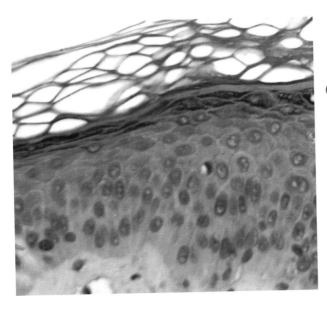

Stratum corneum
(horny layer)

Stratum lucidum
(clear layer, palms/soles)

Stratum granulosum
(granular layer)

Stratum spinosum
(spiny layer)

Stratum basale
(basal layer)

Name	Key Features	Clinical Example	Histopathology
Major tissue reaction patterns			
Lichenoid	• Epidermal basal cell damage ("interface dermatitis") • Band-like infiltrate of inflammatory cells in superficial dermis, pigment incontinence; Civatte bodies (shrunken, eosinophilic, degenerating basal cells)	• Lichen planus • Lichen nitidus • Vitiligo • Erythema multiforme	 Lichen planus
Psoriasiform	• Epidermal hyperplasia, rete ridge elongation uniformly, regular acanthosis ("squirting dermal papilla")	• Psoriasis • Lichen simplex chronicus • Mycosis fungoides • Pityriasis rosea	 Psoriasis

Spongiotic	• Intraepidermal intercellular edema	• Pityriasis rosea
		• Bullous pemphigus
		• Atopic dermatitis
		• Contact dermatitis
		• Five patterns:
		  1. Neutrophilic
		  2. Eosinophilic
		  3. Miliarial (acrosyringial)
		  4. Follicular
		  5. Haphazard
			
			Allergic contact dermatitis

Vesiculobullous	• Blistering within or beneath epidermis or at DE junction
	• Assess:
	  1. Level of split
	  2. Underlying mechanism
	  3. Nature of inflammatory cells in dermis
		• Pemphigus vulgaris
		• Impetigo
		• Epidermolysis bullosa
			
			Pemphigus vulgaris

Name	Key Features	Clinical Example	Histopathology
Granulomatous	• Chronic granulomatous inflammation • Aggregate of histiocytes	• Granuloma annulare • Tuberculosis • Types: 　1. Epithelioid 　　a. sarcoidal 　　b. tuberculoid 　2. Palisading = necrobiotic 　3. Mixed cells 　　a. suppurative 　　b. foreign body	 Granuloma annulare
Vasculopathic	• Pathological changes in cutaneous blood vessels • Vasculitis: 　1. Infiltrate in vessel wall 　2. Fibrin deposition 　3. Endothelial necrosis	• Leukocytoclastic vasculitis • Granuloma faciale • TTP • Sweet's syndrome • Herpes zoster	 Leukocytoclastic vasculitis

Minor tissue reaction patterns

Name	Key Features	Clinical Example	Histopathology
Epidermolytic hyperkeratosis	• Hyperkeratosis with granular and vacuolar degeneration	• Epidermolytic hyperkeratosis • Bullous ichthyosiform erythroderma • Palmar–plantar keratoderma	 Epidermolytic hyperkeratosis
Acantholytic dyskeratosis	• Suprabasilar clefts with acantholytic/dyskeratotic cells	• Darier's disease • Grover's disease • Solar keratosis	 Darier's disease

Name	Key Features	Clinical Example	Histopathology
Cornoid lamellation	• Column of parakeratotic cells with absence of underlying granular layer	• Porokeratosis	 Porokeratosis
Papillomatosis	• "Church-spire" • Undulations and protrusions of epidermis with a fibrovascular core	• Seborrheic keratosis • Acrokeratosis verruciformis • Solar keratosis	 Acrokeratosis verruciformis of Hopf
Angiofibromas	• Increased dermal vessels with surrounding fibrosis	• Periungual fibroma • Pearly penile papules • Adenoma sebaceum (tuberous sclerosis)	 Pearly penile papule
Eosinophilic cellulitis with possible "flame figures"	• Dermal eosinophils and eosinophilic material adherent to collagen bundles	• Wells' syndrome • Arthropod reaction • Parasitic infection • Bullous pemphigoid	 "Flame figure" in Wells' syndrome
Transepithelial elimination	• Elimination of material via the epidermis or hair follicles ("epidermal vacuum cleaner")	• "Black heel" (calcaneal petechiae or talon noir) • Necrobiotic xanthogranuloma	 Talon noir Calcinosis cutis

Patterns of inflammation	1. Superficial perivascular inflammation:
	   • If without spongiosis or other reaction = drug reaction, viral exanthems, chronic urticaria
	2. Superficial and deep dermal inflammation
	3. Folliculitis and perifolliculitis
	4. Panniculitis:
	   • Categories = septal panniculitis, lobular panniculitis, panniculitis secondary vasculitis involving large vessels		

Name	Predilection and Key Clinical Features	Histopathology
Basic epidermal descriptions		
Acanthosis	• Thickening of the epidermis resulting in papules/plaques (thickened malpighian or spinous layer)	
Parakeratosis	• Retention of nuclei in stratum corneum	
Orthokeratosis	• Formation of a thick, anuclear, keratin layer • Hyperkeratosis without parakeratosis (hyperkeratosis = thickened stratum corneum)	
Grenz zone	• Narrow area of uninvolved dermis between the epidermis and a dermal inflammatory or neoplastic infiltrate	 Granuloma faciale with grenz zone

Name	Predilection and Key Clinical Features	Histopathology
Types of white blood cells and complement system		

Neutrophils	• Multilobed nucleus (up to 5 lobes), pink cytoplasm, "fragmented" appearance
	• Circulating cells (motile and free to migrate)
	• 2 weeks to mature in bone marrow; half-life 6–7 hours
	• Stimulated by IL-3, IL-6, GM-CSF
	• Three types of granules:
	  1. Primary (20%) = myeloperoxidase, peroxidase
	  2. Secondary (80%) = lysozyme, lactoferrin
	  3. Tertiary = gelatinase (degrades collagen)
		Examples: Sweet's syndrome, Chediak–Higashi syndrome, chronic granulomatous disease

Eosinophils	• Bilobed nucleus (up to 3 lobes), eosinophilic with granules • 2–6 days to mature in bone marrow • Recruited by IL-4/stimulated by IL-5 • Attracted by RANTES • Fx = engulf and kill bacteria, parasites	*Examples:* Wells' syndrome, Schulman's syndrome, Kimura's disease, granuloma faciale
Basophils	• Large purple granules • Stimulated by IL-3 • Produce IL-4 (mast cells produce also)	• Circulating in blood (related to mast cells and produce heparin/histamine)
Lymphocytes [CD45RO]	• Small, round, basophilic cells with scant cytoplasm • Lymphocytes are triggered by a specific antigen to produce antibodies (B cells), cytokines (CD4+ T cells) or cause direct cytotoxicity (CD8+ T cells) • NK cells = destroy cells • B cells = bone marrow and migrate to lymph nodes (MHC II) • T cells = bone marrow and migrate through thymus	
Monocytes	• Monocyte = largest WBC in a blood smear (can become macrophage, Langerhans cell, etc.) • Called a macrophage in tissue [CD68+]; • Not CD-1a and no Birbeck granules	• Macrophages derived from monocytes when enter tissue, large vacuolated cells (phagocytosis) • Macrophages may become epithelioid or foreign body giant cells

Name	Predilection and Key Clinical Features	Histopathology
Other cells		
Plasma cell [CD78, methyl green pyronin stains the cytoplasm red]	• Basophilic cytoplasm with eccentric nucleus, chromatin along periphery ("cartwheel" appearance) and perinuclear halo (or "hof") • Differentiate from B cells upon stimulation by CD4+ cells • Secrete antibodies	
Mast cell [CD17, CD34, toluidine blue, alcian blue, Giemsa]	• "Fried egg" appearance • Round, centrally-located nucleus, grayish granules in basophilic cytoplasm, bone marrow • Granules contain histamine and heparin • Produce IL-4 • Degranulators = NSAIDs, ASA, opiates, etc.	
Langerhans cell [CD1a, Birbeck granules] (not same as Langhans giant cell, see below)	• Immature dendritic cells found in epidermis (suprabasal) and mucosa • Bone derived, mesenchymal origin • Migrate to regional lymph nodes upon Ag capture, undergoing maturation to become antigen-presenting cell • High density = face, trunk • Low density = palm/sole, anogenital, chronic UV, age	• Reniform or "coffee-bean" nucleus (differentiates from macrophages) • EM = Birbeck granules ("tennis racket" shaped structures)
Multinucleate giant cells of granulomas	• Formed by histiocytes that fuse Types of multinucleate giant cells in granulomas: • Langhans giant cell = nuclei form horseshoe shape • Foreign body giant cell = nuclei dispersed more evenly • Touton cell = foamy cytoplasm with circular nuclei around non-foamy core	 Langhans giant cell Foreign body giant cell Touton cell

Name	Predilection and Key Clinical Features	Histopathology
Melanocyte [MITF, Melan-A]	• Neural crest derived (seen in skin at 8 weeks' gestation) • If nevi, then nucleus with pseudoinclusions (vacuoles) • Produce melanin in melanosomes, which move to keratinocytes by dendrites; synthesize tyrosinase • Basal keratinocytes: melanocytes ratio = 10:1 • Epidermal melanin unit = 1 melanocyte to 36 keratinocytes (transfer melanosomes)	• Vacuole around melanocytes that are without bridging but with a whisky appearance (dendritic processes collapsing) • E-cadherin is the main mediator of adhesion between melanocytes and keratinocytes
Merkel cell [CK20, neuron-specific enolase; TTF1 negative]	• Large oval, violet–blue cells that appear "smudgy" • Responsible for touch/mechano-reception • Normally seen at the base of rete ridges in contact with nerve receptors	 Merkel cell carcinoma Merkel cells stained with CK20
Glomus body	• The glomus body consists of an arteriovenous anastomosis surrounded by a capsule of connective tissue (dermis layer, involved in temperature regulation) • Arterial portion = Sucquet–Hoyer canal	 Glomus cells in glomangioma
Histiocyte	• Large vacuolated nucleus • Derived from bone marrow (develop into macrophage [CD-68] or dendritic, Langerhans cell [CD-1a])	

Name	Predilection and Key Clinical Features	Histopathology
Muscle	• Contraction cell	Smooth muscle Skeletal muscle
Nerve [Neuroma = S100, Bodian stain; Neurofibroma = Bodian negative]	• Whisky, delicate, fusiform nuclei • Neuroma = bundles of nerves • Neurofibroma (NF) = sheets of nerves	
Pacinian corpuscle	• A mechanoreceptor, responsible for deep pressure touch and high-frequency vibration • Located on fingers, toes, nipple, anogenital • Remember: Pacinian = P = Pressure	
Meissner corpuscle	• Receptors of low-frequency tactile stimuli; located on hairless skin • Only located on ventral side of hands and feet, near dermal papillae	

Name	Predilection and Key Clinical Features	Histopathology	
Glands			
Sebaceous gland	• Central nucleus with vacuoles in cytoplasm • In mid-dermal region, association with hair follicles; located everywhere but palms/soles • Holocrine secretion = entire cell disintegrates and releases sebum into duct • Androgen-responsive gland (i.e. hormones) • Lipid released is mainly triglycerides (50%)		*Note:* ducts of apocrine and eccrine are indistinguishable Only glandular features are different
Eccrine sweat gland	• Cuboidal coil of cells; empties onto epidermis • Numerous in the skin of the palms, soles, and forehead (not glans, clitoris, labia minora, lips, EAC) • Merocrine secretion = no part of cell is lost during secretion (reverse pinocytosis) • Innervated by cholinergic fibers (acetylcholine) • Function = heat regulation	 "Donut-shaped" tubules; pale cells	
Apocrine sweat gland	• Cells with globules in lumen; empties into infundibulum • In the axillae and in the anogenital region, usually open to pilosebaceous unit (maybe direct to surface) • Apocrine secretion = the apical portion of the cell breaks off to form part of the secretion ("decapitation") • Innervated by adrenergic fibers • Function = scent glands (pheromones)	 "Decapitation" secretion	

Name	Predilection and Key Clinical Features	Histopathology
Epidermal layers		
Layers of epidermis	1. Horny layer (stratum corneum) 2. Clear layer (stratum lucidum) – palm/soles (resist pressure) 3. Granular layer (stratum granulosum) 4. Prickle-cell layer (stratum spinosum) 5. Basal layer (stratum basale) 6. Basement membrane *Keratinocyte granules*: • Keratohyaline granules – contain loricrin (main component of cornified envelope) and profilaggrin • Odland bodies – membrane-coating granules that discharge contents into extracellular space; contain cerumides and other lipids	 • Stratum corneum (horny layer) • Stratum lucidum (clear layer, palms/soles) • Stratum granulosum (granular layer) • Stratum spinosum (spiny layer) • Stratum basale (basal layer)

2 Diagnostic Clues and "Need-to-know" Items

Name	Pearl	Comments	
Acronyms			
Painful subcutaneous nodules	• "Blue ANGEL" or "BENGAL"	• Blue = blue rubber bleb nevus syndrome (compressible, venous lesions, GI involvement possible) • A = angiolipoma/angioleiomyoma • N = neurilemmoma/schwannoma • G = glomus • E = eccrine spiradenoma ("blue balls in the dermis") • L = leiomyoma	
Pink–red papules	• "Me SPACE"	• Me = Merkel • S = Spitz nevus • P = pyogenic granuloma • A = amelanotic nevus • C = clear cell acanthoma • E = eccrine poroma	
Criteria for SLE (4 of 11)	• "SOAP BRAIN MD"	• S = serositis (pleuritis, pericarditis) • O = oral ulcers (painless) • A = arthritis • P = photosensitivity • B = blood (hemolytic anemia, leukopenia) • R = renal disorder (proteinuria, cellular casts) • A = antinuclear antibodies • I = immunologic disorder (anti-DNA, Sm or phospholipid) • N = neurological disorder (seizures, psychosis) • M = malar rash (fixed erythema, spare nasolabial) • D = discoid rash (follicular plugs, atrophic scar)	
Drug-induced SLE	• "My HIP"	• My = minocycline • H = hydralazine • I = INH • P = procainamide	• Antihistone antibodies are highly characteristic for drug-induced SLE • *Note:* penicillamine may cause a lupus-like syndrome but has +dsDNA, +ANA, and not antihistone antibodies
Drug-induced subacute cutaneous LE (SCLE)	• "GATCH"	• G = griseofulvin • A = ACE inhibitors • T = terbinafine • C = calcium-channel blockers • H = hydrochlorathiazide	

Name	Pearl	Comments
Fixed drug eruption	• "PABA"	• P = phenolphthalein • A = aspirin • B = barbiturates • A = antibiotics (Sulfa, TCN, PCN)
Stain of choice	• Plasma cells = methyl green pyronin (stains cytoplasm red) • Mast cells = tryptase, CD117, toluidine blue, Giemsa stain	

Common exanthems	• "Many Senior Residents Dig Exanthems Redness"	• M = measles/rubeola (1st disease):
		  • red rash (7 days), Koplik spots
		• S = scarlet fever (2nd disease)/Group A *Strep.*:
		  • rash, strawberry tongue, sore throat
		• R = rubella/German measles (3rd disease):
		  • 3-day rash, mild fever
		• D = Duke's disease (4th disease)
		• E = erythema infectiosum (5th disease)/parvovirus B1:
		  • "slapped cheek" appearance
		• R = roseola (6th disease)/HHV-6:
		  • rose-appearing rash with white halos

Elastosis perforans serpignosum associated disorders and causes	• "DERMA POPS"	• D = Down syndrome (most common association) • E = Ehlers–Danlos syndrome • R = Rothmund–Thompson syndrome • M = Marfan's syndrome • A = acrogeria • P = pseudoxanthoma elasticum (PXE) • O = osteogenesis imperfecta • P = penicillamine therapy for Wilson's disease • S = scleroderma
Markers to differentiate	• T cell = CD3+ • Mononuclear cell = CD6+ • B cell = CD20+ • NK cells = CD56+ • Macrophage = CD68+, lysozyme • Mast cells = CD117+ • Dermal dendrocytes = factor XIIIa • Indeterminate cells = S100+, CD1a+, but no Birbeck granules • Langerhans cells = S100+, CD1a+, and Birbeck granules	
Leonine facies	• "A Lion PALMS you"	• P = Paget's disease of bone • A = amyloidosis • L = leishmaniasis/lipoid proteinosis/leprosy/lymphoma • M = mastocytosis/mycosis fungoides • S = sarcoid/scleromyxedema
Red groin common etiologies	• Red groin is quite a "CITE" (sight)	• C = Candida and contact dermatitis • I = inverse psoriasis • T = tinea • E = erythrasma: • Often *Corynebacterium minutissimum* = coral-red color with Wood's lamp caused by porphyrin production (coproporphyrin III)
Nevus sebaceous growth risk	• "TBS" for nevus sebaceous	• T = trichoblastoma • B = basal cell carcinoma • S = syringocystadenoma papilliferum

Name	Pearl	Comments
Multiple facial tumors	• "ANTTSS" on the face	• A = adenoma sebaceum (tuberous sclerosis) • N = neurofibromas (von Recklinghausen's disease) • T = trichilemmoma (Cowden's disease) • T = trichoepithelioma (Rombo, Brooke–Spiegler syndromes) • S = syringoma (Down syndrome) • S = sebaceous hyperplasia (sun exposure, cyclosporine)
Café-au-lait macules	• "Cheerleader with a Café-au-lait spins the BATANS"	• B = Bloom's syndrome • A = Albright's syndrome • T = tuberous sclerosis • A = ataxia telangiectasia • N = neurofibromatosis • S = Silver–Russell syndrome
Acute attack porphyrias	• "VAH"	• V = variegate porphyria • A = acute intermittent porphyria • H = hereditary coproporphyria (HCP)
Porphyria acute attack triggers	• "FIG BEANS"	• F = fever • I = infection • G = griseofulvin • B = barbiturates • E = estrogen • A = alcohol • N = nutrition/NPO • S = sulfonamides
Disorders with an infiltrate filling the papillary dermis	• "LUMP" in the papillary dermis	• L = lichenoid disease • U = urticaria pigmentosa • M = mycosis fungoides • P = pigmented purpuric dermatoses
Mounds of parakeratosis differential	• "PEGS" of parakeratosis	• P = pityriasis rosea (contain spongiosis) • E = erythema annulare centrifugum/EAC ("coat-sleeve" look) • G = guttate psoriasis (neutrophils also) • S = small plaque parapsoriasis (SPP)
Subepidermal blister with neutrophils (especially in dermal papillae)	• "Herpetic LIPS"	• Herpetic = dermatitis herpetiformis • L = lupus (bullous) • I = linear IgA bullous dermatosis • P = pemphigoid • S = Sweet's syndrome (and neutrophilic dermatosis)
Subepidermal blister, cell-poor	• "Blistering APE"	• B = bullous pemphigoid (cell-poor) and ischemic blister • A = amyloidosis (bullous) • P = PCT (porphyria cutanea tarda) • E = epidermolysis bullosa

Name	Pearl	Comments
Malignant spindle cell tumors	• "SLAM DUNK"	• S = squamous cell carcinoma • L = leiomyosarcoma • A = angiosarcoma • M = melanoma • D = DFSP • U = undifferentiate pleomorphic sarcoma (MFH) and AFX • N = nodular fasciitis • K = Kaposi's sarcoma
Superficial and deep dermal lymphocytic infiltrate causes	• "8-Ls" or "DRUGS"	• 8-Ls: 1. light reactions 2. lupus 3. lues (syphilis) 4. leprosy 5. lichen striatus 6. lymphocytic (lymphomas, Jessner's, etc.) 7. lipoidica (NLD and GA) 8. lepidoptera (arthropod bites and parasite infestations) • DRUGS: • D = dermatophyte infections • R = reticular erythematosus mucinosis • U = urticaria (chronic urticaria and urticarial stages of BP and HG) • G = gyrate erythemas • S = scleroderma
Septal panniculitis differential	• "ASPEN Migration" or "Always Make Septal Panniculitis Easy Nowadays"	• A = alpha 1-antitrypsin deficiency • S = scleroderma/morphea • P = polyarteritis nodosa (vasculitis) • E = erythema nodosum • N = necrobiosis lipiodica • Migration = migratory thrombophlebitis
Associations with erythema nodosum	• "NoDOSUM"	• No = no cause found • D = drugs (iodide, sulfonamide) • O = OCPs • S = sarcoid, Löfgren's syndrome • U = ulcer (Behçet's, UC, Crohn's) • M = microbiology (chronic infections)
Pale epidermis differential	• "SHARP Migration of Pale Cells" in the epidermis"	• S = syphilis • H = Hartnup's disease (neutral amino acids, especially tryptophan) • A = acrodermatitis enteropathica (zinc) • R = radiodermatitis • P = pellagra and psoriasis • Migration = necrolytic migratory erythema (glucagonoma) • Pale = Paget's/pagetoid • Cells = clear cell acanthoma

Name	Pearl	Comments
Multiple umbilicated "molluscum contagiosum-like" lesion differential	• "CHiP-off-the-old-Molluscum-block"	• C = cryptococcus (opportunistic) and coccidioidomycosis (HIV) • H = histoplasmosis • P = *Penicillium marneffei* (penicilliosis), *Pneumocystis jiroveci* (PCP) and pox viruses (smallpox, monkey pox) • Molluscum = Molluscum contagiosum
Papillomatosis differential	• "CAVES" in the epidermis	• C = CRP (confluent and reticulated papillomatosis) • A = acanthosis nigricans, acrochordon, acrokeratosis verruciformis • V = verruca vulgaris • E = epidermal nevus • S = seborrheic keratosis (hypertrophic), syringocystadenoma papilliferum
Deep nodule differential	• Still be "GLAM-N-Hot" even with deep nodules	• G = giant cell tumor of tendon sheath • L = liposarcoma • A = angioleiomyoma • M = malignant fibrous histiocytoma • N = nodular fasciitis, neurilemmoma • Hot = hibernoma

Intracellular parasites on H & E	• "Pretty Histo GIRL"	• Pretty = penicilliosis:
		  • *Penicillium marneffei* infection
		• Histo = histoplasmosis:
		  • *Histoplasma capsulatum* (soil fungus)
		  • spores surrounded by clear halo in cells
		• GI = granuloma inguinale:
		  • *Klebsiella granulomatis* (bacterial STD)
		  • Donovan bodies
		  • painless ulcer without lymphadenopathy
		• R = rhinoscleroma:
		  • *Klebsiella rhinoscleromatis* bacterial infection of nares
		  • not rhinosporidiosis (fungi with huge sporangia; often nares)
		  • Russell bodies and Mikulicz bodies
		• L = leishmaniasis:
		  • flagellate protozoan parasite
		  • kinetoplast = mitochondria body near flagella

Teeth and jaw abnormalities	• Peg teeth = incontinentia pigmenti, anhidrotic ectodermal dysplasia • Anodontia = hypomelanosis of Ito, incontinentia pigmenti • Odontogenic cysts = Gorlin syndrome • Retention of primary teeth = Job syndrome (hyper-IgE syndrome) • Enamel pits = tuberous sclerosis	
Wiskott–Aldrich syndrome	• "Three Ps"	• P = pruritus • P = purpura • P = pyogenic infections (deficiency of IgM)
Marked papillary dermal edema	• Dermis "SLUMP" from massive edema	• S = Sweet's syndrome • L = lichen sclerosis et atrophicus • U = urticaria pigmentosa • M = mycosis fungoides • P = PMLE and pigmented purpuric dermatosis (PPD)
Superficial perivascular lymphocytic infiltrate with no epidermal involvement	• "MEET the VP"	• M = morbilliform drug • E = EAC ("coat-sleeving") • E = erythrasma • T = tinea • V = vitiligo (no melanocytes) and viral • P = PIPA, minocycline pigmentation, Schamberg's, etc.

Name	Pearl	Comments
Disorders with bone and calcification presentation clues	• Polyostotic fibrous dysplasia = McCune–Albright syndrome (GNAS mutation) • Calcification of falx cerebri = Gorlin's syndrome (PATCH mutation) • Osteopoikilosis = Buschke–Ollendorf syndrome (associated with LEMD3 mutation) • Stippled epiphyses: • CHILD syndrome (congenital hemidysplasia, ichthyosiform erythroderma, limb defects), Conradi–Hunermann (form of chondrodysplasia punctata), congenital warfarin exposure, trisomy 21, congenital hypothyroidism, Zellweger syndrome (absence of peroxisomes), Smith–Lemli–Opitz syndrome (defect cholesterol synthesis) • Osteopathia striata = focal dermal hypoplasia • PORCN mutation • Ehrlenmeyer flask deformity = Gaucher disease (type I)	
Erythroderma causes	• "ID-SCALP"	• I = idiopathic • D = drugs • S = seborrheic dermatitis • C = contact dermatitis • A = atopic dermatitis • L = lymphoma (i.e. MF) and leukemia • P = psoriasis and PRP
X-linked dominant syndromes	• "BIG Child" with an X-linked dominant syndrome	B = Bazex syndrome (BCCs, follicular atrophoderma) • I = incontinentia pigmenti • G = Goltz syndrome (focal dermal hypoplasia) • Child = CHILD syndrome and Conradi–Hunermann syndrome
Causes of leukocytoclastic vasculitis	• "VASCULITIS"	V = viral (especially hepatitis B and C) • A = autoimmune (SLE, RA) • S = *Staph.*, *Strep.* • C = cryoglobulin, cryofibrinogens, Churg–Strauss • U = ulcerative colitis, urticarial vasculitis • L = lymphomas • I = infection (meningococcemia, RMSF) • T = thiazides and other drugs • I = immune complex reaction, idiopathic • S = sulfa drugs and other antibiotics
Collodion baby differential	• Lamellar ichthyosis (#1) • Congenital ichthyosiform erythroderma • Sjögren–Larsson syndrome • Conradi–Hunermann syndrome • Trichothiodystrophy • Ectodermal dysplasia • Infantile Gaucher disease • Hay–Wells' syndrome • Neutral lipid storage disease	
X-linked recessive syndromes	• "CHAD's Kinky WIFE"	• C = chronic granulomatous disease, chondrodysplasia punctata • H = Hunter's disease • A = anhidrotic ectodermal dysplasia (Christ–Siemens) • D = dyskeratosis congenita • S = SCID (severe combined immunodeficiency) • Kinky = Menke's kinky hair • W = Wiskott–Aldrich • I = ichthyosis, X-linked • F = Fabry's disease • E = Ehlers–Danlos V and IX

Name	Pearl	Comments
DNA viruses	• "HAPPy" DNA virus	• H = herpes virus (HSV, VZV, CMV, EBV) • H = hepadnavirus (hepatitis B) • A = adenovirus • P = papovavirus (HPV) • P = poxvirus (molluscum, smallpox, Orf, milker's nodule) • P = parvovirus B19: • single-stranded DNA virus, while others listed above are double stranded

Conditions often associated with a monoclonal gammopathy	• "ASPEN" mountain looks like a gammopathy spike	• A = amyloidosis
		• S = scleromyxedema (IgG), scleredema (IgG)
		• S = Sneddon–Wilkinson disease (IgA)
		• S = Schnitzler's syndrome (IgM):
		  • non-pruritic urticaria, fever, IgM gammopathy
		• P = pyoderma gangrenosum (IgA)
		• P = POEMS syndrome (IgG or IgA):
		  • polyneuropathy, organomegaly, endocrinopathy, monoclonal gammopathy, skin changes (hyperpigmentation, edema, and glomeruloid hemangiomas)
		• E = erythema elevatum diutinum (IgA)
		• N = necrobiotic xanthogranuloma (IgG)

Drugs often associated with acral erythema	• "BaD Fingers And Toes"	• B = bleomycin • D = doxirubicin • F = 5-FU • A = ara-C (cytarabine) • T = taxol
Neutrophilic dermatosis	• "Sweet BuRPS"	• Sweet = Sweet's syndrome • B = Behçet's syndrome, bowel bypass • R = rheumatoid neutrophilic • P = pyoderma gangrenosum • S = Sneddon–Wilkinson disease (subcorneal pustular dermatosis)
Fluorescent-positive ectothrix fungal infections (Wood's lamp)	• "Dogs And Cats Fight and Growl Sometimes"	• Dogs = *Microsporum **d**istortum* • And = *Microsporum **a**udouinii* • Cats = *Microsporum canis* • Fight = *Microsporum **f**errugineum* • Growl = *Microsporum **g**ypsium* • Sometimes = *Trichophyton **s**choenleinii*
Polarizable conditions	• "Federal Government TAX"	• F = Fabry's disease (urine shows "Maltese crosses") • F = foreign bodies (splinter, talc, silica) • G = gout (urate crystals) • T = trichothiodystrophy's hair ("tiger-tail") • A = amyloid ("apple green" with Congo red stain) • X = xanthomas with cholesterol esters (tuberous, plane, xanthelasma): • eruptive xanthoma not polarized, since not cholesterol esters
Grenz zone differential	• "LG" for large grenz	• L = leukemia/lymphoma (especially AML and AMML) • G = granuloma faciale and erythema elevatum diutinum

Name	Predilection and Clinical Key Features	Histopathology
"Good-to-know" clinical and dermatopathology clues		
Xanthoma	• Clinical = "yellow–pink tumor" • Associated with increased cholesterol and triglyceride (xanthelasma not associated with elevated cholesterol)	
Cylindroma	• Clinical = "turban-tumor" • Path = "pieces of jigsaw puzzle" • Benign eccrine tumor	
Eccrine poroma	• Clinical = "Great Wall of China" around red lesion (especially on side of foot) • Path = small sweat ducts and cuboidal or basaloid "poroid" cells	
Syringoma	• Proliferation of eccrine ductal structure (seen in Down syndrome) • Path = "tadpole" appearance	

Name	Predilection and Clinical Key Features	Histopathology
Dermatofibrosarcoma protuberans (DFSP)	• Clinical = "infected keloid" appearance	
Acquired digital fibrokeratoma	• Path = "vertical-aligned" fibrovascular core	
Supernumerary digit	• Similar to acquired digital fibrokeratoma, but peripheral nerves (resemble Meissner corpuscles for tactile) seen in upper dermis	
Pilomatricoma	• Path = cyst-like with "shadow" or "ghost cells" (ghost of a nucleus in center of swollen cells; attempt to produce a hair shaft); benign tumor of hair follicle matrix • Clinical = "tent sign" with stretching of skin, or "teeter-totter" with depression of one side	

Name	Predilection and Clinical Key Features	Histopathology
Sclerotic fibroma	• Path = "plywood pattern"	
Dermatofibroma	• Large bundles of collagen ("keloidal" collagen) with spindled fibroblasts around bundles ("collagen trapping")	
Schwannoma	• Path = Verocay bodies and alternating hypocellular and dense cells	
Scabies	• Path = "brown nuggets" in cornified layer, or ovoid/pyramidal spaces	
Pityriasis rubra pilaris	• Path = "checkerboard" appearance (alternation of orthokeratotic and parakeratotic cells in both horizontal and vertical directions) • Similar to "P" alternating with "R" in the name "PRP"	

Name	Predilection and Clinical Key Features	Histopathology
Scurvy	• Follicular plugging with perifollicular RBC extravasation • Clinical = perifollicular purpura with "corkscrew" hair; gingival hemorrhage; periungual hemorrhage	
Grover's disease	• Path = various patterns, such as spongiosis in association with focal acantholytic dyskeratosis	
Lichen planus	• Path = band-like infiltrate of lymphocytes; wedge-shape hypergranulosis; saw-tooth lower epidermis; multiple, scattered Civatte bodies	
Lichen nitidus	• Path = "ball-in-claw" appearance	
Dermatophytosis	• Path = "sandwich sign" (two patterns of cornification arranged parallel to skin)	

Name	Predilection and Clinical Key Features	Histopathology
Actinic (solar) keratosis	• Path = alternating columns of parakeratosis (broader) and orthokeratosis	
Psoriasis	• Path = rete ridges elongated and of equal length/ thin; neutrophils in the horn	
Fibroepithelioma of Pinkus (variant of BCC)	• Net-like pattern or strands of basaloid cells extending to dermis from multiple epidermal connections	
Herpes simplex virus	• Steel-gray nuclei and margination of chromatin at edge of nucleus	
Verruca vulgaris (HPV infection)	• Koilocytes = superficial keratinocytes with vacuolated, pyknotic raisin-like nuclei	

Name	Predilection and Clinical Key Features	Histopathology
Molluscum contagiosum	• Molluscum bodies (Henderson–Patterson bodies) = pink–purple intracytoplasmic inclusions that push nucleus and granules aside; epidermal hyperplasia creating a crater with "bodies"	
Mycosis fungoides	• Lymphocytes line up along DE junction and epidermotropism of atypical lymphocytes • *Note:* tumor stage of MF does not have epidermotropism	
Granuloma annulare	• Palisading granuloma around necrobiosis (connective tissue degeneration) and mucin	
Paget's disease	• Pale-staining cells scattered in epidermis (groups may occur and compress basal cells); fuzzy cytoplasm in suprabasal cells	

Name	Predilection and Clinical Key Features	Histopathology
Epidermolytic hyperkeratotic acanthoma	• Bluish, "moth-eaten" keratinocytes (loss of nuclei) below hyperkeratosis • *Note:* not the same as acantholytic acanthoma which has acantholysis of epidermis	
Acanthosis nigricans	• "Church-spire" papillomatosis (not acanthosis)	
Scar	• Fibroblasts parallel to epidermis (instead of swirling); blood vessels perpendicular to epidermis	
Hypertrophic scar	• Nodular, swirls of benign fibroblasts and small collagenous stroma • More cells than keloid	

Name	Predilection and Clinical Key Features	Histopathology
Keloid	• Broad bundles of pink collagen; fewer cells than hypertrophic scar • Increased TGF-β, increased type III and VI collagen	
Electrodesiccation artifact	• Elongated, spindly, "fibroblast-like" epithelial cells	
Freeze artifact	• Numerous vacuoles in the epidermis and dermis	
Gelfoam	• Purple, angled deposits	
Invisible dermatoses differential	• "VITAMin U"	• V = vitiligo • I = ichthyosis vulgaris • T = tinea versicolor and TMEP • A = argyria • M = macular amyloid • U = urticaria

Spindle cell tumor differential
SLAM DUNK

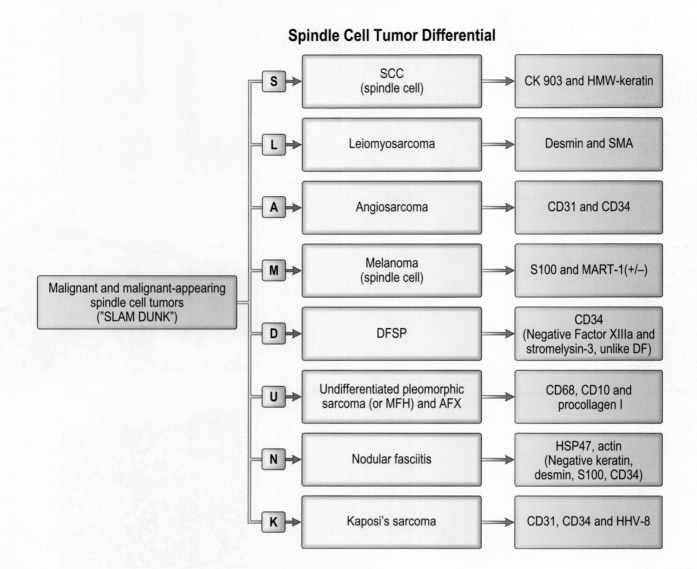

Spindle Cell Tumor Differential

S	SCC (spindle cell)	CK 903 and HMW-keratin
L	Leiomyosarcoma	Desmin and SMA
A	Angiosarcoma	CD31 and CD34
M	Melanoma (spindle cell)	S100 and MART-1(+/−)
D	DFSP	CD34 (Negative Factor XIIIa and stromelysin-3, unlike DF)
U	Undifferentiated pleomorphic sarcoma (or MFH) and AFX	CD68, CD10 and procollagen I
N	Nodular fasciitis	HSP47, actin (Negative keratin, desmin, S100, CD34)
K	Kaposi's sarcoma	CD31, CD34 and HHV-8

Malignant and malignant-appearing spindle cell tumors ("SLAM DUNK")

Dermoscopy classic images

Solar lentigo

- Moth-eaten borders

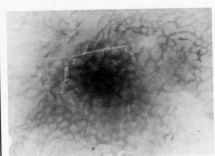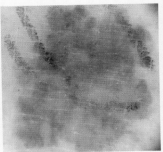

Seborrheic keratosis

- Milia or comedo openings; crypts; hairpin vessels

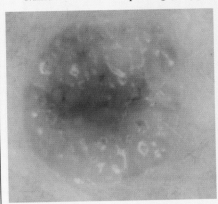

Congenital melanocytic nevus

- Regular pigment network pattern; hair in lesion

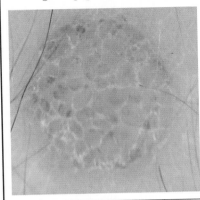

Benign melanocytic nevi

- Homogeneous pattern, comedo-like openings, comma-like vessels

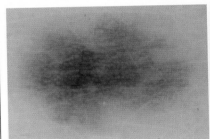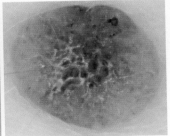

Junctional nevus   Compound nevus

Dermatofibroma

- Most common appearance = central white or scar-like area with peripheral pigment network

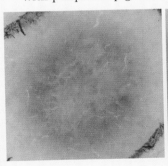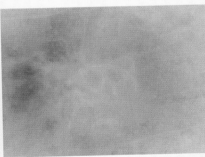

Dysplastic nevus

- Atypical pigment network; branched streaks; network fade at periphery

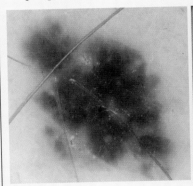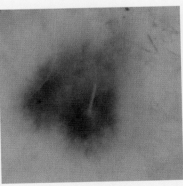

Melanoma

- Irregular pigment network; aggregated globules; asymmetry of color/structure; blue–white structures; pink veil

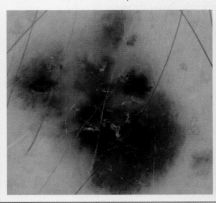 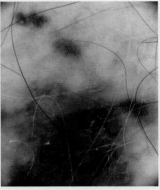

Spitz nevus

- Classic Spitz nevus = "starburst" pattern (grey–blue center with symmetrical streaks radiating outwards)

Benign acral pigment

- Most commonly, the "parallel furrow" pattern (pigment in valleys) or "lattice" pattern (below)

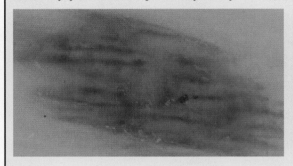

Basal cell carcinoma

- Arborizing vessels; ulceration; pink–white shiny area; blue–gray globule

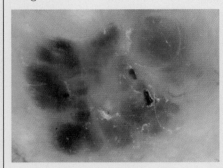

Nail abnormalities overview

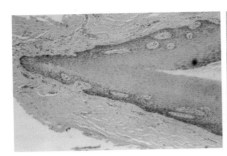 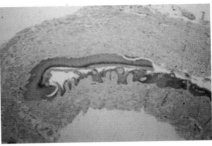

Nail Abnormality	Description	Common Associated Conditions	Clinical Image
Shape or growth change of nail			
Pitting	• Abnormality in the proximal matrix, causing parakeratotic cells in dorsal nail plate that easily detach (leaving pits)	• Psoriasis, Reiter's syndrome, alopecia areata, incontinentia pigmenti	

Beau's lines	• Transverse, indented, linear depressions at the same location on multiple nails due to matrix's growth arrest	• Systemic illness, trauma
		• Clues to trauma severity:
		  • depth = extent of matrix damage
		  • width = duration of insult	

Yellow nail syndrome	• Yellow color to multiple nails, loss of lunula color and cuticle (due to nail growth arrest)	• Lymphedema, pleural effusion/bronchiectasis	
Koilonychia	• Spoon-shaped nail	• Iron deficiency anemia, hemochromatosis, SLE, alopecia areata	
Onycholysis	• Separation from the nail bed	• Psoriasis, infection, hyperthyroidism (Plummer's nails)	
Clubbing	• Rounding of the nail due to soft tissue beneath proximal plate (Lovibond's angle >180 normally 160), Schamroth sign = opposing nails lose diamond shape at proximal end when nails "back-to-back"	• IBD, pulmonary malignancy, cirrhosis, COPD	

Nail Abnormality	Description	Common Associated Conditions	Clinical Image
Trachyonychia	• "Sandpaper nails" = nail roughness with sandpapered look in a longitudinal direction	• Alopecia areata, lichen planus, psoriasis	
Anonychia	• Absent nails	• Ectodermal dysplasia, lichen planus, infection, ichthyosis, drugs (etretinate)	
Onychoschizia	• "Brittle nails" with distal splitting along fracture plane (dehydration)	• Frequent hand washing, normal variant of nails (elderly), vascular psoriasis, lichen planus	
Onychorrhexis	• Excess longitudinal ridging	• Excessive hand washing, normal variant of nails (elderly)	
Onychomadesis	• Shedding of nail from proximal end (due to complete arrest of matrix)	• Keratosis punctata palmaris et plantaris, thrombosis, PCN allergy, drug reaction	
Onychogryphosis	• Nail plate hypertrophy, "oyster-like" appearance	• Normal aging, pressure, trauma • Also seen in Haim–Munk syndrome (PPK + periodontitis + acroosteolysis, associated with cathepsin C mutation)	
Onychauxis	• Thickening of nail plate without significant deformity	• Trauma, psoriasis, infection, PRP, acromegaly, Darier's disease	

Nail Abnormality	Description	Common Associated Conditions	Clinical Image
Color change of nail			
• True leukonychia = white opaque discoloration of nail plate such as Mees' lines • Apparent leukonychia = white discoloration that fades with applied pressure such as Terry's nails, Muehrcke's nails, Lindsay's nails (half-and-half nails) • *Note:* fingernail growth = 3 mm/month; toenail growth = 1 mm/month			
Terry's nails	• Nail plate appears white in colour due to a defect in nail bed (decreased vascularity and increased connective tissue)	• Hepatic failure/cirrhosis, diabetes	
Splinter hemorrhage	• Subungual, red longitudinal lines	• Endocarditis, trauma, SLE, pregnancy, trichinosis infection (worm parasite in uncooked pork/wild game)	
Telangiectasia	• Telangiectasias around cuticle	• Dermatomyositis, RA, SLE	
Half-and-half nails (Lindsay's nails)	• Proximal nail bed portion white and distal portion brown colored (due to nail bed edema)	• Renal failure • (Think of "Leaky Lindsay")	
Mees' lines	• Transverse white bands across the entire nail paralleling lunula (micro-fragmentation in nail) • Line grows out with nail; multiple nail plates involved	• Arsenic poisoning, Hodgkin's disease, carbon monoxide poisoning, CHF	
Muehrcke's lines	• Double pair of fixed-location, transverse white lines extending across the entire nail • Disappears when nail depressed since abnormality of vascular nail bed	• Hypoalbuminemia, malnutrition, liver disease, nephrotic syndrome	

Nail Abnormality	Description	Common Associated Conditions	Clinical Image
Azure (or blue) lunulae	• Blue-colored, non-blanching lunula due to nail matrix defect	• Wilson's disease (or "hepatolenticular degeneration"), silver poisoning (argyria)	
Red lunulae	• Red-colored lunula	• Heart failure, alopecia areata, psoriasis	

Triangular lunulae	• Nail-patella syndrome (hereditary osteo-onychodysplasia or "HOOD") :
	  • hypoplasia of radial side of thumbnails, absent patella, iliac "horns," radial head dysplasia
	  • mutation = LMX1B gene (regulates collagen synthesis)		

Red and white longitudinal lines with V-shaped indentation on distal margin	• Multiple red and white longitudinal streaks with a wedge-shaped subungual hyperkeratosis and fissure on the free margin (corresponding to the white bands)	• Darier's disease ("follicular dyskeratosis")	

Lichenoid Reaction Pattern

3

Lichen planus

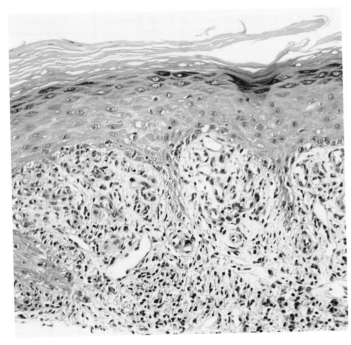

Erythema multiforme

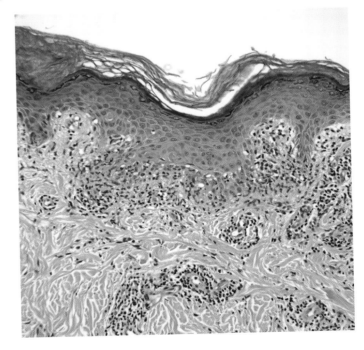

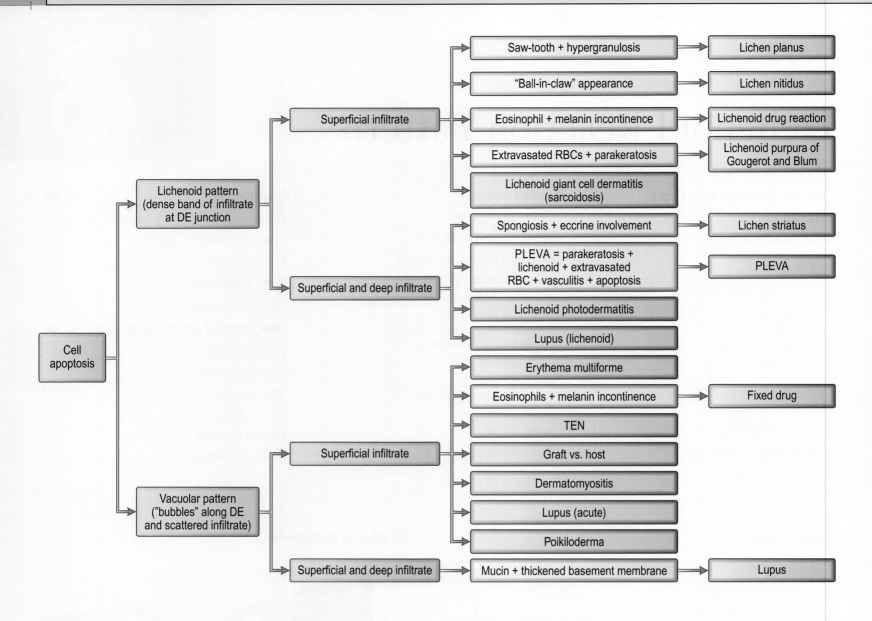

Disorder	Predilection and Clinical Key Features	Histopathology
Lichenoid (interface) dermatoses		
Lichen planus (LP)	• Unknown etiology, possible autoimmune reaction against modified lesional keratinocytes causing apoptosis (perforins/granzyme and Fas/Fas L) • Adults • Wrists (flexor aspect), dorsum hand, sacral area • Violaceous, flat-topped, pruritic papules; Wickham's striae (fine white lines); oral lesions (75%); nail LP (10%) • Associated with hepatitis C (especially oral LP), HHV-6, dental amalgam (mercury), immunodeficiency, malignancy	• Band-like infiltrate of lymphocytes; wedge-shape hypergranulosis (striae clinically); saw-tooth lower epidermis; melanin incontinence; multiple, scattered Civatte bodies and colloid bodies (apoptotic cells with tonofilaments, extruded into papillary dermis) Colloid bodies (above) • DIF = complement and IgM (colloid bodies in papillary dermis) and irregular band of fibrin along basal layer
Lichen planus variants		
Atrophic lichen planus	• May be resolving phase of LP • Lower legs • Resembles porokeratosis clinically with papules of lichen planus at margins	• Epidermis thin; loss of normal rete ridge pattern; less dense infiltrate than LP

Disorder	Predilection and Clinical Key Features	Histopathology
Hypertrophic lichen planus	• "Lichen planus verrucosus" • Usually confined to shins • Pruritic, thick plaques that may have verrucous appearance; often chronic venous stasis present • Associated with HIV • Risk of SCC developing	• "LP + LSC-like" • Prominent hyperplasia overlying orthokeratosis; "vertical-streaked" collagen in papillary dermis (similar lichen simplex chronicus); basal cell damage confined to tips of rete ridges
Ulcerative (erosive) lichen planus	• Ulcerated and bullous lesions on feet • Risk of SCC developing in lesions	• Epidermal ulceration with lichen planus at margins
Erythema dyschromicum perstans	• Macular variant of LP • "Lichen planus pigmentosus" or "ashy dermatosis" • Latin Americans • Symmetric on neck, trunk, extremities (spares palm/soles, scalp, nails, mucosa) • Asymptomatic, ash-colored or brown macular hyperpigmentation on trunk 	 • Vacuolar tissue reaction; prominent melanin incontinence in dermis (causes "ashy" appearance)

Disorder	Predilection and Clinical Key Features	Histopathology
Lichen planus actinicus	• LP that is limited to sun-exposed areas • Young Middle Eastern or Oriental individuals	• Resembles lichen planus but more melanin incontinence; focal parakeratosis

Lichen planopilaris (LPP)	• "Follicular LP"
	• Keratotic follicular lesions; scarring alopecia on scalp
	
	• Related to Graham–Little–Piccardi–Lassueur syndrome:
	  1. Cicatricial alopecia of scalp
	  2. Follicular lichenoid keratosis pilaris
	  3. Non-scarring alopecia of axillae and groins
		• Lichenoid reaction involving upper follicular epithelium (infundibulum and isthmus); dense perifollicular infiltrate (lymphocytes and macrophages); hair follicles replaced by linear tracts of fibrosis (sparing between follicles)
		• DIF = colloid bodies (IgG and IgM) in dermis

Lichen planus pemphigoides	• "LP + BP" (Lichen planus and subepidermal blistering disease resembling bullous pemphigoid) • Possible variant of bullous pemphigoid • Lichen planus patients • Extremities • Tense blister in previously normal skin location; blisters do not necessarily form at location of prior lichen planus lesion (differs from bullous LP which forms in longstanding LP lesions) • Ab = BPAG2 or 180-kDa BP antigen (type XVII collagen)	• Mild perivascular infiltrate (eosinophils and neutrophils beneath blister); occasional Civatte bodies in basal layer at blister margins; subepidermal (cell-poor) bulla with mild, perivascular infiltrate of lymphocytes, neutrophils, and eosinophils • DIF = IgG and C3 in BMZ zone

Disorder	Predilection and Clinical Key Features	Histopathology
Keratosis lichenoides chronica	• Possible chronic variant of LP • Violaceous papular lesions in linear and reticulate pattern on extremities and seborrheic dermatitis-like facial eruption	• Lichenoid reaction pattern with prominent basal cell death and focal basal vacuolar change; superficial dermal telangiectasia
Lichen nitidus	• Children and young adults • Flexor aspect of upper extremities, genitalia, nails • Asymptomatic, eruptions of multiple, small flesh-colored papules (1–2 mm) • Possibly associated with Crohn's disease, LP, atopic dermatitis	• "Ball-in-claw" appearance • Focal, well-circumscribed, subepidermal infiltrate (limited to 1–2 adjacent dermal papillae); "claw-like" acanthotic rete ridges; infiltrate of lymphocytes and multinucleate giant cells; DIF negative (unlike LP)
Lichen striatus	• Unknown etiology, possibly aberrant clone during fetal development migrates along lines of Blaschko and then exposed to infection later • Female children and adolescents • Extremity • Papular eruption on one side of body linearly; usually length of an extremity • Resolves months to years with hypopigmentation	• Lichenoid reaction + spongiosis + eccrine involvement (superficial and deep infiltrate) • Lymphocytes in 3–4 adjacent dermal papillae; acanthosis; intraepidermal vesicles with Langerhans cells; eccrine extension of infiltrate • Dyskeratotic cells at all levels in the epidermis

Disorder	Predilection and Clinical Key Features	Histopathology
Lichen planus-like keratosis	• "Benign lichenoid keratosis" • Arms and presternal area of women • Solitary, discrete, slightly raised, pruritic lesions (3–10 mm) of short duration with violaceous/pink color with rusty tinge Dermoscopy image (photo above)	 • "LP with focal parakeratosis" • Numerous Civatte bodies; mildly vacuolar; pigment incontinence; mild hyperkeratosis; contiguous with a lentigo or a seborrheic keratosis

Lichenoid drug eruptions	• Any age and location
	
	• Eczematous or psoriasiform papule or plaque
	• Numerous drugs indicated (stopping drug then resolves in several weeks)
	• Some associated drugs ("Gold T-BAG"):
	  • Gold
	  • Thiazide (HCTZ)
	  • Beta blockers
	  • ACE inhibitors, antimalarials
	  • Griseofulvin
		• "LP + focal parakeratosis + eosinophils"
		• Focal parakeratosis and mild basal vacuolar change; few eosinophils and plasma cells; melanin incontinence

Disorder	Predilection and Clinical Key Features	Histopathology
Fixed drug eruptions	• Face, lips, groin • Round or oval erythematous lesion (within hours of taking offending drug) • If re-take drug, lesions appear at the same "fixed" spot • Associated with sulfonamides, TCN, nystatin • Major offenders: aspirin, NSAIDs, sulfonamide, maraschino cherry tetracycline, pseudoephedrine (non-pigmented variant)	• "EM-like + eosinophils" • Prominent vacuolar change and Civatte bodies (all levels of epidermis); infiltrate obscures DE interface with extension to mid and upper epidermis; melanin incontinence; eosinophils + neutrophils (similar EM)
Erythema multiforme (EM)	• Self-limited disease with erythematous lesions, may evolve to "target lesions"; distributed symmetrically • Extremities (hands) • Associated with HSV, Orf, *Mycoplasma pneumoniae* and other infections	• Prominent epidermal apoptosis (all levels); basal vacuolar change; lymphocytes infiltrate and obscure DE junction; spongiosis; inflammatory target is keratinocytes (no melanin incontinence neutrophils like fixed drug eruption)

Disorder	Predilection and Clinical Key Features	Histopathology

Toxic epidermal necrolysis (TEN)	• Lyell syndrome
	• Adults
	• Erosive mucosal lesions; extensive blister formation
	• Prodrome syndrome precedes
	
	• Skin resembles "wet cigarette paper"
	• Epidermal detachment:
	  • Stevens-Johnson syndrome (SJS) <10% BSA
	  • SJS/TEN overlap 10–30% BSA
	  • TEN >30% BSA
	• Associated with drugs, 1–3 weeks (especially sulfonamide, NSAIDs, anticonvulsants)
	• SJS = often children; associated with drugs, infections, etc.
	• Possible TX = burn unit and IVIG
		• Subepidermal blister with overlying necrosis; sparse perivascular lymphocytes; full-thickness epidermal necrosis; edge of blister with necrotic keratinocytes
		• TEN apoptosis due to cytokines (i.e., FasL and TNF-α)

Graft-versus-host disease (GVHD)	• Patient with allogeneic, donor immunocompetent lymphocytes in bone marrow transplant (rare in solid organ transplant)
	• Acute: erythematous macular rash with vomiting, diarrhea; histologically similar EM but less infiltrate; "satellite cell necrosis" (lymphocyte next to apoptotic keratinocyte)
	
	• Chronic (>100 days post transplant): early = lichen planus-like histologically; later possibly sclerodermoid phase
	• Biopsy 21 days post transplant to differentiate diagnosis from chemotherapy!
	• Grading of GVHD:
	  • Grade 0 – normal skin
	  • Grade 1 – vacuolar change
	  • Grade 2 – dyskeratotic cells/dermal lymphocytes
	  • Grade 3 – subepidermal microvesicles
	  • Grade 4 – subepidermal blister/epidermal necrosis
		• Basal vacuolation; but not full-thickness epidermal necrosis (often similar EM)

Disorder	Predilection and Clinical Key Features	Histopathology
Eruptions of lymphocyte recovery	• 14–21 days after autologous bone marrow transplant (correspond to return of lymphocytes to circulation) • Especially AML patients • Erythematous eruption, fever	• Resembles mild GVHD with upper dermal perivascular infiltrate of small T-lymphocytes; few apoptotic cells ("satellite cell necrosis")

Lupus erythematosus
[Thick BM = DPAS+; mucin = alcian blue and colloidal iron stains]
	• Chronic inflammatory disease and immune disorder of connective tissue
	• Middle-aged women
		• Three major clinical variants:
		  1. Discoid Lupus Erythematosus
		  2. Subacute Cutaneous Lupus Erythematosus
		  3. Systemic Lupus Erythematosus (SLE)
		• High-specificity Ab = dsDNA and Sm
		• Low-specificity Ab = ANA, ssDNA, U1RNP, Ro, histone (drug-induced SLE), etc.

Discoid lupus erythematosus (DLE)	• "Lupus-involving-only-the-skin" • Adults • Sharply demarcated, erythematous, scaly patches with follicular plugging; scarring alopecia • 5–10% progress to SLE (especially if anti-ssDNA); DLE in 20% of SLE patients • ANA often negative	• Both superficial and deep dermal lymphocytes ("patchy") that accumulate around pilosebaceous follicles; BMZ thickening; vacuolar change and scattered Civatte bodies; keratotic follicular plug; hyperkeratosis • DIF = IgG/IgM at DE junction IgM along the follicle IgG along BMZ

Disorder	Predilection and Clinical Key Features	Histopathology
Tumid lupus erythematosus	• Dermal variant of lupus • Face, upper trunk • Erythematous papules and plaques	• Similar to DLE but increased mucin with subepidermal edema (not involving epidermis) DIF = peri-eccrine IgG

Subacute cutaneous lupus erythematosus (SCLE)	• Variant with unique skin lesions and mild systemic illness
	• Face, neck, upper trunk, extensors of arms
	
	• Recurrent, photosensitive, non-scarring lesions (annular or papulosquamous types); musculoskeletal complaints
	• Associated with "GATCH" drugs:
	  • G = griseofulvin
	  • A = ACE-I
	  • T = terbinafine
	  • C = calcium channel blockers
	  • H = HCTZ
	• Positive Anti-Ro/SSA (75–90%)
	• No antihistone antibodies, like drug-induced SLE
		• Similar DLE but more basal vacuolar change, epidermal atrophy, dermal edema and mucin; less plugging, hyperkeratosis, BMZ thickening
		
		• DIF = granular fluorescence in cytoplasm and nucleus of basal keratinocytes (reflect binding of Ro and La antigens) and in epidermis
		• Deposits in the epidermis, unlike other variants (along DE)
		
		• DIF demonstrating granular anti-Ro antibodies

Disorder	Predilection and Clinical Key Features	Histopathology

Systemic lupus erythematosus	• Diagnosis criteria ("multisystem disease") include:
	  • skin lesions (erythematous, slightly indurated patches with little scale; scarring)
	  • renal involvement (especially if + ds-DNA antibodies)
	  • joint involvement
	  • serositis
	
	• Likely cause of death – renal failure and CNS vascular lesions
	• Associated with "My HIP" drugs (antihistone antibodies):
	  • My = minocycline
	  • H = hydralazine
	  • I = INH
	  • P = procainamide (may not have antihistone Ab)
		• Prominent basal vacuolar change; mild infiltrate of lymphocytes; edema; mucin; usually no Civatte bodies; fibrin deposition around vessels and thickening of BM
		
		• DIF = "full house" (IgG, IgM, IgA, complement) (IgG DIF pictured above)

Neonatal lupus erythematosus	• Transient lupus dermatitis in neonatal period (from mother) • Periorbital, scalp and extremities • Resembles subacute lupus erythematosus; telangiectatic macules; risk of congenital heart block; possible hematologic and systemic abnormalities • Anti-Ro/SSA antibody + (99%); also positive in mother	• Resembles subacute lupus erythematosus

Disorder	Predilection and Clinical Key Features	Histopathology
Other lupus variants		
Bullous lupus erythematosus	• Skin eruption resembles dermatitis herpetiformis	• Subepidermal blister, papillary neutrophils and perivascular lymphocytes
Lupus panniculitis (lupus profundus)	• Firm subcutaneous inflammatory nodules • May precede systemic or discoid LE • Thigh, buttocks, head, neck 	• Lobular panniculitis with lymphocytic infiltrate • One in two cases have epidermal and dermal changes of LE • "Mummified" or hyalinized appearance around fat cells (see p. 359 for more information)
Rowell syndrome	• Lupus patients who develop annular, erythema-like lesions • LE + EM • RF positive, speckled ANA 	• LE + EM-like • DIF = IgG, IgM, etc. in linear band along basement membrane

Disorder	Predilection and Clinical Key Features	Histopathology

Dermatomyositis	• Coexistence of non-suppurative myositis (polymyositis) and inflammatory skin changes
	• Face, shoulder, extensor surface (forearm, thigh)
	
	• Erythematous, slightly scaly lesions; poikiloderma; nail fold changes; heliotrope rash (periorbital edema and purple color); Gottron's papules (atrophic papules over knuckles); proximal muscle weakness
	• Associated with a 10% risk of malignancy (i.e. ovarian cancer, GU cancers, breast, lung, gastric, etc.)
	• Possible positive autoantibodies:
	  • ANA
	  • anti-Jo-1 (antihistidyl transfer RNA synthetase) = correlate pulmonary fibrosis, Raynaud's and polyarthritis
	  • anti-Mi-2 = correlate to classic DM (shawl sign, cuticle change, Gottron's papules/sign, favorable diagnosis)
	  • anti-SRP = correlate cardiac disease, poor prognosis
	  • anti- Ku = correlate sclerodermatomyositis
	  • anti-PL 12 = correlate pulmonary disease
		• "Superficial lupus-like"
		• BMZ thickened and BMZ vacuolar change; superficial perivascular infiltrate (not deep); (i.e. liquefaction); edema and mucin; epidermal atrophy
		
		• DIF usually negative or granular IgG or C5b-9 along BMZ
		
		• Gottron's papules (above) show mild hyperkeratosis, some acanthosis, and basal vacuolar changes. 40% of cases have mucin deposition

Disorder	Predilection and Clinical Key Features	Histopathology
Poikilodermas		
• "HEAT" acronym = Hyper- and hypopigmentation, Erythema, Atrophy of epidermis and Telangiectasia • Histopathology = vacuolar change; telangiectasia; pigment incontinence; later, dermal sclerosis		
Poikiloderma atrophicans vasculare	• Early-stage evolution of mycosis fungoides • Mottled pigmentation, telangiectasias and atrophy	• Atypical lymphocytes in epidermis with atrophy and increased telangiectasias
Rothmund–Thomson syndrome	• "Poikiloderma congenitale" • Autosomal recessive • Multisystem disorder of principally skin, eyes and skeleton • Reticular erythematous eruptions in 1st year of life followed by hyperpigmentation; short stature, cataracts, hypogonadism, mental retardation; alopecia; absent thumbs; risk of osteosarcoma/fibrosarcoma • Mutation = RecQL4 helicase gene	• Poikilodermatous features (hyperkeratosis, atrophy, basal vacuolar change, rare apoptotic keratinocytes in basal layer, telangiectatic vessels, scattered dermal melanophages)
Kindler's syndrome	• Genodermatoses characterized by acral trauma-induced blisters; improves with age • Considered a new category of epidermolysis bullosa classification • Acral area • Photosensitivity, acral bullae, poikiloderma, atrophy • Mutation = KIND1: 　• kindlin-1 protein 　• focal adhesion protein in basal keratinocytes 　• affects the actin–extracellular matrix linkage 　• unlike the keratin–ECM linkage in epidermolysis bullosa	• Hyperkeratosis, epidermal atrophy, basal vacuolar change, numerous telangiectatic vessels, keratotic (warty) lesions, subepidermal bullae

Disorder	Predilection and Clinical Key Features	Histopathology
Bloom's syndrome	• "Congenital telangiectatic erythema" • Autosomal recessive • Telangiectatic, sun-sensitive facial rash; stunted growth; prone to respiratory and GI infections • Risk of adenocarcinoma, lymphoma/leukemias • Mutation = RecQL3 helicase gene	• Dilation of dermal capillaries; mild perivascular lymph infiltrate; basal vacuolar change but does not usually result in pigment incontinence

Dyskeratosis congenita	• Caucasian males
	• First decade develop reticulated hyperpigmentation
	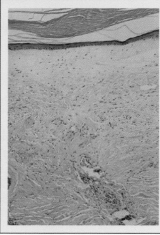
	• Genodermatosis with progressive bone marrow failure, and classic triad:
	1. Reticulate hyperpigmentation:
	  • often poikiloderma
	  • neck, upper chest
	2. Nail dystrophy, pterygiums:
	  • possible absent fingerprints
	3. Leukokeratosis of mucous membranes:
	  • risk of SCC in areas of leukoplakia
	• Lacrimal duct atresia with excessive tearing (epiphora), bone marrow failure (50–90%), including anemia, thrombocytopenia, pancytopenia, etc. (infection risk)
	• Risk of malignancy (AML, Hodgkin's, oral SCC, GI adenocarcinoma)
	• Mutations (telomerase dysfunctions):
	  • X-linked recessive variant = DKC1 gene:
	    • encodes dyskerin (nucleolar ribonucleoprotein)
	  • Autosomal dominant variants = TERC and TERT genes
	  • Autosomal recessive variant = NOP10 gene
		• Mild hyperkeratosis, epidermal atrophy, prominent telangiectasia of superficial vessels and numerous melanophages
		• Hoyeraal Hreidarsson syndrome:
		  • severe variant
		  • dyskeratosis congenita + posterior fossa malformation
		• Clinical DDx:
		1. Naegeli–Franceschetti–Jadassohn syndrome:
		  • Autosomal dominant, reticulated hyperpigmentation, dental anomalies, PPK, hypohidrosis; but lacks leukoplakia and bone marrow failure
		2. Fanconi's anemia:
		  • AR, generalized hypermelanosis + pancytopenia (marrow failure) + risk of leukemia
		  • But also has absent thumbs, radius and tendency for chromosomal breakage

Other lichenoid (interface) diseases		
Lichen sclerosus et atrophicus	• Band-like infiltrate similar to lichen planus (early lesions) • Vacuolar change and apoptotic basal keratinocytes • Infiltrate pushing downward by expanding zone of edema and sclerosis	

Disorder	Predilection and Clinical Key Features	Histopathology

Pityriasis lichenoides	• Acute form = pityriasis lichenoides et varioliformis acute (PLEVA). See Chapter 8 for more information	• Similar to lichen striatus in appearance:
		  • heavy lymph infiltrate that obscures DE interface
		  • focal epidermal cell death and overlying parakeratosis or confluent epidermal necrosis
		  • dermal infiltrate with wedge-shaped distribution

Still's disease (adult onset)	• Adult-onset variant of arthritis • Evanescent, transient rash + high fever + polyarthralgia + lymphadenopathy • Note: Still's disease is more common in children and a variant of juvenile rheumatoid arthritis	• Multiple dyskeratotic cells (mainly in upper epidermis and stratum corneum) • Neutrophils in the dermal infiltrate (no associated lymphocytes)
Late secondary syphilis (lichenoid)	• Develop in untreated syphilis patients (see Chapter 24 for more information) • Cutaneous lesions vary, e.g. maculopapular, psoriasiform, lichenoid, follicular, pustulas, etc.	• Possible lichenoid reaction pattern • Plasma cells usually present • Inflammatory infiltrate extends to mid and deep dermis

Disorder	Predilection and Clinical Key Features	Histopathology
Mycosis fungoides	• Subset of mycosis fungoides patients may have lichenoid changes on biopsy • Erythematons, scaly patches in sun-protected areas • See Chapter 41 for more information	• Pautrier microabscess • BMZ intact with lichenoid infiltrate (lymphocytes line up along BM) • Nuclear atypia in lymphocytes • Eosinophils and sometimes plasma cells
Lichen amyloidosus	• Small, discrete, often pruritic, waxy papules • Extensor surfaces of lower extremities • See Chapter 14 for more information	• Accumulation of filamentous material in basal cells with eventual cell death • Filamentous material extruded into dermis similar to colloid body formation • Gobular oeposits of amyloid in papillary dermis

Psoriasiform Reaction Pattern

"The Big Four" = *Psoriasis, PRP, Lichen Simplex Chronicus, Chronic Eczemas*

4

Psoriasis

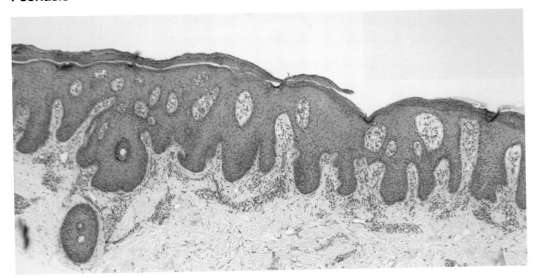

Name	Predilection and Clinical Key Features	Histopathology
Major psoriasiform dermatoses		
Psoriasis	• 2% population (mean 25 years old) • Associated with HLA-Cw6 • Extensor surfaces, extremities, scalp, nails • Well-circumscribed, erythematous patches with silvery white scale; Auspitz's sign (bleeding if remove scale); arthritis • Woronoff ring = white halo around psoriatic plaque due to prostaglandin E2 (PGE2), especially with treatment	• Confluent parakeratosis (not focal); neutrophils in stratum corneum ("Munro microabscesses"); pustule in spinous layer ("pustule of Kogoj"); regular acanthosis (rete ridges same length, but clubbed); hypogranulosis; thin suprapapillary plates with dilated vessels with Rouleaux formation (stack of RBCs in chain); neutrophils in the horn (i.e. stratum corneum)

Basic science of psoriasis

• Th17 > Th1 immune response (IL23 > TNF-α)
• Increased K6, K16, K17; unique cells with K6 and K10 expression
• More CD4 cells in dermis; more CD8 cells in epidermis
• Susceptibility gene = PSOR1 (30%); usually RF negative (80%)
• Epidermal turnover = 3–4 days vs. normally 13 days: causes hypogranulosis due to rapid turnover rate
• Possible triggers or exacerbations: trauma (Koebner Rx), infection, drugs ("BALI" = Beta blockers, ACE inhibitors, Lithium, Interferon)

Name	Predilection and Clinical Key Features	Histopathology
AIDS-associated psoriasiform dermatitis	• Features of AIDS and psoriasis • Associated with initial seroconversion	• Psoriasiform hyperplasia but no thinning of suprapapillary plate; scattered apoptotic keratinocytes

Name	Predilection and Clinical Key Features	Histopathology
Pustular psoriasis	• Acute form of psoriasiform dermatosis characterized by widespread eruption of numerous sterile pustules on an erythematous base and associated with constitutional symptoms. Arthritis, erythroderma and geographical tongue may also develop • Variants include: 　• Von Zumbusch pustular psoriasis: 　　• generalized pustular variant 　　• explosive onset, fever and high mortality (30%); most common variant 　• Acropustulosis = tips of fingers 　• Palmoplantar = palm and plantar areas 　• Impetigo herpetiformis = pustular variant occurring during pregnancy (see below)	• Intraepidermal pustules in various stages of development; neutrophils in papillary dermis and epidermis; subcorneal pustules with a thin roof of stratum corneum; "spongiform pustules of Kogoj" (in spinous layer) • No eosinophils usually

Name	Predilection and Clinical Key Features	Histopathology
Impetigo herpetiformis	• "Pregnancy + pustular psoriasis" • Onset in third trimester • Usually remits after pregnancy • May flare with use of oral contraceptives • Risk of fetal mortality due to placental insufficiency • Subset variant is related to hypoparathyroidism and hypocalcemia 	• Similar to pustular psoriasis histologically
Guttate psoriasis	• Children • Often occurs after illness (i.e. streptococcal pharyngitis) • Trunk • Small, erythematous, drop-like papules with a fine scale	• Focal "mounds" of parakeratosis; less acanthosis than psoriasis; neutrophils

Name	Predilection and Clinical Key Features	Histopathology

Reiter's syndrome	• Males; HLA-B27
	• 30% of reactive arthritis patients develop syndrome
	• Associated with GI infection (*Shigella*, *Yersinia*), genital infections (*Chlamydia*, *Ureaplasma*) and HIV
	• Triad ("can't see, pee or climb a tree"):
	  1. Non-gonococcal urethritis
	  2. Ocular inflammation
	  3. Arthritis
	• Also circinate balanitis, mucosal erosions and red plaques
	• Keratoderma blennorrhagica = feature of Reiter's syndrome with pustular-psoriasis-like cutaneous lesions (feet/palms, genitalia, groin) with a crusted erythematous papule/plaque; heals without scarring
	
		• Histopathology similar to pustular psoriasis (psoriasiform epidermal hyperplasia with thick horny/stratum corneum layer); thick parakeratotic scale crust (often detaches)

Name	Predilection and Clinical Key Features	Histopathology
Pityriasis rubra pilaris (PRP)	• Unknown etiology • Follicular papules with central keratin plug; "islands of sparing"; palmoplantar keratoderma; may become erythrodermic • Clinically similar to phrynoderma (vitamin A deficiency) • Clinical classifications: Type I/classic adult (most common): • "Islands of sparing," waxy PPK; usually clear in 3 years Type II/atypical adult: • Coarse, lamellated PPK, ichthyosiform scale on legs, possibly alopecia; chronic course Type III/classic juvenile: • Similar to type I, but in children Type IV/circumscribed juvenile (most common juvenile): • Elbows and knees; variable course Type V/atypical juvenile: • Scleroderma-like on hands/feet; majority of familial cases; chronic course	• "Psoriasiform + seborrheic dermatitits + keratosis pilaris-like" • "Checkerboard" = alternating orthokeratosis and parakeratosis in vertical and horizontal directions, forms collarette around follicular ostia; acanthosis; hypergranulosis; follicular plugging and parakeratotic lipping of follicle; perivascular infiltrate, mainly lymphocytes (occasional eosinophils and plasma cells) • "Shoulder parakeratosis" (similar to seborrheic dermatitis) • *Note:* the "P" alternating with "R" in "PRP" helps in remembering the alternating ortho- and parakeratosis!

Name	Predilection and Clinical Key Features	Histopathology
Parapsoriasis	• Small plaque parapsoriasis or SPP ("chronic superficial dermatitis"): • resembles mild eczema and spongiotic, but possibly psoriasiform (see p. 79) • no risk of mycosis fungoides • Large plaque parapsoriasis (possibly early mycosis fungoides) may appear psoriasiform	
Lichen simplex chronicus	• Females and atopic dermatitis patients • Neck and distal extremities • Scaly, thickened plaque in response to persistent rubbing of pruritic site	• Prominent psoriasiform hyperplasia; compact orthokeratosis overlying hypergranulosis; vertical streaking of collagen in papillary dermis; papillomatosis appearance • *Note:* differs from PN which has irregular-shaped rete and nodule-like

Other psoriasiform dermatoses

Name	Predilection and Clinical Key Features	Histopathology
Subacute and chronic spongiotic dermatitides	• Eczematous dermatitides (allergic contact, seborrheic dermatitis, nummular dermatitis and atopic dermatitis)	• Subacute = spongiosis with a scale crust (or serum + parakeratosis) • Chronic = eosinophils; progressive psoriasiform hyperplasia; eosinophils and plasma cells in superficial dermis (this is not seen in psoriasis)
Erythroderma	• "Exfoliative dermatitis" • Characterized by erythema, edema and scaling of skin • Associated with pre-existing dermatosis (i.e. psoriasis, PRP, MF, chronic eczema/atopic); drug; or cancer/T-cell lymphoma	• Uniform spongiosis, parakeratosis, dilated vessels and infiltrate • Findings vary and are non-specific (psoriasiform hyperplasia and mild spongiosis possible)

Name	Predilection and Clinical Key Features	Histopathology

Mycosis fungoides	• Men/African-Americans
	• Clones of malignant helper T cells (CD4+)
	
	• *Multiple stages* (see Chapter 41 also):
	  1. Pre-MF (parapsoriasis)
	  2. Patch (eczema-like)
	  3. Plaque (red–brown color)
	  4. Tumor (brown, red–gray)
	  5. Erythrodermic form (Sezary syndrome)
	• Tx = steroids, retinoids (bexarotene), PUVA, chemotherapy with nitrogen mustard, cyclophosphamide, electron beam radiation
		• Psoriasiform hyperplasia; epidermotropism of lymphocytes and variable cytological atypia of lymphocytes; Pautrier's microabscesses

Chronic candidosis and dermatophytoses [methenamine silver stain; PAS stain]	• Scaly plaques and patches on various cutaneous locations 	• "Sandwich sign" = stratum corneum with alternating "compact-basket weave-compact layers"; progressive psoriasiform hyperplasia; rete ridges not too long; neutrophils in parakeratotic scale ("neuts in the horn") with serum

Name	Predilection and Clinical Key Features	Histopathology
Inflammatory linear verrucous epidermal nevus (ILVEN)	• Variant of epidermal nevus • Females • Lower extremities (unilateral) • Pruritic, linear, psoriasiform plaque • Increased involucrin in the orthokeratotic epithelium and minimal amounts in the epidermis below parakeratosis (psoriasis has increased involucrin in all the epidermal layers except the basal layer)	• Papillated psoriasiform hyperplasia with foci of parakeratosis overlying hypogranulosis; alternating orthokeratosis and parakeratosis in horizontal direction; crypt areas may have hypergranulosis; "wart-like" appearance of papillomatosis
Norwegian (crusted) scabies	• Infested with thousands of mites • Associated with mentally/physically debilitated or immunosuppressed • Thick, hyperkeratotic crusts on body	• Marked orthokeratosis and scale crust; numerous mites/larvae/ova in keratinous layer

Name	Predilection and Clinical Key Features	Histopathology
Squamous cell in-situ	• "Bowen's disease" • Crusted, erythematous papule or plaque 	• Variant may show full-thickness keratinocyte atypia; psoriasiform hyperplasia with thick suprapapillary plate
Clear cell acanthoma [PAS+ due to glycogen in cells]	• Lower part of legs • Papulonodular red lesion • Increased glycogen in cells due to defect in phosphorylase (degrades glycogen)	• Well-demarcated psoriasiform epidermal hyperplasia; pallor of keratinocytes without atypia; abundant glycogen; numerous vessels

Name	Predilection and Clinical Key Features	Histopathology
Lamellar ichthyosis	• Autosomal recessive form of ichthyosis • Present at birth • Large plate-like scale, involves palms/soles; collodion baby; scarring alopecia; risk of skin cancers • Mutation = TGM1 (transglutaminase-1) gene Causes excessive turnover with hyperkeratosis	• Mild psoriasiform hyperplasia; prominent orthokeratosis and focal parakeratosis overlying thick granular layer (hypergranulosis)

Pityriasis rosea (PR)	• "Herald patch" only of PR may show psoriasiform tissue reaction
	
	• Typically resolves in 6 weeks
		• Spongiosis + Mild Psoriasiform + Focal parakeratosis
		• Superficial and deep infiltrate with psoriasiform appearance; acanthosis and mild psoriasiform hyperplasia; focal parakeratosis; spongiosis; exocytosis of lymphoctyes leading to "mini-Pautrier simulants"
		
		• DDx for mounds of focal parakeratosis = "PEGS":
		  • P = pityriasis rosea
		  • E = erythema annulare centrifugum
		  • G = guttate psoriasis (neutrophils)
		  • S = small plaque parapsoriasis

Name	Predilection and Clinical Key Features	Histopathology
Pellagra	• Inadequate amount of niacin (nicotinic acid), vitamin B$_3$ • Scaly, erythematous rash in sun-exposed areas that may blister; followed by hyperpigmentation and epidermal desquamation • Casal's necklace = hyperpigmentation around neck	• Mild to moderate psoriasiform hyperplasia; upper epidermis pallor and ballooning progressing to necrosis; confluent parakeratosis

Acrodermatitis enteropathica	• Zinc deficiency
	
	• Periorificial and acral lesions which may be eczematous, vesiculobullous, pustular, or mixed
	• *Triad* of clinical symptoms:
	  1. Acral dermatitis
	  2. Diarrhea
	  3. Alopecia
	• Possible blood test = low alkaline phosphatase level
		• Confluent parakeratosis overlying psoriasiform hyperplasia; upper epidermis pallor with some necrosis or subcorneal clefting
		
		• Possible DDx for pale epidermal cells = "SHARP migration of pale cells":
		  • SHARP = syphilis, Hartnup disease, acrodermatitis enteropathica, radiodermatitis, pellagra/psoriasis
		  • Migration = necrolytic migratory erythemata (see below)
		  • Pale = Paget's
		  • Cells = clear cell acanthoma

Name	Predilection and Clinical Key Features	Histopathology
Glucagonoma syndrome	• "Necrolytic migratory erythema" (cutaneous lesion term) • Perineum, buttocks, groin • Recurrent erythematous patches that blister, crust and heal with hyperpigmentation • Usually a manifestation of glucagon-secreting islet cell pancreatic tumor	• (Similar to acrodermatitis enteropathica) • Psoriasiform hyperplasia, upper epidermal pallor, confluent parakeratosis overlying area; subcorneal clefts; loss of granular layer • Distinct appearance with compact parakeratosis, then vacuolated/ballooning zone, then normal epidermal cells with psoriasiform hyperplasia (unique look); often involves only upper epidermis

Name	Predilection and Clinical Key Features	Histopathology
Secondary syphilis (psoriasiform) [anti-treponema antibody stain, Warthin–Starry stain]	• "Great imitator" • Palms and soles, face, genitals (condyloma lata), mucous patches in mouth 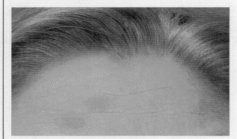 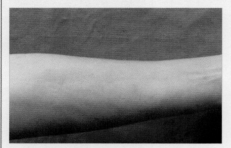 • Non-pruritic morbilliform eruption with constitutional symptoms 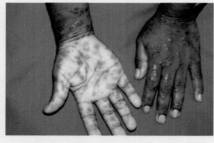 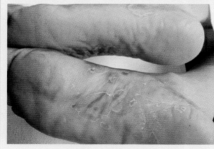	• "Lichenoid + psoriasiform appearance" • Considerable variation; psoriasiform hyperplasia seen in late lesions of secondary syphilis; superficial and deep dermal infiltrate with plasma cells 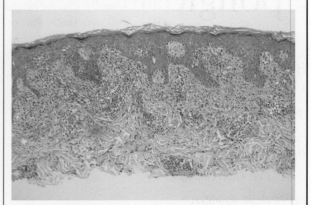 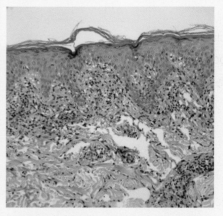 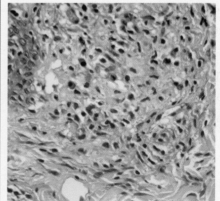 • Numerous plasma cells visible in the dermis

Spongiotic Reaction Pattern

Allergic contact dermatitis

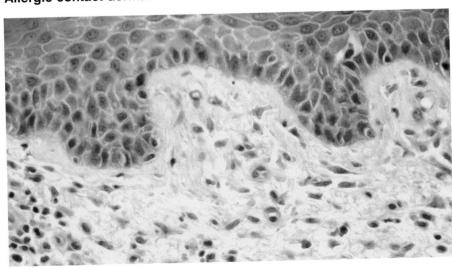

Name	Histopathology	Name	Histopathology
Neutrophilic spongiosis			
Pustular psoriasis and Reiter's syndrome (similar on histopathology)		**IgA pemphigus**	
Acute generalized exanthematous pustulosis (AGEP)		**Dermatophytoses and candidosis**	
Beetle (*Paederus*) dermatitis	• Type of irritant contact dermatosis with pederin, a toxic alkaloid produced by a beetle, such as the rove beetle (*Paederus*) • Usually linear due to crushing of bug		
Eosinophilic spongiosis			
Pemphigus (precursor)		**Pemphigus vegetans**	

Name	Histopathology	Name	Histopathology
Bullous pemphigoid		**Eosinophilic, polymorphic and pruritic eruption**	• "PUPPP of radiation" • Associated with radiotherapy (especially for breast carcinoma)
Drug reactions	• See drug reaction chapter	**"Id" reactions**	• See section below
Allergic contact dermatitis	• See section below	**Arthropod bites**	• Especially scabies (see section below)
Eosinophilic folliculitis ("Ofuji's disease")	• Can involve follicular infundibulum, adjacent epidermis and follicle 	**First stage of incontinentia pigmenti (first stage = vesicles)**	• Eosinophilic spongiosis; necrotic keratinocytes

Name	Predilection and Clinical Key Features	Histopathology
Miliarial spongiosis		
Miliaria	• Miliaria = free flow of eccrine sweat is impeded in distal pore due to accumulation of extracellular polysaccharide substance (EPS) • Miliaria crystallina (miliaria alba); asymptomatic, clear 1–2-mm vesicles • Miliaria rubra (prickly heat) = small, erythematous papulovesicles with a predilection for clothed areas, often pruritic (photos above) • Miliaria profunda = flesh-colored papules (gooseflesh); associated with anhidrosis	• "Spongiosis around the sweat glands" • Miliaria crystallina (photo above) = superficial obstruction with a vesicle within or directly beneath the stratum corneum • Miliaria rubra (photo above) = edema in the papillary dermis near eccrine duct entry to epidermis; variable spongiosis and spongiotic vesiculation related to the sweat duct unit and adjacent epidermis; usually mild lymphocytic infiltrate • Miliaria profunda (photo above) = sweat duct obstruction near dermal-epidermal (DE) junction; subepidermal vesiculation
Follicular spongiosis		

Follicular spongiosis	• Presence of intercellular edema in the follicular infundibulum:
	  • Infundibulofolliculitis = pruritic, follicular papular eruptions on trunk and proximal extremities; young adults, typically black patients
	  • Atopic dermatitis (follicular lesions)
	  • Apocrine miliaria (Fox–Fordyce disease; see below)
	• Eosinophilic folliculitis (Ofuji's disease) = eosinophilic spongiosis centered on follicular infundibulum	

Name	Predilection and Clinical Key Features	Histopathology
Fox–Fordyce disease	• "Apocrine miliaria" • Axilla of young adult females • Small, infundibulocentric papules with intense pruritus • Chronic papular eruption • Result of apocrine duct infundibular rupture • See Chapter 15 also	• Periductal foam cells (specific clue); spongiosis around apocrine duct's entry into follicular infundibulum

Name	Predilection and Clinical Key Features	Histopathology
Pityriasiform spongiosis		
Pityriasis rosea (PR)	• Age 10–35 years old • Trunk, neck and proximal extremities • Acute, self-limited dermatosis with oval, salmon-pink, papulosquamous lesions on trunk, neck and proximal extremities; often have preceding "Herald patch" • Typically resolves in 6 weeks	• Undulating epidermis with focal parakeratosis and spongiosis (may resemble small Pautrier microabscess); lymphocyte exocytosis; perivascular infiltrate; extravasated RBCs • *Note:* Herald patch is more psoriasiform

Name	Predilection and Clinical Key Features	Histopathology
Erythema annulare centrifugum (EAC)	• All ages (infants to elderly) • Annular, erythematous lesions spreading outwards with a fine "trailing" scale (parakeratosis); pruritus • Deep variant = same but advancing edge more elevated; usually no scaling or pruritus • Possibly due to a type IV hypersensitivity reaction such as drug, infection (i.e. dermatophytes) and malignancy; possibly associated with systemic diseases (SLE, liver, Graves')	• Superficial variant = non-specific with mild spongiosis and focal pegs of parakeratosis (associated with trailing edge scale); mild superficial perivascular cuffing by lymphocytes ("coat-sleeve" appearance) • *Reminder:* "EA sleeve in EAC" • Deep variant = deeper perivascular infiltrate and cuffing, with sparing of epidermis (no spongiosis); however, this may be a different condition
Other spongiotic disorders		
Irritant contact dermatitis (ICD)	• Inflammatory condition of skin produced in response to direct toxic effect of irritant (detergents, solvents, acid/alkali) • ICD more common than ACD	• Superficial ballooning, necrosis and neutrophils; mild irritants produce spongiotic dermatitis mimicking ACD, although superficial apoptotic keratinocytes may be present • Necrosis of the epidermis is often present

Name	Predilection and Clinical Key Features	Histopathology
Allergic contact dermatitis (ACD)	• Inflammatory disorder initiated by allergen contact which has previously sensitized the patient • Erythematous papules, vesicles, pruritic, develop 12–48 hours after exposure to allergen (resolve = 2–4 weeks avoid) • Most common allergen = poison ivy/oak • Most common skin patch test allergen = nickel • Rhus dermatitis (due to poison ivy, poison oak, or poison sumac), photo above	• Variable spongiosis and vesiculation at different horizontal and vertical levels with an "ordered" pattern; mild exocytosis; progressive psoriasiform hyperplasia with chronicity; usually eosinophils and edema in superficial dermis, numerous Langerhans cells
Protein contact dermatitis	• Chronic eczema with episodic acute exacerbations a few minutes after contact with agent (fruit, vegetable, plant, grain, enzyme)	• No distinguishing features; possible urticarial component
Nummular dermatitis	• Dorsum of hands, extensor forearm surface, lower legs, outer thighs • Tiny papules and papulovesicles that become confluent into "coin-shaped" lesions; central clearing may occur	• May mimic ACD but usually more "untidy" appearance; neutrophils in dermal infiltrate and epidermis; psoriasiform hyperplasia in chronic cases

Name	Predilection and Clinical Key Features	Histopathology
Sulzberger–Garbe syndrome	• "Oid-oid disease" • Variant of nummular dermatitis • Middle-aged Jewish males • Oval lesions on penis, trunk, face • Syndrome of chronic exudative discoid and lichenoid dermatitis; severe, nocturnal pruritus (a constant feature)	• Similar to nummular dermatitis
Seborrheic dermatitis	• Up to 5% of the population; especially males • Scalp, ears, eyebrows, nasolabial area • Erythematous, scaling papules with greasy yellow appearance in "seborrheic areas" • Associated with *Malassezia furfur* (*Pityrosporum*) • Seborrheic dermatitis also associated with: • HIV • Neurological disorders (especially Parkinson's) • Leiner's disease = infant with generalized seborrheic dermatitis + recurrent infections + failure to thrive • Possible mutation = complement 5	• "Shoulder parakeratosis" (parakeratosis around ostia) with crust containing neutrophils; crust centered on follicle • Variable spongiosis and psoriasiform hyperplasia depending on activity and chronicity

Name	Predilection and Clinical Key Features	Histopathology
Pityriasis amiantacea	• Likely a reaction pattern due to an inflammatory scalp disease, such as psoriasis (most common), seborrheic dermatitis, atopic dermatitis, etc. • Often called "tinea amiantacea," but does not involve tinea • Scalp • "Asbestos-like" sticky scales that bind down hair; possible scarring alopecia results • Often coexists with seborrheic dermatitis	• Spongiosis of follicular and surface epithelium with parakeratotic scale at the follicular ostia; parakeratotic scale is in "onion skin arrangement" around outer hair shafts
Atopic dermatitis	• Onset in infancy or childhood • Chronic, pruritic, inflammatory disease, usually in patient with family history of atopy (asthma, allergic rhinitis and atopic dermatitis) • Initially, a Th2 response (IL-4, IL-10, IL-13, IgE) • As the condition progresses, it switches to a Th1 response	• Similar to other spongiotic diseases; increased "volume" of hyperplasia; prominent vessels in papillary dermis • DDx in infant with atopic dermatitis-like lesions = ichthyosis vulgaris, Wiskott–Aldrich syndrome, ataxia–telangiectasia, phenylketonuria (PKU), atopic dermatitis
Papular dermatitis	• "Itchy red bump" disease • Symmetrically on trunk, extensor surfaces, face, neck, buttocks • Pruritic papular eruption with changes from excoriation	• Variable epidermal spongiosis and focal parakeratosis; excoriation changes

Name	Predilection and Clinical Key Features	Histopathology
Pompholyx	<ul><li>"Dyshidrotic eczema"</li><li>Side of fingers, soles</li></ul> <ul><li>Recurrent, vesicular eruption of palms/soles often with "tapioca-pudding" vesicles between fingers</li><li>Associated with contact dermatitis, infection (tinea), etc.</li></ul>	<ul><li>Thick stratum corneum over fluid-filled vesicles; vesiculation often with peripheral displacement of acrosyringium</li></ul>
Hyperkeratotic dermatitis of the palms	<ul><li>Clinical variant of chronic hand dermatitis</li><li>Adults</li><li>Limited to palms</li><li>Sharply marginated, fissure-prone, hyperkeratotic dermatitis</li></ul>	<ul><li>Chronic spongiotic dermatitis with spongiosis and psoriasiform hyperplasia; overlying compact orthokeratosis; chronic inflammatory cell infiltrate (lymphocytes, no neutrophils)</li></ul>
Juvenile plantar dermatosis	<ul><li>Children 3–14 years old</li><li>Weight-bearing portion of feet</li></ul> <ul><li>Shiny, scaly, erythematous disorder on weight-bearing portion of feet</li><li>Possibly associated with atopy and footwear</li></ul>	<ul><li>Localized around acrosyringium; variable parakeratosis and hypogranulosis overlying psoriasiform acanthosis; spongiosis, mild spongiotic vesiculation</li></ul>

Name	Predilection and Clinical Key Features	Histopathology
Stasis dermatitis	• Middle age and older • Due to impaired venous drainage of legs (most prominent medial malleoli) • Discoloration due to deposition of hemosiderin in dermis	• Mild spongiosis only; proliferation of superficial dermal vessels; extravasation of erythrocytes; abundant hemosiderin (especially in deeper dermis; while pigmented purpura superficial); fibrosis and loss of follicles
Auto-eczematization ("Id" reaction)	• Eczematous reaction pattern due to disseminated inflammation at other skin sites • Associated with dermatophyte infections, scabies, burns, stasis	• Variable spongiosis; edema of papillary dermis and activated lymphocytes present

Papular acrodermatitis of childhood (Gianotti–Crosti syndrome)	• Triad:
	  1. Erythematous papular eruption of several weeks
	  2. Mild lymphadenopathy
	  3. Acute hepatitis (anicteric)
	• Face and extremities (often spares trunk)
	
	• Associated with EBV, hepatitis B, Coxsackie A17, hepatitis A and C
		• Focal parakeratosis; focal spongiosis; papillary edema; perivascular lymphocytes
		
		• Three tissue patterns:
		  1. Lichenoid
		  2. Spongiotic
		  3. Lymphocytic vasculitis

Name	Predilection and Clinical Key Features	Histopathology
Spongiotic drug reactions	• Three major categories: 1. Provocation of endogenous dermatitis (cimetidine) 2. Systemic contact reaction (neomycin) 3. Miscellaneous group (thiazide, calcium channels)	• Spongiosis with conspicuous exocytosis of lymphocytes relative to spongiosis; eosinophils, plasma cells and activated lymphs in superficial dermis
Small plaque parapsoriasis or chronic superficial dermatitis	• Persistent superficial dermatitis • "Digitate dermatosis" variant with finger-like, linear patches on the lateral trunk • Well-defined, round and oval patches (<5 cm) with a fine "cigarette-paper" scale, usually on trunk and proximal extremities	• Only mild spongiosis and focal "mounds" of parakeratosis with variable psoriasiform hyperplasia; superficial perivascular infiltrate with upward extension and mild exocytosis (CD4+ cells)

Name	Predilection and Clinical Key Features	Histopathology
Psoriasis	• Early stages of psoriasis show spongiosis • Palms and soles; erythrodermic psoriasis • Erythematous, scaly patches and plaques	• Spongiosis with lymphocyte exocytosis; mounds of scale crust regularly distributed within the cornified layer
Light reactions	• Include photoallergic dermatitis, phototoxic dermatitis, "eczematous" form of PLE, etc.	• Variable; usually mild spongiosis; superficial and deep perivascular inflammation

Name	Predilection and Clinical Key Features	Histopathology
Dermato-phytoses	• Occur anywhere on body • Scaly patches 	• Neutrophils in stratum corneum; "sandwich sign" meaning compact orthokeratosis/parakeratosis sandwiched between orthokeratotic layers (see below) • If neutrophils are in the stratum corneum, search for hyphae and consider a PAS stain to assist • Neutrophils in stratum corneum • Hyphae in stratum corneum • "Sandwich sign" • PAS stain highlighting hyphae in stratum corneum

Name	Predilection and Clinical Key Features	Histopathology
Arthropod bites	• Epidermal spongiosis common in arthropod bites, especially scabies Ant bites Scabies	• Spongiotic vesicle containing variable number of eosinophils; superficial and deep (often "wedge-shaped"); dermal infiltrate with interstitial eosinophils • ("Eosinophils in the meadow")
Grover's disease	• "Transient acantholytic dermatosis" • Adult males • Trunk area • Rare variant which has spongiosis histologically, indistinguishable clinically from typical Grover's	 • Spongiosis with focal acantholysis in spongiotic variant; "untidy" superficial dermal inflammation

Name	Predilection and Clinical Key Features	Histopathology
Pruritic urticarial papules and plaques of pregnancy (PUPPP)	• Third trimester of pregnancy • Favors striae (does not involve umbilicus) • Intensely pruritic eruption of papules and urticarial plaques towards the end of pregnancy (third trimester) • DDx in pregnancy: • Herpes gestationis ("BP of pregnancy") = second to third trimester (earlier than PUPPP), forms around umbilicus and spreads (unlike PUPPP)	• Subtle superficial perivascular lymphocytic infiltrate with variable edema of papillary dermis; epidermal spongiosis
Pigmented purpuric dermatoses (PPD) [Perls' stain for hemosiderin/iron]	• Purpuric lesions develop from hemosiderin deposition • Young adults; lower extremities • Lower extremities • Multiple variants (see below and Chapter 8, Vasculitis)	• Variable infiltrate (majority CD4+) and infiltrate upper dermis (perivascular); lymphocytic vasculitis; no fibrosis as in stasis dermatitis; hemosiderin in papillary dermis; possible mild epidermal spongiosis present
Schamberg's disease	• Variant of pigmented purpuric dermatosis • "Progressive pigmentary dermatosis" • Pretibial area • Symmetric, punctate purpuric, "cayenne pepper" macules on pretibial area • See Chapter 8, p. 185, for more information	• Upper dermal infiltrate with lymphocytes and histiocytes; RBC extravasation. No epidermal involvement usually
Purpura annularis telangiectodes of Majocchi	• Variant of pigmented purpuric dermatosis • Trunk area • Annular patch with perifollicular, red punctate lesions and telangiectasia • See Chapter 8, p. 185, for more information	• Similar to Schamberg's on HP with spongiosis
Pigmented purpuric lichenoid dermatosis of Gourgerot and Blum	• Variant of pigmented purpuric dermatosis • Lower legs • Symmetric, lichenoid papules/plaques • Associated with hepatitis C • See Chapter 8, p. 185, for more information	• Similar to Schamberg's on HP, but slightly lichenoid-like and spongiosis
Lichen aureus	• Variant of pigmented purpuric dermatosis • Unilateral, grouped macules/papules with rusty, golden, or purple color • See Chapter 8, p. 185, for more information	• The most lichenoid-like, with superficial, heavy infiltrate; no exocytosis or spongiosis (as in others)

Name	Predilection and Clinical Key Features	Histopathology
Eczematid-like purpura of Doucas and Kapetanakis	• Variant of PPD • Lower extremities • Pruritic, eczematous-like and orange color • Case reports associated with infliximab • See Chapter 8, p. 186, for more information	• Spongiosis and similar other variants (hemosiderin, etc.)
Pityriasis alba	• Often atopic individuals • Usually on head and neck • Hypopigmented, scaly patches on head and neck of atopic individuals • Present with a patch of lighter-colored skin at the malar eminence • Usually the preceding eczema has resolved (See p. 225 for more information)	• Mild epidermal spongiosis with minimal parakeratosis in clinically hypopigmented lesions (reduction of melanin in the basal layer). See p. 225 also
Eruption of lymphocyte recovery	• Associated with cytotoxic agents/chemotherapy	• Mild epidermal spongiosis with lymphocyte exocytosis; keratinocyte atypia with impaired maturation; some dyskeratosis • Difficult to distinguish from exanthematous drug reaction, viral infection or acute GVHD

Name	Predilection and Clinical Key Features	Histopathology
Lichen striatus	• Unknown etiology, possible aberrant clone during fetal development migrates along lines of Blaschko and then exposed to infection later • Female children and adolescents • Extremities • Papular eruption on one side of body linearly; usually length of an extremity • Resolves months to years with hypopigmentation	• Lichenoid + spongiotic appearance; melanin incontinence, parakeratosis, hyperkeratosis, heavy infiltrate with lymphocytes in 3–4 adjacent dermal papillae; acanthosis; intraepidermal vesicles with Langerhans cells; eccrine extension of infiltrate; dyskeratotic cells at all levels in the epidermis
Erythroderma	• Common etiologies (ID-SCALP): • I = idiopathic • D = drug allergy • S = seborrheic dermatitis • C = contact dermatitis • A = atopic dermatitis • L = lymphoma and leukemia • P = psoriasis/PRP 	• Mild spongiosis; variable psoriasiform hyperplasia; appearance depends on underlying disease (often biopsy of little value)

Name	Predilection and Clinical Key Features	Histopathology
Mycosis fungoides	• Cutaneous T-cell lymphoma which evolves through several clinical stages (patch, plaque, and tumor). See also Chapter 41	• Mild spongiosis, variable epidermal hyperplasia and epidermal mucinosis; epidermotropism, often with Pautrier microabscess; variable cytological atypia of lymphocytes which extend upwards into papillary dermis

Acrokeratosis paraneoplastica	• Bazex's syndrome
	• Elderly
	• Acral areas, ears
	• Symmetrical, acral, psoriasiform, red-to-violaceous plaques or patches
	• Associated with internal malignancy:
	  • especially SCC of upper aerodigestive tract
	  • often precedes malignancy diagnosis
		• Variable with psoriasiform appearance, or mild spongiosis; hyperkeratosis; focal parakeratosis; exocytosis of lymphoctyes
		• *Note:* Not the same "Bazex's syndrome" which involves multiple BCCs + follicular atrophoderma + hypotrichosis + hypohidrosis (or hyper-) + pili torti

Vesiculobullous Reaction Pattern

6

Vesiculobullous reaction pattern

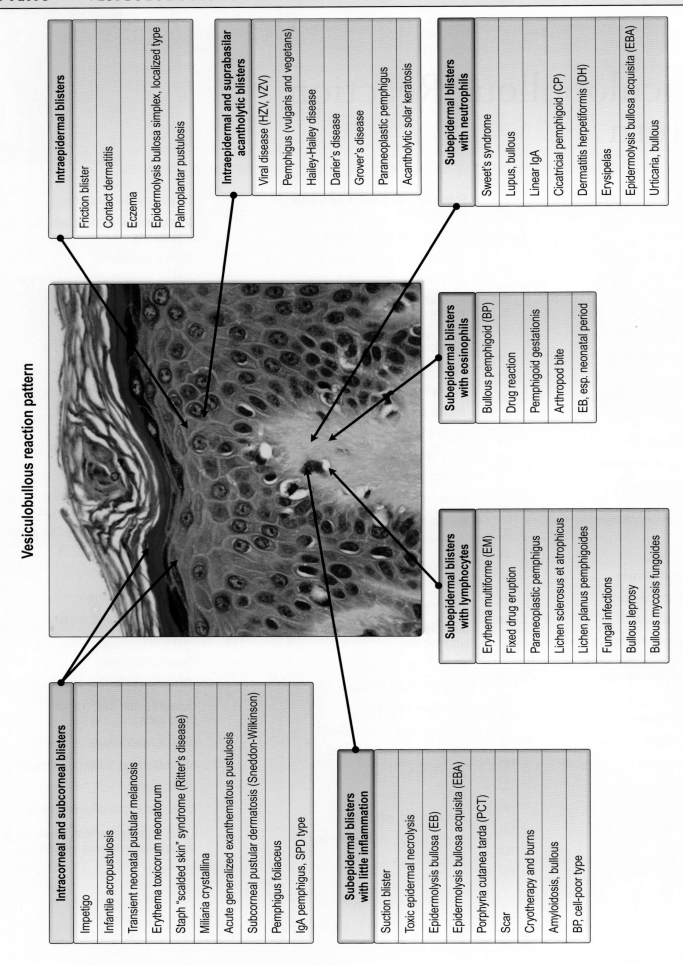

Intraepidermal blisters

Friction blister

Contact dermatitis

Eczema

Epidermolysis bullosa simplex, localized type

Palmoplantar pustulosis

Intraepidermal and suprabasilar acantholytic blisters

Viral disease (HZV, VZV)

Pemphigus (vulgaris and vegetans)

Hailey-Hailey disease

Darier's disease

Grover's disease

Paraneoplastic pemphigus

Acantholytic solar keratosis

Subepidermal blisters with neutrophils

Sweet's syndrome

Lupus, bullous

Linear IgA

Cicatricial pemphigoid (CP)

Dermatitis herpetiformis (DH)

Erysipelas

Epidermolysis bullosa acquisita (EBA)

Urticaria, bullous

Subepidermal blisters with eosinophils

Bullous pemphigoid (BP)

Drug reaction

Pemphigoid gestationis

Arthropod bite

EB, esp. neonatal period

Subepidermal blisters with lymphocytes

Erythema multiforme (EM)

Fixed drug eruption

Paraneoplastic pemphigus

Lichen sclerosus et atrophicus

Lichen planus pemphigoides

Fungal infections

Bullous leprosy

Bullous mycosis fungoides

Intracorneal and subcorneal blisters

Impetigo

Infantile acropustulosis

Transient neonatal pustular melanosis

Erythema toxicorum neonatorum

Staph "scalded skin" syndrome (Ritter's disease)

Miliaria crystallina

Acute generalized exanthematous pustulosis

Subcorneal pustular dermatosis (Sneddon–Wilkinson)

Pemphigus foliaceus

IgA pemphigus, SPD type

Subepidermal blisters with little inflammation

Suction blister

Toxic epidermal necrolysis

Epidermolysis bullosa (EB)

Epidermolysis bullosa acquisita (EBA)

Porphyria cutanea tarda (PCT)

Scar

Cryotherapy and burns

Amyloidosis, bullous

BP, cell-poor type

Bullous disorders along the basement membrane zone (BMZ)

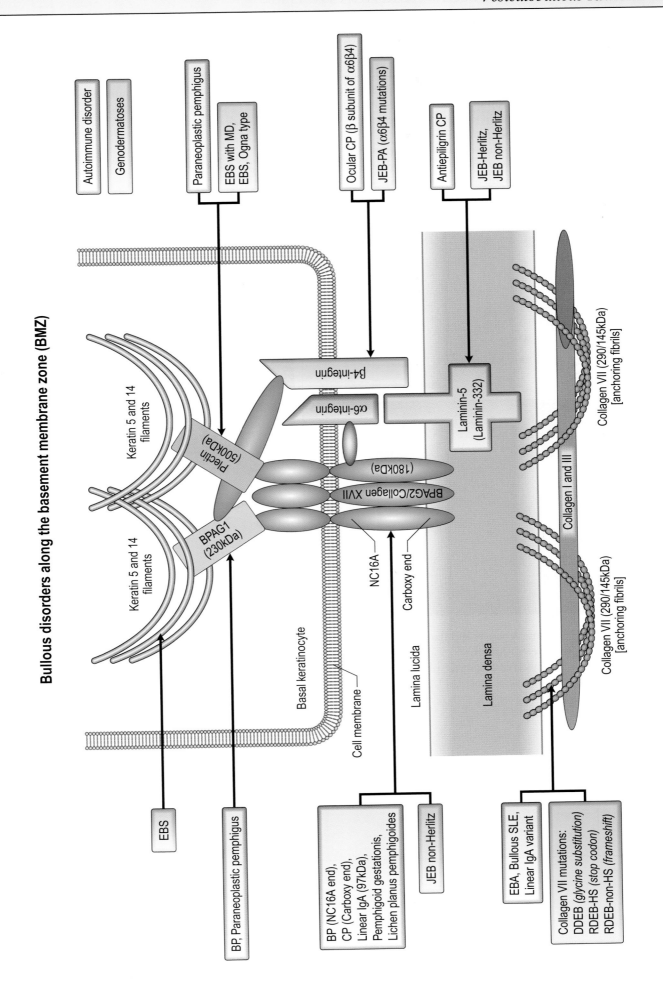

Autoimmune disorder

Genodermatoses

Paraneoplastic pemphigus

EBS with MD, EBS, Ogna type

Ocular CP (β subunit of α6β4)

JEB-PA (α6β4 mutations)

Antiepiligrin CP

JEB-Herlitz, JEB non-Herlitz

Keratin 5 and 14 filaments

Keratin 5 and 14 filaments

Plectin (500kDa)

β4-integrin

α6-integrin

Laminin-5 (Laminin-332)

BPAG1 (230kDa)

BPAG2/Collagen XVII

(180kDa)

NC16A

Carboxy end

Collagen I and III

Collagen VII (290/145kDa) [anchoring fibrils]

Basal keratinocyte

Cell membrane

Lamina lucida

Lamina densa

Collagen VII (290/145kDa) [anchoring fibrils]

Collagen VII (290/145kDa) [anchoring fibrils]

EBS

BP, Paraneoplastic pemphigus

BP (NC16A end), CP (Carboxy end), Linear IgA (97kDa), Pemphigoid gestationis, Lichen planus pemphigoides

JEB non-Herlitz

EBA, Bullous SLE, Linear IgA variant

Collagen VII mutations: DDEB (glycine substitution) RDEB-HS (stop codon) RDEB-non-HS (frameshift)

Name	Predilection and Clinical Key Features	Histopathology
Intracorneal and subcorneal blisters		
Bullous impetigo [Gram stain]	• "Localized form of staphylococcal scalded skin syndrome" resulting from the production in situ of staphylococcal epidermolytic toxin • Premature infants and chronic renal insufficiency adults (due to poor renal function which excretes toxin) • May be localized or more generalized • Shallow erosions and flaccid bullae with an erythematous rim • *Staphylococcus aureus*, phage II, type 71 • Exfoliative toxins A–D target desmoglein 1 (160 kDa)	• Subcorneal collection of numerous neutrophils, acantholytic cells (<pemphigus foliaceus) • Gram+ cocci visible • Gram stain showing bacteria (picture above)

Name	Predilection and Clinical Key Features	Histopathology
Staphylococcal "scalded skin" syndrome (SSSS)	• Called Ritter's disease in neonates • Children <6 years old • Rapid onset of fragile blisters, perioral crusting, diffuse rash (spare mucosa, palm/sole) • Caused by epidermolytic/exfoliative toxin A and B (epidermolysin) from *Staphylococcus aureus*, phage group II strains • Toxins target desmoglein 1 (160 kDa)	• Fragile, subcorneal blister; acantholytic cells; neutrophils; do not see major inflammation since toxin, therefore no organism visible and does not involve mucosa • Due to distant site infection (no organism seen)
Dermatophytosis	• "Bullous tinea" • Dermatophytoses may result in superficial blisters • Often on hands and feet • Vesicles or bullae • *Note:* Candida may uncommonly cause subcorneal blisters also	• Neutrophils in stratum corneum; subcorneal and intraepidermal blisters possible

Name	Predilection and Clinical Key Features	Histopathology
Pemphigus foliaceus (PF)	• Face, trunk initially; then spreads • Recurrent crops of flaccid bullae that easily rupture and cause shallow erosions/crusted plaques • Ab = desmoglein 1 (160 kDa) • Possible drug-induced pemphigus foliaceus (especially captopril, long-term penicillamine)	• Superficial bullae high in granular layer with fibrin, neutrophils and scattered acantholytic cells; no bacteria present like impetigo • DIF = "chicken wire" IgG/C3 (pictured above) • Indirect IF = best on guinea pig esophagus
Endemic pemphigus foliaceus	• Fogo Selvagem or "wild fire" • Children and young adults • Rural areas of South America (Brazil) • PF-like, sunlight can exacerbate • Elevated thymosin levels in patients indicate possible viral cause • Possible transmission by black fly (*Simulium*)	• Same pathology as pemphigus foliaceus

Name	Predilection and Clinical Key Features	Histopathology
Pemphigus erythematosus	• "Senear–Usher syndrome" • Systemic LE + pemphigus foliaceus (variant of pemphigus foliaceus) • Erythematous, scaly, crusted plaques in butterfly distribution (nose/malar) and "seborrheic areas" • Possibly drug induced (especially heroin, captopril, penicillamine) • Associated with myasthenia gravis and thymoma	• Subcorneal blister with occasional acantholytic cells (histology similar to pemphigus foliaceus) • DIF = IgG at intracellular and granular BMZ
Herpetiform pemphigus	• "Dermatitis herpetiformis clinically, but pemphigus-like on DIF" • Erythematous, urticarial plaques and vesicles in herpetiform arrangement; severe pruritus • Ab = desmoglein 1 (160 kDa)	• Eosinophilic spongiosis with formation of intraepidermal vesicle; minimal/no acantholysis • DIF = IgG on keratinocytes, similar to pemphigus
Subcorneal pustular dermatosis (SPD)	• "Sneddon–Wilkinson disease" • IgA pemphigus but negative DIF • Chronic, relapsing, vesiculopustular dermatosis • Women (40–50 years old) • Trunk, especially intertriginous areas and flexor aspect of limbs (spares face, mucosa) • Associated with IgA gammopathy, but DIF negative	• Similar to SPD variant of IgA pemphigus, but negative DIF • Subcorneal pustule filled with neutrophils; typically, pustule "sits" on the epidermis with no depression • DIF = negative

Name	Predilection and Clinical Key Features	Histopathology

IgA pemphigus	• Vesiculobullous eruption with deposits of IgA in epidermis (not IgG)
	• Types:
	  1. Subcorneal pustular dermatosis (SPD):
	  • subcorneal pustule; does not involve mucosa
	  • DIF = IgA in upper epidermis
	  • Ab (IgA) = desmocollin 1
	  2. Intraepidermal neutrophilic (IEN):
	  • pustule and neutrophils mid-stratum
	  • DIF = IgA in all of epidermis
	  • possible Ab (IgA) = desmoglein 1 or 3?
		• Neutrophils "attracted" and found inside blister, do not see many outside of blister
		
		• DIF = IgA in epidermis

Infantile acropustulosis	• Onset at 3–6 months of age • Black males • Distal extremities and acral areas • Recurrent crops of intensely pruritic vesiculopustules • Resolves/stops recurring = 2–3 years	• Intraepidermal pustule with neutrophils (some eosinophils) that progress to subcorneal pustule; sparse perivascular infiltrate • Smear of pustule shows mainly neutrophils (no bacteria or fungi)

Name	Predilection and Clinical Key Features	Histopathology
Erythema toxicum neonatorum [Wright's stain]	• 50% of full-term neonates (rarely premature infants) • First few days of life • Face, trunk area (spares palms/soles unlike infantile acropustulosis) • Benign disorder • Erythematous macules, wheals, papules and pustules • Resolves 1–2 days 	• Subcorneal or intraepidermal pustules with eosinophils; close to pilosebaceous follicle orifice • Wright's stain of pustule shows numerous eosinophils • Eosinophils in dermis and epidermis

Name	Predilection and Clinical Key Features	Histopathology
Transient neonatal pustular melanosis	• Usually 3–6 months of age (may occur in utero) • Black newborns (4–5%) • Widespread = head and neck (below chin); palms/soles; trunk • Pustules resolve in days (pigment slowly fades) • Continuum of three phases: 1. 2–10-mm vesiculopustules: not pruritic or recurring 2. Fine collarette of scale at ruptured sites 3. Hyperpigmented brown macules	• Vesiculopustules with intracorneal or subcorneal neutrophils with fibrin and only a few eosinophils • Pigmented macules have increased melanin within basilar keratinocytes (not located in dermis)

Name	Predilection and Clinical Key Features	Histopathology
Acute generalized exanthematous pustulosis (AGEP)	• Fever; peripheral leukocytosis; rapidly evolving pustular eruption with sterile, miliary pustules on erythematous background; non-follicular lesions • Resolve rapidly after stopping drug • Confirm by patch test • Usually associated with drugs (beta-lactam antibiotics/penicillin; cephalosporin, diltiazem, furosemide) • "Toxic pustuloderma" 	• Subcorneal or superficial intraepidermal pustule with mild spongiform pustulation at margins; exocytosis of neutrophils adjacent to pustule; edematous papillary dermis • Heavy mixed infiltrate with eosinophils (unlike pustular psoriasis)

Name	Predilection and Clinical Key Features	Histopathology
Miliaria crystallina	• "Prickly heat" • Obstruction of eccrine sweat ducts • May be present at birth • Forehead, neck, upper trunk • Small 1–2-mm vesicles which rupture easily • Resolve with cooling	• Vesicle forms within or directly beneath stratum corneum with neutrophils and lymphocytes; centered on the acrosyringium
Intraepidermal blisters (within Malpighian/spiny layer)		
Spongiotic blistering disease	• Allergic contact dermatitis, nummular dermatitis, pompholyx, polymorphic light eruption, insect bite, first stage of incontinentia pigmenti, miliaria rubra, etc. • Hint: look for spongiosis adjacent to vesicle	
Palmoplantar pustulosis	• Possibly form of psoriasis or "bacterial-Id-reaction" • Women (40–60 years old) • Erythematous scaly plaque with recurrent sterile pustules symmetrically on palms/soles; sternocostoclavicular ossification (10%); lytic, sterile bone lesions • Possible autoantibodies to thyroid antigens • Possible Tx = low-dose cyclosporine	• Unilocular, well-delimited pustule within epidermis and extending upwards to undersurface of stratum corneum; focal parakeratosis; eosinophils (unlike pustular psoriasis)
Amicrobial pustulosis associated with autoimmune disease (APAD)	• Females • Associated with autoimmune diseases • Chronic relapsing eruption involving mainly cutaneous flexures, external auditory canal and scalp	• High intraepidermal spongiform pustule in an acanthotic epidermis; parakeratosis • Possible improvements with zinc supplement

Name	Predilection and Clinical Key Features	Histopathology
Viral blistering diseases	• Seen in herpes simplex, herpes zoster, varicella, etc. • Herpes simplex virus (above)	• Ballooning degeneration (intracellular edema); nuclear margination (slate-gray nucleus)
Friction blister	• Sites where epidermis thick and firmly attached to dermis • Palms, soles and heels	• Intraepidermal blister just beneath stratum granulosum in the epidermis (vs. suction blister which is a subepidermal blister)

Name	Predilection and Clinical Key Features	Histopathology
Suprabasilar blister		
Pemphigus vulgaris (PV)	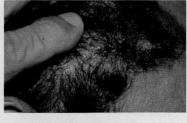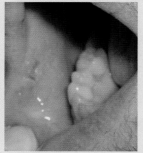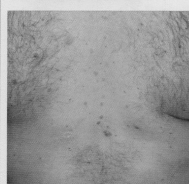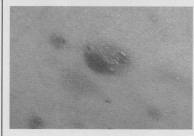<ul><li>Initially oral blisters, ulcers followed in weeks/months by cutaneous, flaccid blisters; Nikolsky's sign (side pressure leads to blister extension)</li><li>Mortality = 5–15% (infection)</li><li>Ab = desmoglein 3 (130 kDa) and desmoglein 1 (160 kDa)</li><li>Mucosa-dominant form = Ab to desmoglein 3 only</li><li>Possibly due to trauma, drugs (captopril, penicillamine)</li></ul>	<ul><li>"Row of tombstones" (specific), since impact desmosomes and not hemidesmosomes; follicular involvement common</li></ul>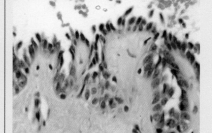<ul><li>Suprabasal bullae with acantholysis; "tombstone appearance" at basal cells; edema and disappearance of intercellular bridges</li></ul>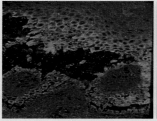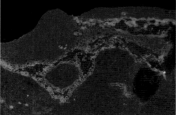<ul><li>DIF = intercellular IgG4 and IgG1 in "chicken-wire" appearance (cutaneous PV pictured above left, mucosal PV above right)</li><li>Indirect IF (pictures below) = best with monkey esophagus</li></ul>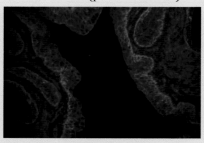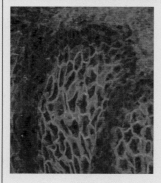

Name	Predilection and Clinical Key Features	Histopathology
Pemphigus vegetans	• Variant of PV • Vegetating erosions; flexural areas; tongue cerebriform pattern; blood eosinophilia • Associated with drugs (captopril, heroin) • Variants: 1. Hallopeau type = pustular lesions initially (more benign, few relapses) 2. Neumann type = vesicular and erosive lesions initially • Ab = Desmoglein 3 (130 kDa)	• Vegetating lesion: hyperkeratosis, papillomatosis, prominent acanthosis with downward proliferation of rete ridges; likely see acanthosis easiest around follicles • Early lesions: • Hallopeau = eosinophilic spongiosis and eosinophilic microabscesses • Neumann = intraepidermal vesicles, no eosinophil abscesses • DIF = IgG like PV • Differ from pyodermatitis–pyostomatitis vegetans which has negative DIF and is associated with IBD

Name	Predilection and Clinical Key Features	Histopathology
Paraneoplastic pemphigus (PNP)	 • Chronic stomatitis; polymorphous skin lesions with features of EM and PV; mucosal erosions, corneal melting • May develop bronchiolitis obliterans • Disorder affects all types of epithelium in body • Associated with non-Hodgkin's lymphoma (#1 in adults), CLL, Hodgkin's, thymoma, Castleman's disease (#1 in children) • Targets desmogleins and plakin family: • Desmogleins: • desmoglein 1 (160 kDa) • desmoglein 3 (130 kDa) • Plakin family: • desmoplakin 1 (250 kDa) • desmoplakin 2 (210 kDa) • desmocollins 2 and 3 • envoplakin (210 kDa) • periplakin (190 kDa) • BPAG1 (230 kDa) • plectin (500 kDa) • Ab usually present = desmoglein • Unique bullous disease that is B-cell and cytotoxic T-cell mediated	• Variable histology • DIF = IgG and C3 on BMZ • Indirect IF (picture above) on murine bladder epithelium (best tissue)

Name	Predilection and Clinical Key Features	Histopathology
Hailey–Hailey disease	• "Familial benign chronic pemphigus" • Autosomal dominant genodermatosis • Axilla, genital area, chest, neck • Recurrent, erythematous, vesicular plaques that progress to small flaccid bullae that rupture/crust • Gene mutation = ATP2C1 (Golgi Ca^{2+} pump)	• Suprabasilar clefting with acantholytic cells lining clefts; "dilapidated brick wall" appearance (partial acanthosis at different epidermal levels); does not involve follicle • DIF = negative • Rarely corp ronds and grains (as in Darier's disease)
Darier's disease	• "Keratosis follicularis" • Autosomal dominant • Onset adolescence (teenagers) • Head, neck and trunk (seborrheic areas) • Greasy, crusted papules and papulovesicles; cobblestone oral papules; mental retardation; odor; skin-colored or brownish papules on dorsum of hands, feet; red and white bands on nails with "V-shape" defects distally • Gene = ATP2A2 (endoplasmic reticulum Ca^{2+} pump in keratinocyte, encodes SERCA2) • Depletion of ER's Ca^{2+} stores causes acantholysis due to loss of cell adhesion and dyskeratosis due to apoptosis • *Note:* worsens with lithium intake, sweat, heat	• Acantholytic dermatosis; suprabasilar clefts with acantholysis + dyskeratotic cells forming corps ronds (upper epidermis) and grains (stratum corneum); keratin plug with orthokeratosis and parakeratosis • DIF = negative • Corp ronds = vacuolated perinuclear halo in upper epidemis • Grain = premature aggregate of tonofilaments; cells have small "cigar-shaped" nuclei

Name	Predilection and Clinical Key Features	Histopathology

Grover's disease	• "Transient acantholytic dermatosis"
	• Elderly men
	• Upper trunk
	
	• Sudden onset of small, crusted, erythematous papules and papulovesicles ("heat rash" like)
		
		• Four histological pattern types:
		  1. Darier's-like
		  2. Hailey–Hailey-like
		  3. Pemphigus vulgaris-like
		  4. Spongiotic
		(May contain >1 type of histological pattern)
		
		• Spongiotic Darier's-like
		
		• Pemphigus vulgaris-like

Acantholytic solar keratosis	• May resemble a superficial BCC clinically • Suprabasilar clefting with acantholytic cells in cleft and margins; atypical (dysplastic) keratinocytes present	

Name	Predilection and Clinical Key Features	Histopathology
Subepidermal blisters with little inflammation		
Epidermolysis bullosa overall	• Mechanically fragile skin from gene mutations in structural proteins • DIF is negative • Diagnosis with electron microscopy or immunomapping (light microscope of little value)	
Epidermolysis bullosa simplex (EBS)	• Intraepidermal skin split • Usually autosomal dominant, except EBS with MD is AR	
Generalized type or Kobner EBS	• Autosomal dominant • Blisters at birth or infancy • Blisters, palmoplantar hyperkeratosis; worse in warm weather • Defect in K5/K14	
Localized type or Weber–Cockayne	• Autosomal dominant • Onset age of 2 years • Hyperhidrosis; thick-walled blisters on hands/feet after exercise/friction; worsen with heat • Defect in K5/K14	
Dowling–Meara or EB herpetiformis	• Autosomal dominant • Hemorrhagic blisters in first few months of life; heal with transitory milia/pigmentation; herpetiform arrangement; diffuse PPK; heat does not exacerbate • EM feature = clumping tonofilaments (not specific) • Defect in K5/K14	• Separation level low in epidermis; keratin in lower part of blister
EBS with muscular dystrophy	• Autosomal recessive (only EBS that is autosomal recessive) • Decayed teeth, alopecia, palmoplantar hyperkeratosis, late-onset muscle dystrophy • Often consanguineous marriage • Defect in plectin (found in hemidesmosome and muscle)	

Name	Predilection and Clinical Key Features	Histopathology
Junctional epidermolysis bullosa (JEB)	• Heals without scarring usually • All lack uncein/19-DEJ-1 (associated with anchoring filaments)	
JEB, Herlitz	• Autosomal recessive • Erosions/bullae at birth • Anemia, affects organ's epithelium • Usually die in infancy • Significant involvement of all epithelial mucosal surfaces (GI, GU); hoarse cry as infant indicates laryngeal involvement (may be first sign) • Defect = laminin-5 (LAMA3, LAMB3, LAMC2 gene)	• Split in the lamina lucida/central basement membrane zone (BMZ)
JEB, non-Herlitz	• Autosomal recessive • Generalized form, heals with atrophy and scarring (no milia/constrictions); alopecia, absence of pubic and axillary hair • Multiple SCC risk; scalp and nail lesions • Defect = BPAG2/type XVII collagen or laminin-5; (COL17A/BPAG2 and laminin-5 gene)	
JEB with pyloric atresia	• Autosomal recessive • Blisters; pyloric atresia; may present with aplasia cutis congenita or ureterovesical junction obstruction • Defect = α6β4 integrin (ITGB4 and ITGA6 gene)	

Name	Predilection and Clinical Key Features	Histopathology
Dystrophic (dermolytic) epidermolysis bullosa (DEB)	• Defect in anchoring fibril type VII collagen (COL7A1 gene) • Trauma-induced blisters with scars and milia formation	
Dominant dystrophic EB (DDEB)	• Autosomal dominant • Two variants: 1. Cockayne–Touraine: • blisters at birth/child on extensor surfaces likely, scarring/milia • not debilitating (no "mitten deformity") 2. Pasini/Albopapuloid variant: • extensive blisters at birth • flesh-color, scar-like lesions on trunk spontaneously form ("albopapuloid lesions") • Defect = usually glycine-to-arginine substitution in collagen VII (impacts anchoring fibril's helix)	
Recessive dystrophic EB, Hallopeau–Siemens	• Autosomal recessive • Large flaccid bullae at birth, "mitten deformities" from digital fusion, usually debilitating; sparse hair; SCC in scars • Defect = usually termination codon in collagen VII (most severe type, lacks fibrils)	
Recessive dystrophic, non-HS	• "Dermolytic EB inversa" • Blisters usually in acral areas; nail dystrophy; minimal mucosa blisters • Defect = missense/frameshift in collagen VII (defective fibrils)	
Transient bullous dermolysis of newborn	• Rare DDEB variant in newborns • Blisters only for 1–2 years • Possibly due to a short delay in transporting type VII collagen from basal keratinocytes to lower BMZ	• Cell-poor subepidermal blister
Other inherited BMZ bullous disorders	• Bart syndrome: • any form of EB + aplasia cutis congenita (or congenital localized absence of skin) • Shabbir syndrome (laryngo-onycho-cutaneous syndrome): • autosomal recessive disorder • mutation = laminin 5 (α3 gene or LAMA3 gene) • Cutaneous erosions + nail dystrophy + exuberant vascular granulation tissue (especially conjunctiva, larynx)	

Name	Predilection and Clinical Key Features	Histopathology
Epidermolysis bullosa acquisita [PAS+ mostly on "roof" of blister]	• Autoimmune condition (not hereditary) • Mid-adult age • Non-inflammatory bullae in areas of minor trauma, especially extensor surface of limbs; mucosa (30-50%); ocular involvement • Heals leaving atrophic scars and milia • Associated with systemic diseases (SLE, Crohn's disease, RA, amyloidosis, etc.) • Ab = Type VII collagen (290/145 kDa) of anchoring fibrils (similar to bullous LE)	• Subepidermal bulla with fibrin and only few inflammatory cells; roof of blister intact; upper dermal infiltrate with neutrophils • DIF = linear IgG >> C3 along BMZ • Salt-split = Ab to the dermal "floor" (BP will show Ab on "roof" side)

Name	Predilection and Clinical Key Features	Histopathology
Porphyria cutanea tarda (PCT) [PAS+ in vessel walls]	• Deficient disorders of the heme synthetic enzyme • PCT = uroporphyrinogen decarboxylase (UROD); mutation = UROGEN decarboxylase gene 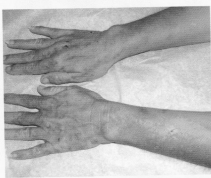 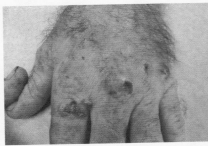 • Blisters form in light-exposed areas, especially dorsa of hands; malar hypertrichosis; diabetes • Elevated urinary porphyrin (coral-pink with Wood's light) • Associated with hepatitis C, alcohol, liver disease • Tx = phlebotomy • *Note:* check for possible hemochromatosis (acute intermittent porphyria – no skin lesions; abdominal pain, neurologic issues; Scandinavians; PBGD gene)	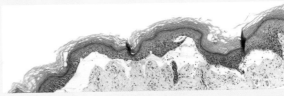 • Subepidermal bulla with preservation of dermal papillae in lesion floor ("festooning"); no inflammatory infiltrate; "caterpillar bodies" (eosinophilic, linear BMZ material; collagen IV) 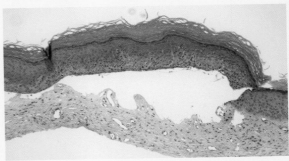 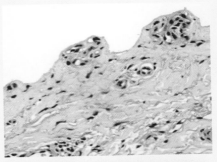 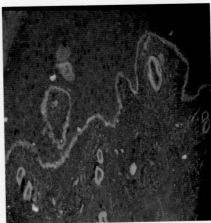 • DIF = IgG/C3 around vessels and BMZ (likely due to "trapping" of antibodies); pseudo-PCT is the same

Name	Predilection and Clinical Key Features	Histopathology

Bullous pemphigoid (cell-poor type)	• Autoimmune, subepidermal, blistering skin disease (rarely involves mucosa)
	• Bullous lesion without an erythematous base
	• See section below on BP also
	• Antibodies:
	  • BPAg2/BP180 (especially NC16A portion): transmembrane protein
	  • BPAg1/BP230: cytoplasmic protein
		• Subepidermal blister formation; few inflammatory cells in the dermis (neutrophils and eosinophils)
		
		• DIF = along BMZ and salt-split = "roof" side

Name	Predilection and Clinical Key Features	Histopathology
Burns and cryotherapy	• Thermal burn (photo below) • Chemical burn (photo below) • Cryotherapy bulla (photo below) 	• Electrocautery results in epidermis necrotic; elongation of keratinocytes; fusion of collagen bundles in upper dermis; basket-weave stratum corneum
Toxic epidermal necrolysis (TEN)	• Erosive mucosal lesions; extensive blister formation • TEN is on a spectrum with Stevens-Johnson Syndrome (SJS) • Epidermal detachment: • SJS <10% body surface area (BSA) • SJS/TEN overlap 10–30% BSA • TEN > 30% BSA • Associated with drugs (sulfonamide, anticonvulsants)	• Subepidermal bulla with confluent necrosis of overlying epidermis

Name	Predilection and Clinical Key Features	Histopathology
Suction blisters	• Subepidermal blister • Dermal papillae preserved ("festooning")	
Blisters overlying scars	• Scar tissue in base of blister in association with history of surgery or trauma	
Bullous solar elastosis	• Intradermal blister that occurs in areas of severe solar elastosis; thin grenz zone of papillary dermis overlies blister • Due to damaged, poorly-adherent dermal collagen	
Bullous amyloidosis [Congo red, crystal violet, thioflavin T]	• Associated with systemic amyloidosis 	• Bullae form above amyloid deposits in skin • Hyaline deposits of amyloid in base of blister
Bullosis diabeticorum	• Rare condition associated with diabetes mellitus • Lower extremities • Asymptomatic blisters that often develop "overnight" • Associated with peripheral neuropathy • Heals usually within 2–6 weeks	• Intraepidermal or subepidermal blister; spongiosis; bullae contain fibrin and few inflammatory cells (no acantholysis and DIF negative)
Bullous drug reaction	• Various drugs implicated 	• Variable infiltrate seen in dermis; rare eosinophil seen

Name	Predilection and Clinical Key Features	Histopathology

Kindler's syndrome	• Poikilodermatous genodermatosis
	• Acral bullae, poikiloderma, atrophy
	• KIND1 gene mutation = encodes kindlin-1:
	  • Focal adhesion protein in basal keratinocytes
	  • Affects the actin–extracellular matrix linkage (unlike the keratin-ECM linkage in epidermolysis bullosa)
		• Subepidermal, cell-poor bullae

Subepidermal blisters with lymphocytes

Erythema multiforme (EM)	• Extremities (hands); mucosal involvement 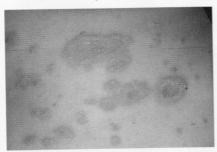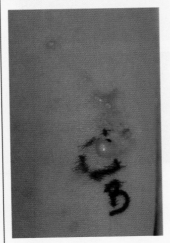 • Self-limited disease with erythematous lesions, may evolve to "target lesions"; distributed symmetrically • May develop vesiculobullous lesions due to damage to basal cells of the epidermis • Often association with HSV	• Lichenoid pattern; subepidermal blister has mild–moderate infiltrate; apoptotic keratinocytes; may have necrosis 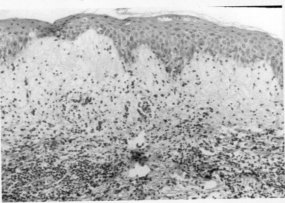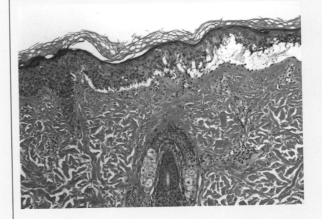

Name	Predilection and Clinical Key Features	Histopathology
Paraneoplastic pemphigus (PNP)	 • See PNP section earlier in chapter 6, p. 102	• Variable histology depending on pathology • DIF = IgG and C3 on BMZ • Indirect IF (picture above) on murine bladder epithelium (best tissue)

Name	Predilection and Clinical Key Features	Histopathology
Fixed drug eruptions	• Bullous variant of fixed drug eruption (similar to EM) • Drugs (half hour to 8 hours after taking medication) • Eruptions occur in same, "fixed" area, if drug re-taken • Circular, violaceous, edematous plaques; resolve with macular hyperpigmentation • Associated with pseudoephedrine (non-pigmented variant), NSAIDs, etc.	• Eosinophils; melanin in macrophages; deep inflammatory cells; obscure DE interface
Lichen sclerosus et atrophicus (LsetA)	• Bullous variant of LsetA • Middle-aged and elderly women • Anogenital region and extragenital areas • Initially translucent, shiny papules/plaques that become white in appearance	• Broad edema or sclerotic collagen in base of blister (homogenized superficial dermis); telangiectatic vessels and some hemorrhage; mainly perivascular infiltrate below possible blister

Name	Predilection and Clinical Key Features	Histopathology
Lichen planus pemphigoides	• "LP + BP" (lichen planus and subepidermal blistering disease resembling bullous pemphigoid) • Possible variant of bullous pemphigoid • Lichen planus patients • Extremities • Tense blister in previously normal skin location; blisters not necessarily form at location of prior lichen planus lesion (differs from bullous LP which forms in long-standing LP lesions) • Ab = BPAG2 or 180-kDa BP antigen (type XVII collagen)	• Mild perivascular infiltrate (eosinophils and neutrophils beneath blister); occasional Civatte bodies in basal layer at blister margins; subepidermal (cell-poor) bulla with mild, perivascular infiltrate of lymphocytes, neutrophils, and eosinophils • DIF = IgG and C3 in BMZ zone

Name	Predilection and Clinical Key Features	Histopathology
Bullous lichen planus	• Bullous variant of LP • Lichen planus patients • At sites of lichen planus papules	• "Lichen planus lesion + bullae" • Heavy, superficial, band-like infiltrate; numerous Civatte bodies in overlying and adjacent basal keratinocytes • Lichen planus DIF = complement and IgM (colloid bodies in papillary dermis) and irregular band of fibrin along basal layer

Name	Predilection and Clinical Key Features	Histopathology
Polymorphic light eruption (PMLE)	• Most common form of idiopathic photodermatoses • Develops several hours after sun exposure (UVA > UVB or visible) • Typically occurs in Spring more often • Papules, plaques or "erythema-like" lesions in sun-exposed areas	• Subepidermal edema leading to blister; cobweb-like appearance with collagen fibers separated by edema; superficial and deep perivascular lymphocytic infiltrate
Bullous fungal infection	• Fungal infection may cause significant edema and blister formation • Anywhere on body • Vesicles • May be seen in autoeczematous reaction (or "Id reaction") to fungus	• Possible neutrophils in the stratum corneum; fungal organisms found; pronounced subepidermal edema that leads to vesiculation
Dermal allergic contact dermatitis	• May result from contact with neomycin, zinc, and nickel salts	• Pronounced subepidermal edema leading to vesiculation; epidermal spongiosis
Bullous leprosy	• Rare manifestation of borderline lepromatous leprosy	• Acid-fast bacilli present within macrophages; subepidermal bullae with dermal infiltrate (lymphs and macrophages)

Name	Predilection and Clinical Key Features	Histopathology
Bullous mycosis fungoides	• Rare manifestation of MF (cutaneous T-cell lymphoma) • See also Chapter 41 for more information on mycosis fungoides	• Usually subepidermal blister; atypical lymphocytes in dermis; Pautrier microabscesses in epidermis

Name	Predilection and Clinical Key Features	Histopathology
Subepidermal blisters with eosinophils		

Bullous pemphigoid (BP)	• Elderly
	• Lower abdomen, inner thighs, flexor forearms
	
	• Multiple, tense bullae arising on pruritic/ urticarial lesions (erythematous, pruritic lesions may precede weeks before); occasional oral lesions
	• Nikolsky sign usually negative (since split is at the basement membrane)
	• Ab = hemidesmosomes at BPAG2/ 180 kDa (especially NC16A) and BPAG1/230 kDa
	• Possible drug etiology triggers condition (especially diuretics, such as furosimide)
	• Variants:
	  • Vesicular pemphigus
	  • Pemphigoid vegetans
	  • Polymorphic pemphigus
	  • Pemphigoid excoriée
	  • Pemphigoid nodularis
		• Unilocular subepidermal blister, mainly eosinophils in lumen and upper dermis (unlike bites and ACD involves upper and lower dermis)
		
		• DIF = linear C3 (above left) > IgG (above right) along BMZ (When complement C3 present, it leads to blister formation)
		• Salt-split = epidermal or "roof" side (unlike EBA, which highlights the "floor")

Name	Predilection and Clinical Key Features	Histopathology
Bullous pemphigoid, urticarial stage	• Precedes blistering stage of BP • Pruritic, urticarial lesions	• Numerous eosinophils, which often "line-up" along DEJ; do not see blister if early • DIF = IgG along BMZ (mainly IgG4 > IgE) (Minimal C3 complement present, so no blister formation yet)

Name	Predilection and Clinical Key Features	Histopathology
Pemphigoid gestationis	• "Gestational pemphigoid" or "herpes gestationis" • "BP of pregnancy" variant • Rare, pruritic vesiculobullous dermatosis of pregnancy • Second to third trimester • Initially localized to periumbilical region that spreads to trunk/extremities • Possibly associated with autoimmune conditions (especially Grave's disease) • Ab = BPAg2/180 kd • Clinical DDx: PUPPP is located clinically in the striae, and does not involve the periumbilical region; occurs during the third trimester	• Appear similar to bullous pemphigoid with subepidermal clefting with neutrophils and eosinophils in dermal infiltrate • DIF = linear C3 > IgG along BMZ (identical to BP's DIF)

Name	Predilection and Clinical Key Features	Histopathology
Bullous arthropod bites	• Bullous lesion in susceptible individuals after arthropod bite 	• Eosinophils; dermal infiltrate of lymphs and eosinophils (often "wedge-shaped"); may be subepidermal blister or mixed intraepidermal and subepidermal lesions with thin strands of keratinocytes bridging the bulla
Bullous drug reactions	• Vesiculobullous eruptions resembling bullous pemphigoid; often photo-exacerbated • Especially with second-generation quinolones (especially ciprofloxacin and levofloxacin)	• Mixed infiltrate including eosinophils
Epidermolysis bullosa	• See EB section (p. 105)	• Eosinophils found in bullae of all three major subtypes, especially in neonatal period biopsies

Name	Predilection and Clinical Key Features	Histopathology
Subepidermal blisters with neutrophils		
Dermatitis herpetiformis (DH)	• "Duhring's disease" • Cutaneous manifestation of celiac disease (20% have clinical CD, but >90% have some gluten-sensitive enteropathy) • Men (North European origin) • Mean age 40s • Extensor surfaces of extremities, buttocks • Excoriations and pruritic papulovesicles with herpetiform grouping • Associated with gluten sensitivity; HLA-DQ2 (90%) and HLA-DR 3 • Ab = epidermal transglutaminase (TG), likely TG3 • Also endomysial antibody to tissue transglutaminase, which cross-reacts and relates to degree of enteropathy • Associated with thyroid disease (especially Hashimoto's) and enteropathy-associated T-cell lymphoma (especially MALT) • Tx = dapsone (also sulfapyridine) and gluten-free diet (oat, corn, rice, potato, tapioca; avoid wheat, rye, barley) • Iodide will worsen symptoms (stimulates neutrophils) • DDx of subepidermal blister + neutrophils predominantly (Herpetic LIPS): • Herpetic = DH • L = lupus (bullous) • I = linear IgA • P = pemphigoid (BP) • S = Sweet's syndrome	• Neutrophilic infiltrate of dermal papillae with vesicles at DE junction; vesicles with fibrin, neutrophils/eosinophils; "ragged-lined" blister • Difficult to differentiate from linear IgA on histology; but with DIF, DH has granular in papillae vs. linear IgA • DIF = granular IgA in normal skin adjacent lesion, especially in dermal papillae

Name	Predilection and Clinical Key Features	Histopathology
Linear IgA bullous dermatosis	• Bimodal = adults (60s); children (age 5) • Vesiculobullous lesion in herpetiform arrangement on erythematous or normal skin ("crown of jewels") • Associated with autoimmune, infection, drugs (especially vancomycin, furosemide, TMX/SMZ) • Ab = 97 kDa of BPAG2 (child variant) and 285 kDa of type VII collagen (adult variant) • Tx = dapsone, possibly steroids • Childhood variant is called "chronic bullous disease of childhood" 	• Neutrophils along BMZ and dermal papillae with vacuolar change • DIF = linear IgA deposition along BMZ (pictured below left) • Salt-split of type VII variant = "floor" of split (pictured above right) • Indirect IF = linear IgA along BMZ (70% of cases) • Chronic bullous disease of childhood (pictured below) • Salt-split of 97 kDa of BPAG2 = "Roof" side (pictured below)

Name	Predilection and Clinical Key Features	Histopathology
Cicatricial pemphigoid (CP)	• "Benign mucous membrane pemphigoid" • Elderly; females • Associated with HLA-DQw7 • Mainly involves oral and ocular mucous membranes, 25–30% cases involve skin • Erosions, ulcers in the mouth; tendency to scar, blindness • Ab = laminin-5, BP180/BPAG2 (especially NC-1 segment or carboxy end of BPAG2), laminin-6, integrin β4, type VII collagen • Antibody to laminin 5 (anti-epiligrin) associated with cancer risk (e.g. colon cancer)	• Subepidermal and "smooth-lined" blister; lymphocytes, eosinophils, neutrophils; sebaceous gland in blister; scarring • DIF = linear IgG/C3 along BMZ
Ocular cicatricial pemphigoid	• Ocular variant of CP • Ab = integrin β4 subunit (hemidesmosomes) • Think: "Four-eyes" for β4 and ocular CP • Ocular involvement; possible symblepharon (scarring on eye)	 • DIF = linear IgG or IgA along conjunctival BMZ

Name	Predilection and Clinical Key Features	Histopathology
Localized cicatricial pemphigoid (Brunsting–Perry)	• Variant of cicatricial pemphigoid • Elderly males • Temple (localized to head/neck area) • Erosions or bullous lesions; scarring alopecia • No mucosal membrane involvement	• Subepidermal blister with lymphocytes, eosinophils, and neutrophils • DIF = linear IgG and C3 along BMZ
Deep lamina lucida (anti-p105) pemphigoid	• Unique non-scarring, subepidermal bullous dermatosis • Extensive bullae and erosions of mucous membrane and skin	• Subepidermal blister with neutrophils in papillary dermis • DIF = linear IgA and C3 along BMZ • Ab = 105-kDa antigen in lower lamina lucida
Anti-P200 pemphigoid	• Clinical appearance of BP, DH, or linear IgA • May be associated with psoriasis • Ab = 200-kDa protein in lower lamina lucida (distinct from laminin-5 or type VII collagen)	• Subepidermal blister with dermal papillary microabscesses; mainly neutrophils and some eosinophils
Bullous urticaria	• Uncommon manifestation of urticaria resulting from severe papillary dermal edema • Neutrophils and eosinophils in upper dermis	
Bullous acute vasculitis	• Acute vasculitis forming bullae that are sometimes hemorrhagic • Vessels with acute vasculitis; leukocytoclasis	

Name	Predilection and Clinical Key Features	Histopathology
Bullous lupus erythematosus	• Uncommon eruption in SLE • Herpetiform vesicles to large hemorrhagic bullae; may be limited to sun-exposed area • Antibodies = type VII collagen (similar to EBA)	• Subepidermal "smooth-edged" splitting; papillary microabscesses; nuclear dust prominent in papillae and superficial vessels; neutrophils extend deep in dermis • DIF = IgG, C3, IgA, ANA (DIF for ANA pictured above left) • Salt-split = highlight the "floor," similar to EBA (pictured above right)

Name	Predilection and Clinical Key Features	Histopathology
Erysipelas	<ul><li>St Anthony's fire</li><li>Superficial bacterial skin infection that characteristically extends into the cutaneous lymphatics</li><li>May form as a result of massive edema in upper dermis</li></ul> 	<ul><li>Elongated rete ridges bridge blister and connect with underlying dermis; mild neutrophilic infiltrate; numerous extravasated erythrocytes</li></ul>
Sweet's syndrome	<ul><li>Acute febrile neutrophilic syndrome</li><li>Females</li><li>Drug-induced variant seen typically in women; while malignancy-related variant has no predilection</li><li>Face, extremities; heal without scarring</li></ul> <ul><li>Abrupt onset of painful dark red crusted plaques/nodules; fever, malaise</li><li>Sudden onset of fever, leukocytosis, and tender, erythematous, well-demarcated papules and plaques</li><li>May recur (30–50%)</li><li>Vesiculobullous variant is often associated with myelogenous leukemia</li><li>Associated with:<ul><li>post-infection (especially URI, *Strep.*)</li><li>malignancies: leukemia-AML, solid tumors</li><li>immunologic diseases: rheumatoid arthritis, IBD)</li><li>pregnancy</li><li>drugs: G-CSF therapy, furosemide, minocycline, OCP, all-*trans*-retinoic acid</li></ul></li><li>Marshall syndrome = complication of Sweet's syndrome (rare); destruction of elastic tissue produces acquired cutis laxa</li></ul>	<ul><li>"Dense neutrophil infiltrate in upper half of dermis; epidermis spared (usually); superficial dermal edema; not a true vasculitis with vessel wall necrosis/fibrinoid; RBC extravasation</li><li>"Papillary dermal edema + neutrophilic dermal infiltrate"</li></ul>

Name	Predilection and Clinical Key Features	Histopathology
Epidermolysis bullosa acquisita	• See EBA section above • Autoimmune disorder affecting trauma-prone areas; may be associated with systemic diseases • Milia and scarring from skin fragility possible • Ab = type VII collagen of anchoring fibrils	

Subepidermal blisters with mast cells

| Bullous mastocytosis | • Uncommon manifestation in mastocytosis in neonates and infants
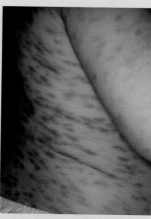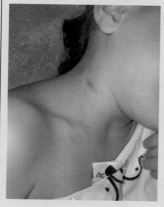
• Tan-brown lesions, may have systemic involvement; may cause blisters | • Numerous mast cells in dermis beneath blister
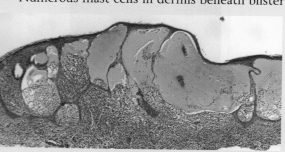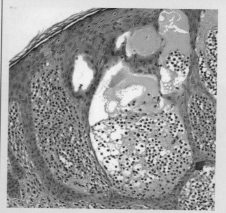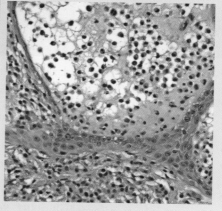
• Giemsa stain (below)
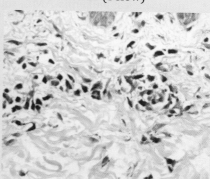 |

Name	Predilection and Clinical Key Features	Histopathology
Miscellaneous blistering diseases		
Coma blister	• Overdose patients in coma • Occur at pressure points • Blisters form due to pressure and drug overdoses (i.e., comas, barbiturate overdose)	• Intraepidermal or subepidermal blister; sparse infiltrate; necrosis of eccrine glands (look like "EM of the sweat glands")

Notes on immunofluorescence (IF)

- Biopsy placed in Michel's solution (contains ammonium sulfate)
- DIF = detect tissue-bound immunoreactant, while indirect IF = detect circulating autoantibodies
- Usually use fluorescein isothiocyanate to fluoresce = absorbs at 490–495 nm (blue) and peak emission at 510–517 nm (green color)

Name	Histopathology	Name	Histopathology
Table of major bullous disorders and immunofluorescence results (DIF images courtesy of Carlos H. Nousari, MD)			
Pemphigus foliaceus [Ab = desmoglein 1 (160 kDa)]		Pemphigus vulgaris [Ab = desmoglein-3 (130 kDa), desmoglein-1 (160 kDa)]	
Bullous pemphigoid [Ab = BPAG2/ 180 kDa and BPAG1/230 kDa]		EBA [Ab = collagen VII (290/145 kDa)]	
Cicatricial pemphigoid [Ab = laminin 5, BPAG2, etc.]		Paraneoplastic pemphigus [Ab = plakins and desmogleins]	
Dermatitis herpetiformis [Ab = TG3 (transglutaminase)]		Linear IgA pemphigus [Ab = BPAG2 and collagen VII]	

Granulomatous Reaction Pattern

7

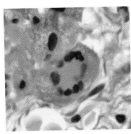

Touton cell
Foamy cytoplasm with circular nuclei and non-foamy center

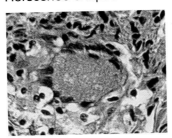

Langhans giant cell
Horseshoe-shaped nuclei

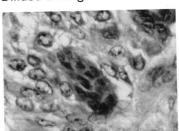

Foreign body giant cell
Diffuse arrangement of nuclei

Type of Granuloma Classification	Another Type of Granuloma Classification	Granulomatous Pattern
Sarcoidal	Epithelioid	Discrete nodular pattern
Tuberculoid		
Necrobiotic	Palisading	Irregular and nodular
Suppurative	Mixed	Diffuse pattern
Foreign body		

Name	Predilection and Clinical Key Features	Histopathology
Sarcoidal granulomas (Epithelioid granuloma with paucity of surrounding lymphocytes/plasma cells, usually without "caseation" necrosis)		

Sarcoidal granulomas

(Epithelioid granuloma with paucity of surrounding lymphocytes/plasma cells, usually without "caseation" necrosis)

Sarcoidosis

- Multisystem granulomatous disease due to a Th1 response with CD4+ T-helper cells
- Adults; Irish, Afro-Caribbean origin
- Bimodal age (ages 25–35 and 45–65)

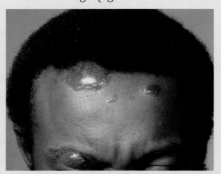

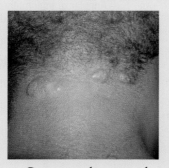

- Cutaneous lesions only in one-third of patients
- Non-specific erythema nodosum-like lesion (3–25%), but highly variable appearance; red–brown papules and plaques; may appear "apple jelly" color under diascopy (blanch with pressure); nail changes (clubbing, onycholysis); leonine facies
- Also lung disease (90%), lymph nodes (mediastinal and peripheral LN), liver, spleen, eyes
- Associated with HLA-1, HLA-B8, HLA-DR3
- ACE level may be useful
- In past, used Kveim–Siltzbach skin test to diagnose

Histopathology:

- Non-caseating, well-demarcated dermal granulomas with sparse lymphoid cells (i.e. "naked" granuloma); normal epidermis

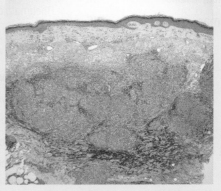

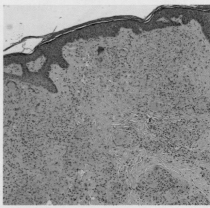

- Langhans giant cells may contain:
  - conchoidal bodies (or Schaumann bodies) = round blue, calcified laminated protein inclusion, possibly due to degenerating lysosomes
  - asteroid body (stellate collagen inclusion), pictured below

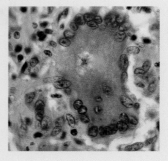

Name	Predilection and Clinical Key Features	Histopathology
Sarcoid variants	• Löfgren's syndrome = "HEFA Löfgren" (hilar lymphadenopathy + erythema nodosum + fever + arthritis) • Heerfordt's syndrome = parotid gland enlargement + cranial nerve palsy (especially facial) + uveitis, fever • Lupus pernio = papules on face, especially "beaded-like" along nasal rim (see below) • Darier–Roussy disease = subcutaneous sarcoidosis (see below)	
Lupus pernio	• Variant of sarcoidosis • Nasal rim • "Beaded-like" papules along the nasal rim and on the face • Often associated with chronic lung sarcoidosis	• Same histology as sarcoidosis
Nodular subcutaneous sarcoidosis	• "Darier–Roussy disease" • Variant of sarcoidosis that involves the subcutis and fat • Adults • Extremities (especially forearms) • Firm, subcutaneous, indurated nodules and linear-like bands • Often associated with systemic disease	• "Naked" granulomas limited to the subcutis without any dermal extension; lobular infiltrate with little or no septal involvement; discrete foci of necrosis present in center of some granulomas
Blau's syndrome	• Autosomal dominant: • may be early-onset familial form of sarcoid • Familial sarcoid-like granulomatous disease with cutaneous sarcoid + uveitis + synovial joint cysts: • possible camptodactyly (or flexion contracture of PIP on third to fifth fingers) • does not involve lungs or viscera • Defect in CARD15 gene • Some patients with Crohn's diseases have same mutation	

Name	Predilection and Clinical Key Features	Histopathology

Reactions to foreign bodies	• Foreign bodies may produce granulomatous dermatitis due to glass, tattoo pigment, zinc, beryllium, etc.:
	  • birefringent in polarized light ("spiny TAZS") = Sea urchin Spines, Talc, Arthropod parts, Zinc (rhomboidal crystals) and Silica (windshield), suture
	  • non-birefringent: zirconium (underarm deodorant), beryllium, aluminum, tattoo (most commonly red ink, especially if it contains mercury sulfide/cinnabar; see photo below)	

Other causes of sarcoidal lesions	• Herpes-zoster scars, secondary syphilis, Sézary syndrome, systemic lymphomas, common variable immunodeficiency, lepromatous leprosy	
Tuberculoid granulomas (Epithelioid granulomas with rim of lymphocytes/plasma cells, often central "caseation" necrosis)		
Tuberculosis (TB)	• Cause = *Mycobacterium tuberculosis* (acid-fast organisms) • See Chapter 23, Bacterial and Rickettsial Infections, for more information	• Confluent and poorly formed granulomas with substantial rim of lymphocytes and plasma cells; possible caseation; occasional asteroid and Schaumann bodies present in multinucleate giant cells

Tuberculids	• Group of cutaneous disorders associated with TB infection elsewhere in the body (do not see organism, but detected with PCR methods):
	  • Lichen scrofulosorum = superficial inflammatory reaction at hair follicles/sweat ducts; caseation rare
	  • Papulonecrotic tuberculid = vasculitis and dermal coagulative necrosis (resembles granuloma annulare)
	  • Erythema induratum-nodular vasculitis = lobular panniculitis; tuberculoid granulomas may extend to deep dermis	

Name	Predilection and Clinical Key Features	Histopathology

Leprosy (Hansen's disease)	
	
	• Leprosy groups:
	  1. Tuberculoid leprosy (TT) = epithelioid granuloma, rim of lymphs; caseation; may destroy basal layer; around neurovascular bundles and arrectores pilorum muscles; do not see organism usually (Wade–Fite method, modified Ziehl–Neelsen stain by addition of peanut oil)
	  2. Borderline tuberculoid (BT) = fewer lymphs, no caseation or destruction of epidermis; foreign body giant cells > Langhans cells
	  3. Borderline (BB) = poorly-formed granulomas; epithelioid cells separated by edema; minimal nerve involvement; see organism
		• Tuberculoid leprosy

Late syphilis [Warthin–Starry stain]	• Late secondary and nodular lesions of tertiary syphilis	• Superficial and deep dermal infiltrate with tuberculoid granulomas; plasma cells; organism rarely found

Name	Predilection and Clinical Key Features	Histopathology
Leishmaniasis [Wright–Giemsa stain]	• Red plaques, nodules or ulcers • Vector = *Phlebotomus* or *Lutzomyia* sand flies (female) • Amastigote organism (possesses kinetoplast = mass of circular DNA in mitochondria, paranuclear rod shape) • Tx = amphotericin or antimony	• Diffuse mixed granulomatous dermal infiltrate; occasional caseation; intracytoplasmic inclusions (tend to go towards outer portion) • Kinetoplast seen in organism (seen as a purple dot, intracytoplasmic inclusions next to the nucleus; mitochondria-like function)
Granulomatous variant of rosacea	• Cheeks, chin, nose, forehead • Persistent erythema and telangiectasia	• Tuberculoid-type granuloma with folliculitis; follicular and perifollicular pustules; marked vascular dilation (telangiectasias) • Difficult differentiating from lupus vulgaris, but rosacea has marked vascular dilation
Perioral dermatitis	• Young women • Chin, nasolabial folds with clear zone around lips • Symmetric red papules, papulovesicles with erythema	• Histopathology identical to rosacea

Name	Predilection and Clinical Key Features	Histopathology
Lupus miliaris disseminatus faciei	• Adolescents/young adults • Central part of face including eyebrows and eyelids • Yellow–brown papules; resolve in months without scarring • Proposed new name: FIGURE (facial idiopathic granulomas with regressive evolution)	• Dermal necrosis surrounded by epithelioid histiocytes, may appear related to ruptured pilosebaceous unit
Crohn's disease	• Dusky, erythematous plaques often on buttock and genital area; may develop oral lesions (differentiates from Melkersson–Rosenthal syndrome) • "Metastatic" = if lesions not contiguous with intestinal Crohn's disease • May develop non-caseating granulomas of tuberculoid type (rarely)	

Necrobiotic granulomas (or palisading granulomas)

Necrobiosis = blurring and loss of definition of collagen bundles, possibly due to mucin, fibrin, lipids, etc.

Granuloma annulare (GA) overall	• Females and young adults • Multiple clinical variants = localized (classic), generalized, perforating, subcutaneous (deep) • Three main histological variants = necrobiotic granulomas, interstitial type, and granulomas of sarcoidal or tuberculoid type • DIF = C3, IgM, fibrin in vessel walls [Mucin stains with colloidal iron (blue–green) or alcian stain] • Associated with sarcoidosis, hepatitis C, AIDS, tattoos, lymphoma, etc. • Possible triggers = insect bites, trauma, warts, sunlight, erythema multiforme, etc. • Tendency to regress spontaneously (but also recur)	

Name	Predilection and Clinical Key Features	Histopathology

Localized (classic) GA	• Majority of GA patients
	• Young adults
	• Hands and arms
	
	• Annular, grouped papules (skin color, pink, or violaceous)
		• GA histology may be one of three variants:
		  1. Necrobiotic granulomas (see below)
		  2. Interstitial variant (see p. 141)
		  3. Sarcoidal or tuberculoid variant (see p. 141)

Generalized GA	• 15% of GA patients • Adults • Trunk and limbs • Multiple papules/nodules • Associated with HLA-BW35, allopurinol, diabetes	

GA with necrobiotic granulomas
 	
[Colloidal iron and alcian blue stain mucin]
	• Necrobiotic granulomas (25% of cases):
	  • Palisading granuloma with central necrobiosis; no fibrosis; abundant mucin [stain with colloidal iron and alcian blue] in central area
	  • No plasma cells seen (unlike necrobiosis lipoidica)
	
	• Photo on left shows mucin in blue with a colloidal iron stain	

Name	Predilection and Clinical Key Features	Histopathology
Interstitial form of GA [colloidal iron and alcian blue stain mucin]	• Interstitial or "incomplete" (most common pattern, 70% of cases): • "Busy" look to dermis due to increased number of inflammatory cells (histiocytes and lymphocytes) arranged around vessels and between collagen bundles; palisade or single file of histiocytes around collagen fibers with a basophilic hue • No necrobiosis seen 	
GA of sarcoidal or tuberculoid type histologically	• Uncommon pattern of GA • Sarcoidal or tuberculoid type appearance • Eosinophils and mucin present (not seen in sarcoid type)	
Perforating GA	• High incidence seen in Hawaii • Dorsal hands, extremities • Grouped papules with central crust or umbilication	 • Central transepidermal elimination of collagen, which communicates with an underlying necrobiotic granuloma

Name	Predilection and Clinical Key Features	Histopathology
Subcutaneous GA	• "Deep" variant of GA • Children (5–6 years old) • Lower legs (anterior tibia), hands, palms • Firm, non-tender, skin-colored nodule	• Large areas of "necrobiosis" surrounded by a palisade of lymphocytes and histiocytes; foci distributed in the deep dermis and subcutis

Name	Predilection and Clinical Key Features	Histopathology
Necrobiosis lipoidica [Sudan stains lipids in necrobiotic areas]	• "Necrobiosis lipoidica diabeticorum"(NLD) • Females in 30s • Some cases associated with diabetics • Legs (especially shins); 75% bilateral • Red papules with atrophic, shiny yellow–brown center and well-defined raised red-to-purple edge • May develop SCC in older lesions • Possibly decreased sensation, hypohidrosis in plaques • Areas of sclerotic collagen show GLUT-1 protein (glucose transporter)	• Granuloma with necrobiosis paralleling epidermis; perivascular infiltrate including plasma cells; necrotizing vasculitis; involves full dermis and diffuse/broad area; fibrosis; lipids in necrobiotic areas (Sudan stain); no mucin • DIF = IgM and C3 in vessel walls Numerous plasma cells visible (photo above)

Name	Predilection and Clinical Key Features	Histopathology
Necrobiotic xanthogranuloma (NXG)	• Periorbital area, trunk, limbs • Elderly (often in 60s) • Violaceous-to-red, partly xanthomatous plaques and nodules • Often associated with paraproteinemia • See Chapter 40 for more information	• Palisading granuloma with focal hyaline necrobiosis; numerous giant cells, foam cells and bizarre histiocytes; cholesterol clefts • May be similar to NLD, but significantly different clinically • Cholesterol clefts and giant cells

Name	Predilection and Clinical Key Features	Histopathology
Rheumatoid nodules [fibrin stains with PTAH (blue color)]	• 20% of RA patients; SLE (5%) (possibly due to vasculitic process) • Hands, feet • Multiple nodules; persist for months to years • *Note:* accelerated rheumatoid nodulosis = methotrexate patients who develop multiple nodules on hands and feet	• Deep in dermis/subcutis with palisading granuloma with irregular areas of necrobiosis with palisade of elongated histiocytes; obvious fibrin in homogeneous, eosinophilic necrobiotic area; eosinophils and lymphocytes; no mucin (different from GA)

Name	Predilection and Clinical Key Features	Histopathology
Rheumatoid nodules	• 20% of RA patients; SLE (5%) (possibly due to vasculitic process)	• *Note:* epithelioid sarcoma may appear histologically similar

Name	Predilection and Clinical Key Features	Histopathology
Rheumatic fever nodules	• Children with rheumatic fever • Associated with acute rheumatic carditis • Asymptomatic, symmetric nodules over bony prominences (especially elbows) • Involute in short period of time (differs from rheumatoid nodules)	• Subcutis or deeper with palisading granuloma; separation and swelling of collagen bundles and increased eosinophilia; scattered inflammatory cells
Reactions to foreign materials and vaccines	• May form necrobiotic granulomas, as well as suppurative granulomas • Seen in bovine collagen injections, splinters, *T. rubrum* infections, etc.	
Suppurative granulomas (Epithelioid histiocytes and multinucleate giant cells with central collection of neutrophils)		
Chromomycosis	• "Chromoblastomycosis" • Caused by *Fonsecaea* (#1 cause), *Phialophora*, *Cladosporium* species • Often follows superficial trauma • Extremities 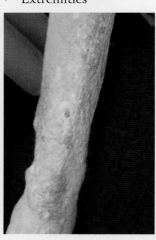 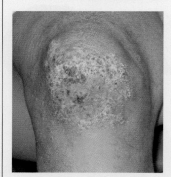 • Scaly papule slowly expands to annular, verrucous plaques • Systemic infections rare	• Pseudoepitheliomatous hyperplasia; mixed dermal infiltrate; no caseation; clusters of brown spores ("copper pennies" or Medlar/sclerotic bodies) 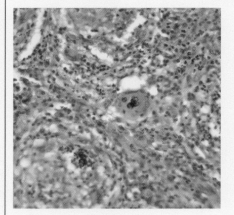

Name	Predilection and Clinical Key Features	Histopathology
Pheohypho-mycosis	• "Dark-filamentous-fungi" • Distal extremities • Often follows superficial trauma (especially wood splinter or vegetable matter) • Solitary subcutaneous cyst or nodular, cystic or verrucous lesion	• Brown hyphae (not copper penny); walled-off cystic space; suppurative granulomatous reaction; may see foreign body (such as a wood splinter)
Sporotrichosis	• "Rose gardener's disease" • *Sporothrix schenckii* (yeast form causes lesions) • Nodules and pustules on hands, forearms after inoculation (rose thorns, sphagnum moss) • *Note:* epitheloid sarcoma may appear clinically similar	• Pseudoepitheliomatous hyperplasia; diffuse mixed dermal infiltrate; granulomas (tuberculoid, histiocytic and suppurative); extracellular "sporothrix asteroid" (hyaline material is immune complexes on fungal surface); round/oval/cigar-shaped spores (difficult to see even with PAS, GMS stain)

Name	Predilection and Clinical Key Features	Histopathology
Non-tuberculous (atypical) mycobacterial infections	• *Mycobacterium marinum, Mycobacterium chelonae* • Crusted lesion, often on extremity; may have "sporotrichoid-like" appearance • *Mycobacterium marinum* (pictured above)	• Epidermis hyperplastic; diffuse dermal mixed infiltrate; tuberculoid granulomas without caseation; prominent fibrosis
Blastomycosis [PAS, silver methenamine]	• "Gilchrist's disease" • *Blastomyces dermatitidis* (dimorphic fungus) • Adults, face • Southeastern USA • Crusted verrucous plaques with annular pustular border, possible central healing • Causes lung infections (#1 symptom) • See Chapter 25 for more information	• Pseudoepitheliomatous hyperplasia; microabscesses; diffuse mixed infiltrate • Spores have broad-based bud (seen in giant cell or tissue)

Name	Predilection and Clinical Key Features	Histopathology
Paracoccidioido-mycosis [Grocott silver methenamine stain]	• "South American blastomycosis" • *Paracoccidioides brasiliensis* (dimorphic fungus in soil) • Latin America • Mucocutaneous areas • Causes lung infection, regional lymphadenopathy, mucocutaneous ulcerations, verrucous plaques • Clinical variants: 1. Primary pulmonary disease with subsequent mucocutaneous ulcerations (if disseminated) 2. Primary mucocutaneous (especially if chewed on stick/leaves) 3. Primary cutaneous (verrucous plaques) • See Chapter 25 for more information	• Pseudoepitheliomatous hyperplasia; dermal infiltrate; granulomas • Spores have multiple buds ("mariner's wheel") • GMS stain (photo above) • Difficult to see fungi or "mariner's wheel" without staining
Coccidioido-mycosis [PAS, silver methenamine; not mucicarmine]	• "Valley fever" • *Coccidioides immitis* (dust-borne, "barrel-shaped" arthrospores) • One of the most virulent fungi (extremely infectious arthroconidium) • Southwest USA • Face • Typically self-limiting, flu-like lung infection • Red, verrucous nodules (especially on face); erythema nodosum occurs in 20% with pulmonary infections • See Chapter 25 for more information	• Pseudoepitheliomatous hyperplasia; diffuse suppurative granulomatous reaction (non-caseating granulomas); large, thick-walled spherules (average 50 μm) with granular cytoplasm or endospores

Name	Predilection and Clinical Key Features	Histopathology
Blastomycosis-like pyoderma	• Large verrucous plaque studded with multiple pustules and draining sinuses • *Staphylococcus aureus* and *Pseudomonas* are often isolated from tissue	• Heavy infiltrate with small abscesses; few granulomas; pseudoepitheliomatous hyperplasia; intraepidermal microabscesses; usually severe solar elastosis
Actinomycosis, mycetomas, and nocardiosis (bacteria)	• Actinomycosis = draining sinus tract, nodule; results in massive enlargement and bony deformity; feet common • Actinomycosis ("lumpy jaw") • Mycetoma	• Abscess of neutrophils, mixed infiltrate, granules (sclerotia), bacteria granules (sulfur granules are clumps of basophilic organisms) PAS stain Gram stain • Splendore–Hoeppli phenomenon = eosinophilic border due to immunoglobulins (Ab); also seen with *Staph. aureus*, *Proteus*, *Pseudomonas* and *E. coli*

Name	Predilection and Clinical Key Features	Histopathology
Cat-scratch disease	• *Bartonella henselae* (bacteria) • Painful lymphadenopathy develops weeks after cat scratch or bite	• Suppurative granuloma and zone of necrosis surrounded by palisade of epithelioid cells; stellate granuloma
Lympho-granuloma venereum (LGV)	• *Chlamydia trachomatis* (bacteria) • Usually men • Groin area; STD that infects lymphatics • 2–3-mm papules or erosions on penis or vulva; subsequent buboes develop (enlarged LN) • "Groove sign" (due to lymph nodes on both sides Poupart's ligament enlarged)	• Diffuse mixed infiltrate including plasma cells; regional nodes with suppurative and centrally necrotic granulomas
Superficial pyoderma gangrenosum (variant of PG)	• Unknown etiology • Trunk • Site of surgical incisions, trauma • Superficial ulcer, usually solitary; draining sinus	• Suppurative granulomas and giant cells associated with irregular hyperplasia, sinus formation, fibrosis, and heavy mixed infiltrate

Name	Predilection and Clinical Key Features	Histopathology
Ruptured cysts and follicles	• Suppurative granuloma may form adjacent to ruptured cysts and inflamed hair follicles that rupture 	• Suppurative granuloma around cyst or hair follicle; foreign body giant cells; possible scar tissue with horizontal orientation • Ruptured follicle (pictured above) • Ruptured cyst (pictured below)

Name	Predilection and Clinical Key Features	Histopathology
Foreign body granulomas		
Exogenous material	• Foreign body granuloma formation around starch, talc, tattoo material, suture, wood splinters, pencil lead, glass • Birefringent = silica, zinc, talc, starch granules ("Maltese cross"), suture • Non-birefringent = beryllium, zirconium	• [PAS+] = plant likely Wood splinter Tattoo granuloma Suture granuloma Gelfoam Silica

Name	Predilection and Clinical Key Features	Histopathology
Silicone granuloma	• Due to injection of silicone, often for cosmetic reasons • Breasts, calves 	• May form granulomatous reaction (see Chapter 14, Cutaneous Deposits, for more information) • Vacuoles of various sizes surrounded by foreign body cells and macrophages
Endogenous material	• Form due to reaction from calcium deposits, urates, oxalate, keratin, and hair • Most common = keratin (i.e. ingrown nails or hair as in pseudofolliculitis)	Hair granuloma Gout (tophus), urate crystals Amyloid (especially nodular amyloidosis, see photo below)

Name	Predilection and Clinical Key Features	Histopathology
Miscellaneous granulomas		
Cheilitis granulomatosa	 • Episodic lip swelling • May be associated with Melkersson–Rosenthal syndrome (see below)	• Widely dilated lymphatics with inflammatory cells; marked dermal edema with perivascular infiltrate; variable granulomas ("naked" collections, loose tuberculoid granulomas, or isolated giant cells)

Melkersson–Rosenthal syndrome	• Unknown etiology
	 • Occurs in 20s usually
	 • Associated with sarcoidosis, infection/foreign material reaction
	 • *Triad ("TSP")*:
	   • Tongue = fissured tongue (lingua plicata)
	   • Swelling = chronic orofacial swelling, especially lips
	   • Paralysis = recurrent facial nerve paralysis
	   • DDx: tuberculosis cutis orificialis, oral Crohn's disease	

Elastolytic granulomas	• Granulomatous conditions that have annular lesions on sun-exposed areas with granulomatous rim and loss of elastic fibers centrally
	 • [Verhoeff-van Gieson stain = elastic is black, collagen is red, muscle/nerve is yellow]
	 • Main variants which may be part of spectrum of "annular elastolytic giant cell granuloma" group:
	   • actinic granuloma
	   • atypical necrobiosis lipoidica
	   • granuloma multiforme	

Name	Predilection and Clinical Key Features	Histopathology
Actinic granuloma of O'Brien	<ul><li>May be considered part of the group called annular elastolytic giant cell granulomas</li><li>Possible variant of granuloma annulare (GA) on sun-damaged skin</li><li>Middle-aged women</li><li>Often on sun-damaged face</li></ul> <ul><li>Annular plaques with red, elevated borders and atrophic, hypopigmented central area in sun-damaged areas</li></ul>	<ul><li>Diffuse granulomatous infiltrate; no mucin or necrobiosis (differs from granuloma annulare and NLD)</li><li>Three zones horizontally:<ol><li>Solar elastosis</li><li>Granuloma in rim with elastic fiber phagocytosis (elastophagocytosis) by large giant cells (up to 12 nuclei)</li><li>Central zone of absent elastic fibers</li></ol></li></ul> <ul><li>Verhoeff-van Gieson (VVG) stain (pictured above):<ul><li>VVG stains elastic tissue black and collagen stains red</li></ul></li></ul>

Name	Predilection and Clinical Key Features	Histopathology
Atypical necrobiosis lipoidica	• Females in 30s • Upper face and scalp • Annular lesions • Resolve without scarring or alopecia	• Zones: 1. Central healing zone with loss of elastic tissue 2. Peripheral raised edge with infiltrate between collagen bundles • VVG stain shows lack of elastic fibers (pictured above)

Name	Predilection and Clinical Key Features	Histopathology
Granuloma multiforme	• Africa; Indonesia • Adults • Annular lesion on sun-exposed trunk/arms (may resemble tuberculoid leprosy clinically)	• Similar to actinic granuloma
Annular granulomatous lesions in hydroquinone-induced ochronosis	• Ochronosis *rarely* forms granuloma • Individual applying hydroquinone cream • South Africa • Face • Annular eruption in ochronotic areas of face with hydroquinone-induced ochronosis • Resembles actinic granuloma with a zonal appearance and peripheral hyperpigmented ochronotic zone, elevated rim and central hypopigmented area • May be associated with systemic sarcoidosis	• Granulomatous lesion: hyperpigmented ochronotic zone with elevated rim with central hypopigmentation; resembles actinic granuloma; central zone with atrophic epidermis with underling absence of elastotic material and ochronotic fibers together with mild fibrosis

Name	Predilection and Clinical Key Features	Histopathology

Interstitial granulomatous dermatitis	• "Palisaded and neutrophilic granulomatous dermatitis"
	
	• Skin-colored or erythematous papules with umbilication, crusting or perforation; possible "rope sign" (skin-colored or erythematous linear cords, papules on lateral trunk)
	• May present with arthralgias
	• Associated with autoimmune (rheumatoid arthritis, SLE) or malignant lymphoproliferation (lymphoma)
		• Different patterns, such as:
		  • resembles granuloma annulare (lacks mucin)
		  • mixed infiltrate including more neutrophils
		  • small granulomas with palisading granulomas; accentuation especially in lower dermis
		  • palisade of histiocytes around individual collagen bundles
		  • possibly vasculitis and DIF show C3, IgM in vessels

Name	Predilection and Clinical Key Features	Histopathology
Interstitial granulomatous drug reaction	• Inner aspect of arms, medial thighs, intertriginous areas, trunk • Erythematous to violaceous, non-pruritic plaques with an annular configuration • Associated with calcium channel blockers, beta-blockers, ACE inhibitors, antihistamines, etc.	• "GA-like" (incomplete form) with "busy" appearing dermis; eosinophils; epidermotropism (50%); usually a mild lichenoid interface reaction with vacuolar change seen
Granulomatous mycosis fungoides	• "Granulomatous slack skin" is a variant of MF, and presents with "slack skin" clinically	• Granulomatous infiltrate in the dermis (Disorder destroys the elastic fibers)

Name	Predilection and Clinical Key Features	Histopathology
Traumatic ulcerative granuloma	• "Riga–Fede disease" • Elderly • Lateral tongue, buccal mucosa • Painless ulcer • Likely associated with history of trauma	• Ulcerated epidermis with granulation tissue and deep infiltrate (lymphocytes, eosinophils, plasma cells) around muscles; inflammation surrounds muscle with degeneration

8

Vasculopathic Reaction Pattern

Non-inflammatory purpura   **163**

Senile purpura   163

Vascular occlusive diseases   **164**

Warfarin necrosis   164

Atrophie blanche   165

Disseminated intravascular coagulation   166

Purpura fulminans   166

Thrombotic thrombocytopenic purpura   166

Thrombocythemia   166

Cryoglobulinemia   167

Cutaneous cholesterol embolism   168

Antiphospholipid syndrome   168

Factor V Leiden mutation   168

Sneddon's syndrome   168

CADASIL   169

Miscellaneous conditions causing vascular occlusion   169

Urticaria   **169**

Papular urticaria   169

Chronic urticaria   169

Angioedema   170

Acute vasculitis   **170**

Leukocytoclastic (hypersensitivity) vasculitis   170

Henoch–Schönlein purpura   171

Acute hemorrhagic edema of childhood   171

Eosinophilic vasculitis   171

Rheumatoid vasculitis   172

Urticarial vasculitis   172

Mixed cryoglobulinemia   173

Waldenström's macroglobulinemia   174

Hypergammaglobulinemia D syndrome   174

Septic vasculitis   174

Erythema elevatum diutinum   175

Granuloma faciale   176

Microscopic polyangiitis   176

Polyarteritis nodosa   177

Kawasaki syndrome   177

Superficial thrombophlebitis   178

Neutrophilic dermatoses   **179**

Sweet's syndrome   179

Pustular vasculitis of the hand   180

Bowel-associated dermatosis–arthritis syndrome   180

Rheumatoid neutrophilic dermatosis   180

Behçet's disease   180

Chronic lymphocytic vasculitis   **181**

Toxic erythema   181

Collagen vascular disease   181

PUPPP   181

Prurigo of pregnancy   181

Erythema annulare centrifugum   182

Erythema gyratum repens   182

Erythema marginatum   182

Erythema chronicum migrans   183

Pityriasis lichenoides et varioliformis acuta   183

Pityriasis lichenoides chronica   184

Pigmented purpuric dermatoses   184

Progressive pigmentary dermatosis   185

Purpura annularis telangiectodes of Majocchi   185

Pigmented purpuric lichenoid dermatosis of Gourgerot and Blum   186

Lichen aureus   186

Eczematid-like purpura of Doucas and Kapetanakis   186

Miscellaneous pigmented purpura dermatosis   187

Malignant atrophic papulosis   187

Perniosis   187

Rickettsial and viral infections   187

Pyoderma gangrenosum   188

Polymorphic light eruption   189

TRAPS   189

Sclerosing lymphangitis of the penis   189

Leukemic vasculitis   189

Vasculitis with granulomatosis   **190**

Wegener's granulomatosis   190

Lymphomatoid granulomatosis   190

Churg–Strauss syndrome   191

Giant cell (temporal) arteritis   192

Takayasu's arteritis   192

Miscellaneous vascular disorders   **192**

Erythromelalgia   192

Granuloma faciale

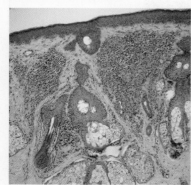 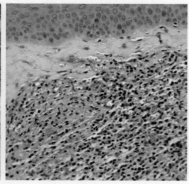

Name	Predilection and Clinical Key Features	Histopathology
Non-inflammatory purpura (Includes senile purpura, idiopathic thrombocytopenic purpura, autoerythrocyte sensitization syndrome, traumatic and drug purpura)		
Senile purpura	• "Bateman's purpura" • UV light causes loss and fragmentation of dermis collagen and extracellular matrix • Elderly • Forearms and hands • Well-demarcated, dark purple patches; does not usually show the color changes of bruising	• Extravasation of RBCs mostly in upper dermis/perivascular; marked solar elastosis; thinning of dermis with atrophy of collagen

Name	Predilection and Clinical Key Features	Histopathology
Vascular occlusive diseases		
Warfarin necrosis	• Patients with acquired protein C deficiency (a vitamin K-dependent plasma protein with anticoagulant properties, inactivates Va and VIIIa); warfarin (vitamin K inhibitor) • Obese, middle-age women; loading-dose treatment • Fatty areas (thighs, buttocks, breasts) • Well-defined ecchymotic changes that rapidly develop to blistering and necrosis • *Note:* Vitamin K-dependent proteins = VII, IX, X, prothrombin, protein C and S	• Fibrin–platelet thrombi in deep dermis/subcutis; possible subepidermal blister; variable hemorrhage; epidermal necrosis; sparse infiltrate

Name	Predilection and Clinical Key Features	Histopathology
Atrophie blanche (or livedoid vasculopathy)	• Atrophie blanche means = "white atrophy" • Vasculopathy with occlusion of small dermal vessels by fibrin thrombi (possibly due to decreased fibrinolytic activity from defective tissue plasminogen activator) • Middle-age females • Lower part of legs (ankles/dorsum of feet) • Telangiectatic, purpuric papules that form crusting ulcers that heal in months to form atropic stellate scars • Possible association with lupus-type anticoagulant, protein C deficiency, factor V Leiden mutation, etc.	• Hyaline thrombi in lumen of upper dermis; fibrin in vessel walls; ulceration; sparse infiltrate (no vasculitis); later lesion if it shows bands around vessels • DIF = perivascular IgM

Name	Predilection and Clinical Key Features	Histopathology
Disseminated intravascular coagulation (DIC)	• Activation of coagulation system results in thrombi and subsequent consumption of platelets and fibrin causing hemorrhage (seen in infection, neoplasms, massive tissue injury, liver disease, snake bite)	• Fibrin thrombi in capillaries and venules; hemorrhage; NO vasculitis
Purpura fulminans	• Rare cutaneous manifestation of DIC with rare organ involvement • Extensive purpura in severely ill patients, especially infancy and early childhood. Often associated with infectious illness (streptococcal, meningococcal, viral, etc.) • Lower extremities, buttocks • Erythematous macules rapidly enlarge and develop central purpura that becomes necrotic and ulcerates; hypotension; fever • Rarely visceral symptoms (uncommon)	• Fibrin thrombi fill most of venules and capillaries in skin; no vasculitis (mild perivascular infiltrate); extensive hemorrhage; may form subepidermal blister; develops epidermal necrosis
Variants of purpura fulminans	• Neonatal purpura fulminans (congenital protein C or S deficiency) • Purpura fulminans of sepsis (possibly acquired protein C dysfunction/deficiency) • Purpura fulminans in children recovering from infection (acquired protein S dysfunction)	

Thrombotic thrombocytopenic purpura	• Variants:
	 • Idiopathic TTP (autoimmune):
	  • antibodies to ADAMTS13 enzyme, which is a metalloproteinase responsible for the breakdown of von Willebrand factor (vWF), which links platelets
	 • Secondary TTP:
	  • possibly due to prostacyclin inhibition and impaired fibrinolysis
	  • usually no causal event or underlying disease found, but may be associated with drugs (antiplatelet drugs, especially ticlopidine and clopidogrel/Plavix), infection, cancer, pregnancy, etc.
	 • Possible Tx = plasmapheresis
		• Platelet-rich thrombi mixed with fibrin in vessels at level of arteriocapillary junction; extravasation of blood; no vasculitis
		• Clinical features = "FATRN"
		F = fever
		A = anemia
		T = thrombocytopenia (petechiae/ecchymoses)
		R = renal disease
		N = neurological symptoms

Thrombocythemia	• Myeloproliferative disorder with an increased platelet count • 20% patients show livedo reticularis, erythromelalgia, ischemic manifestations	• Erythromelalgia areas = fibromuscular intimal proliferation involving arterioles and small arteries • Ischemic areas = vascular thrombosis, infarction of dermis/epidermis

Name	Predilection and Clinical Key Features	Histopathology
Cryoglobulinemia	<ul><li>Cryoglobulin = immunoglobulin that reversibly precipitates from serum/plasma on cooling</li><li>Types:<ul><li>Type I (monoclonal, 25%) = presence of monoclonal IgG or IgM (precipitate and occlude vessels); associated with myeloma, CLL, Waldenström's macroglobulinemia; lower extremities<ul><li>clinical = purpura</li></ul></li><li>Type II and III (mixed, 75%) = cryoglobulins attached to polyclonal IgG<ul><li>type II = monoclonal IgM against polyclonal IgG</li><li>type III = polyclonal IgM against IgG</li></ul></li><li>Typically an underlying cause: RA, SLE, hepatitis C (75–90%), hepatitis B, HIV, etc.<ul><li>clinical = ulcers, urticaria, digital necrosis; renal disease, neurological symptoms</li><li>low C4 level (consumes); +RF without RA</li><li>IgM/C3 mediated</li></ul></li></ul></li></ul>	<ul><li>Type I (pictured below) = no vasculitis, a vascular occlusive disorder; homogeneous, eosinophilic material (thrombi) in upper dermal vessels, usually below epidermal ulceration; extravasated RBCs</li></ul><ul><li>Type II/III (pictured below) = vasculitis; sparse infiltrate; extravasated RBCs, possibly hemosiderin (old lesion); DIF shows immunoglobulins and complement in vessels</li></ul>

Name	Predilection and Clinical Key Features	Histopathology

Cutaneous cholesterol embolism	• 35% patients with cholesterol crystal emboli show cutaneous involvement, due to atheromatous plaque in major blood vessel (especially abdominal aorta)
	• High mortality
	• Three clinical settings for cholesterol emboli:
	  1. Cauterizations
	  2. Prolonged anticoagulation
	  3. Acute thrombolytic therapy
	• Distal extremities
	
	• Livedo reticularis, gangrene, ulceration, cyanosis, purpura
		• Acicular clefts (site of cholesterol crystals in arteriole); fibrin thrombus surrounds cholesterol; foreign body giant cells and sparse infiltrate
		
		DDx: atrial myxoma may cause occlusions with a myxoid stroma, but no cholesterol clefts

Antiphospholipid syndrome	• Repeated episodes of thrombosis, fetal loss, and thrombocytopenia • Antibodies to lupus anticoagulant or to anticardiolipin • Associated with SLE (20–50% have antibody but only half have syndrome), RA, infections or is "primary antiphospholipid syndrome" if no associated disease • Livedo reticularis, Raynaud's, thrombophlebitis, gangrene of digits, subungual splinter hemorrhage	• Prominent dermal edema and hemorrhage with thrombi in arteries/veins; mild infiltrate; no vasculitis • In later lesions, hemosiderin
Factor V Leiden mutation	• Hypercoagulable state due to a mutation involving glutamine for arginine in factor V, which makes it resistant to degradation by activated protein C (APC) • 2–5% of US population have mutation • Increased risk of venous thrombosis (10-fold increase); venous leg ulcers	

Sneddon's syndrome	• Neurocutaneous disorder with idiopathic livedo reticularis + cerebrovascular accidents (i.e. strokes)
	• Young to middle-aged females
	• Widespread livedo reticularis, ischemic cerebrovascular manifestations
		• Small and medium arteries at the dermal–subcutaneous junction:
		• Stages:
		  • Endothelitis (detachment of endothelium)
		  • Occlusion of lumen by a plug of fibrin with inflammatory cells
		  • Plug replaced by proliferating subendothelial cells (have markers of smooth muscle)
		• Atrophy of vessels

Name	Predilection and Clinical Key Features	Histopathology
CADASIL	• Cerebral autosomal dominant arteriopathy with subcortical infarcts and leukoencephalopathy (CADASIL) • NOTCH3 gene mutation, a transmembrane receptor Vascular disorder associated with migraines, recurrent ischemic stroke, early-onset dementia (no skin signs) • Best location for biopsy = forearm	• Luminal obliteration of small leptomeningeal and intracerebral arteries; no vascular occlusion of the skin • EM diagnostic – granular, electron-dense osmiophilic material in basement membrane of vascular smooth muscle cells ("black blobs" in vessel wall)
Miscellaneous conditions causing vascular occlusion	• Hypereosinophilic syndrome, renal failure with hyperparathyroidism, protein C or S deficiency, drugs (dopamine, vasopressin, Depo-Provera, heparin, cocaine), ulcerative colitis, bacterial endocarditis	
Urticaria		
Papular urticaria	• Clinical variant of urticaria • Possible hypersensitivity reaction to arthropod bites (especially fleas) • Usually occur in crops on exposed skin (more persistent than usual urticarial wheals)	• Heavy superficial and deep infiltrate of lymphocytes and eosinophils in a perivascular location; often wedge-shaped
Chronic urticaria	• Urticaria lasting >6 weeks • One-third of patients have antibodies to FcεRIα (high-affinity IgE receptor) causing histamine release from mast cells (more severe disease) • Variants: • Physical urticaria (15%) = heat, cold, light, water, vibration, or contact (i.e. stinging nettle/Urtica dioica) with chemical; wheals with short duration; exposed areas • Cholinergic = exercise, heat, emotion; young adults; 2–3-mm wheals surrounded by large erythematous flares; blush areas • Cold urticaria (pictured above) • Urticaria due to histamine-releasing agents = opiates, strawberries, egg white, lobster cause mast cells to release histamine • IgE mediated = mast cell degranulation due to antigen-specific IgE from foods, drugs, pollens, parasite infestations, stings • Immune complex mediated = often due to hepatitis, mononucleosis, SLE, serum sickness-like illness • Idiopathic = 75% of chronic urticaria • Schnitzler's syndrome: chronic, non-pruritic urticaria + recurrent fever, bone pain, arthralgia/arthritis + monoclonal IgM gammopathy	• Dermal edema (especially upper dermis); normal epidermis; sparse perivascular infiltrate (presence of neutrophils/eosinophils in vessel lumens in upper dermis); dilated blood vessels and lymphatics

Name	Predilection and Clinical Key Features	Histopathology

Angioedema	• Causes non-pitting edema, not a chronic urticarial disorder
	
	• Face, genitalia
	• Abrupt swelling of skin, mucous membranes
	• Variants:
	  • Angioedema: due to high bradykinin levels (affect skin, GI, airway):
	    • severe colicky abdominal pain; painless, non-pitting edema, and laryngeal edema with absence of urticaria (C4 low during attacks)
	  • Hereditary angioedema (HAE): autosomal dominant:
	    • type 1 = low C1-INH production (80–85% HAE)
	    • type II (decreased function) = normal or high C1-INH
	    • labs = normal to slightly low C1q and LOW C4 level
	    • Possible Tx = Danazo
	  • Acquired angioedema (AAE):
	    • due to low C1-INH (lymphoma, CLL or antibodies)
	    • labs = low C1q level (C4, C2, C1-INH are low)
	  • Drug-induced angioedema: ACE inhibitors
		• Edema and vascular dilation involving deep dermis and/or subcutis
		• In HAE, usually no inflammatory cell infiltrate present

Acute vasculitis (Presence of fibrin in vessel wall)		

Leukocytoclastic (hypersensitivity) vasculitis (LCCV)	• Involves deposition of immune complexes in walls of cutaneous post-capillary venules with activation of the complement system
	• Predilection to lower legs
	
	• Possible causes (40% with no apparent cause):
	  • Infections (*Strep.*, URI, influenza)
	  • Drugs (penicillin, furosemide)
	  • Chemicals (nicotine patch)
	  • Cancer (lymphoma, MF)
	  • Systemic disease (SLE, celiac, IBD)
	  • Erythematous macules or palpable purpura; vesicles, crusted ulcers 20% have extracutaneous symptoms (arthralgia, low-grade fever, malaise)
	• No new lesions at 2–3 weeks typically
	• Best time to biopsy a site = 18–24 hours old
		• Infiltration of vessel wall by neutrophils with leukocytoclasis and nuclear dust; swollen endothelial cells; edema and extravasation of RBCs; thrombosis; DIF = IgM+ (possibly C3)

Name	Predilection and Clinical Key Features	Histopathology

Henoch–Schönlein purpura (HSP)	• IgA vasculitis
	• Variant of leukocytoclastic vasculitis due to IgA-dominant deposits
	• Self-limited course
	• Children
	• Lower legs; buttocks
	• Preceded by URI that forms IgA
	  • In children, usually infection
	  • In adults, usually drug
	
	• Purpuric rash; usually one or more features including arthritis, abdominal pain, cardiac, or neurological manifestation; worse if spreads to trunk and involves kidneys
	• Possible Koebner phenomenon = linear purpura in areas of excoriation (due to damage of papillary dermal tip vessel from IgA)
		• Indistinguishable from LCCV histologically
		
		• DIF = IgA in vessel walls

Acute hemorrhagic edema of childhood (AHEC)	• Possible variant of HSP in infants with no systemic symptoms • Children <2 years old, usually recent URI or antibiotics • Annular, targetoid purpuric plaques on the head and distal extremities (no extracutaneous/systemic) involvement; facial edema; resolves in 1–3 weeks	• Same as HSP histologically • DIF = IgA in vessel walls
Eosinophilic vasculitis	• Eosinophil-predominant necrotizing vasculitis of small dermal vessels • Pruritic, erythematous, purpuric papules • Associated with connective tissue disease or hypereosinophilic syndrome typically	• Necrotizing, eosinophil-rich vasculitis of small dermal vessels; deposition of eosinophil granule major basic protein in vessel walls

Name	Predilection and Clinical Key Features	Histopathology
Rheumatoid vasculitis	• Patients with long-standing seropositive, erosive RA • Acute vasculitis involving large and small blood vessels • Often recurrent • Mortality 30% • Palpable purpura; digital gangrene; ulcers; digitial nail fold infarction	• Acute vasculitis of small and large vessels • Chronic IgM mediated (not short acting because rheumatoid factor (RF) activated)
Urticarial vasculitis	• Clinical variant of leukocytoclastic vasculitis • Associated with hepatitis, SLE, pregnancy, drugs (diltiazem, cocaine); methotrexate may exacerbate • Urticarial wheals and/or angioedema last >24 hours and resolve with ecchymoses • Two forms: 1. Normocomplement variant: • DIF = IgM+ • lower extremities • urticarial variant of hypersensitivity vasculitis 2. Hypocomplementemic variant: • women • DIF = granular IgG/C3+ • trunk, proximal extremities • systemic symptoms (renal, GI, respiratory) • may be a spectrum of SLE (anti-C1q antibodies)	• Prominent edema in upper dermis; mild infiltrate; similar to leukocytoclastic vasculitis • Hypocomplementemic vasculitis DIF = granular IgG (pictured below)

Name	Predilection and Clinical Key Features	Histopathology
Mixed cryoglobulinemia	• See p. 167 for more information • Associated with hepatitis C and connective tissue diseases (SLE, RA, Sjögren's syndrome)	• Acute vasculitis resembling leukocytoclastic vasculitis

Name	Predilection and Clinical Key Features	Histopathology
Waldenström's macroglobulinemia	• Also known as "hypergammaglobulinemic purpura" • Recurrent purpura, anemia, elevated ESR, polyclonal hypergammaglobulinemia • Associated with autoimmune diseases such as SLE, Sjögren's (+ antifodrin antibodies), etc.	• Similar to leukocytoclastic vasculitis histologically; often have antibodies to Ro/SSA
Hypergamma-globulinemia D syndrome	• Autosomal recessive • Mutation mevalonate kinase (MVK) (sterol biosynthesis) • Early childhood • Erythematous macules, or urticarial/erythematous nodules; recurrent febrile attacks with abdominal distress, headache, arthralgias	• Demonstrate mild acute vasculitis
Septic vasculitis	• Septicemic cause (meningococcal, *Pseudomonas*, *Staph*. endocarditis) • Accomplish blood cultures, if suspected	

Name	Predilection and Clinical Key Features	Histopathology
Erythema elevatum diutinum (EED)	• Variant of small vessel vasculitis with fibrosing LCV histologically • Middle age • Extensor extremities (especially elbows, knees); symmetric • Persistent, firm red-to-yellow–brown plaques; persistent lesions over joints • Associated with lymphoma, multiple myeloma, IBD and IgA monoclonal gammopathy • Possible Arthus-type reaction due to bacterial/viral antigen • Possible Tx = dapsone	• Epidermis normal; neutrophilic infiltrate mainly (less eosinophils than granuloma faciale); leukocytoclastic vasculitis • Older lesions = fibrosis or lipid deposits (extracellular cholesterosis); possible "storiform" spindle cell appearing proliferation with neutrophils

Name	Predilection and Clinical Key Features	Histopathology
Granuloma faciale (GF)	• Misnomer, actually no granuloma formations • White, middle-aged males • Nose, face • Well-circumscribed, asymptomatic brown–red plaques on face; dilated follicular pores in lesion	• Grenz zone above diffuse mixed infiltrate (lots of eosinophils) and surround pilosebaceous units; leukocytoclastic vasculitis; hemosiderin • DIF = IgG/complement at BMZ and around vessels • DDx: GF has eosinophils > neutrophils around pilosebaceous unit; but in EED has neutrophils > eosinophils, no grenz zone
Microscopic polyangiitis (polyarteritis)	• Small vessel vasculitis with glomerulonephritis and circulating p-ANCA antibodies (antimyeloperoxidase) • Middle-aged males • Lower legs; possible pulmonary and kidney involvement • Palpable purpura on lower legs; tender erythematous nodules • DDx: Wegener's granulomatosis which involves upper airway but c-ANCA (proteinase-3) > p-ANCA (myeloperoxidae)	• Acute neutrophilic vasculitis involving arterioles and capillaries; extravasation of RBCs; p-ANCA+

Name	Predilection and Clinical Key Features	Histopathology
Polyarteritis nodosa (PAN)	• Inflammatory disease of medium arteries primarily • May involve multiple organs (kidney, liver, GI) and skin (10–15%) • Lower legs • Associated with hepatitis B (50%), hepatitis C; cryoglobulinemia • Possible cutaneous PAN only form (lacks systemic involvement) • Urticarial lesions; palpable purpura; painful, red nodules/ulcers; livedo reticularis, digital infarctions; fever, arthralgia, myalgia	• Thickening of vessel walls; leukocytoclastic vasculitis of small to medium arteries in deep dermis and subcutaneous fat; thrombi; fibrosis in older lesions
Kawasaki syndrome	• "Mucocutaneous lymph node syndrome" • Infancy and childhood • Criteria = fever for 5 days (>104°C) plus four out of five: • Bilateral conjunctival changes • Oral mucosal changes • Hand/foot edema then desquamation (starts at tips) • Polymorphous, erythematous skin eruption • Cervical lymphadenopathy • Risk of possible coronary artery aneurysm development • Possible Tx = IVIG and high-dose aspirin (corticosteroids contraindicated since may favor coronary aneurysm development)	• Non-specific histological pattern (edema, perivascular infiltrate)

Name	Predilection and Clinical Key Features	Histopathology
Superficial thrombophlebitis	• Chest, lower legs • Tender, erythematous swellings of cord-like thickenings of the subcutis on the lateral chest • Associated with Behçet's disease, Buerger's disease (thromboangiitis obliterans), cancer (pancreas, stomach) • Mondor's disease = thrombophlebitis of breast or anterolateral chest (history of breast trauma/surgery)	• Involves veins in upper subcutis; intramural abscesses; mixed infiltrate • Histological assessment of the smooth muscle pattern is the most reliable method to differentiate an artery (continuous wreath of concentric smooth muscle) vs. a vein (bundled smooth muscle fibers with intermixed collagen)

Name	Predilection and Clinical Key Features	Histopathology
Neutrophilic dermatoses (Predominant neutrophils with no significant fibrinoid necrosis of vessel walls)		
Sweet's syndrome (acute febrile neutrophilic dermatosis)	<ul><li>Females (Drug-induced variant seen typically in women; while malignancy-related variant has no predilection)</li><li>Face, extremities; heals without scarring</li></ul>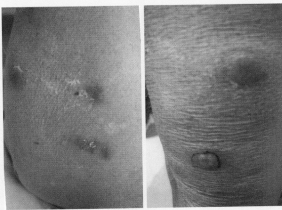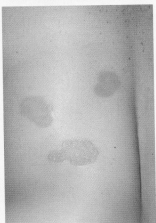<ul><li>Abrupt onset of painful dark red crusted plaques/ nodules; fever, malaise. Sudden onset of fever, leukocytosis, and tender, erythematous, well-demarcated papules and plaques</li><li>May recur (30–50%)</li><li>Vesiculobullous variant is often associated with myelogenous leukemia</li><li>Associated with:<ul><li>Post-infection (especially URI, *Strep.*)</li><li>Malignancies: leukemia-AML, solid tumors</li><li>Immunologic diseases: IBD, rheumatoid arthritis</li><li>Pregnancy</li><li>Drugs: G-CSF therapy, furosemide, minocycline, OCP, all-trans-retinoic acid</li><li>Marshall syndrome = complication of Sweet's syndrome; destruction of elastic tissue produces acquired cutis laxa</li></ul></li></ul>	<ul><li>Dense neutrophil infiltrate in upper half of dermis; epidermis spared (usually); superficial dermal edema; not a true vasculitis with vessel wall necrosis/fibrinoid; RBC extravasation; leukocytoclasis</li><li>"Papillary dermal edema + neutrophilic dermal infiltrate"</li></ul>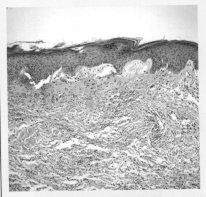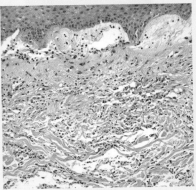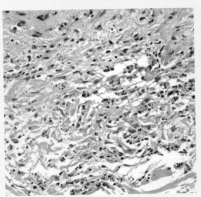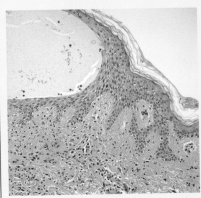

Name	Predilection and Clinical Key Features	Histopathology
Pustular vasculitis of the hand	• Variant of Sweet's syndrome • Hemorrhagic and edematous papules and large plaques limited to dorsum of radial side of hands and first three digits	
Bowel-associated dermatosis–arthritis syndrome	• 10–20% of intestinal bypass surgery patients (possibly due to bacteria overgrowth in blind loop and immune complex deposition) • Upper extremities and trunk • Small pustular lesions on upper extremities and trunk with influenza-like illness with malaise, fever and polyarthritis • Possible Tx = antibiotics, surgery, steroids	• Similar to Sweet's syndrome with subepidermal edema and heavy neutrophil infiltrate
Rheumatoid neutrophilic dermatosis	• Cutaneous manifestation of RA • Joints of extremities • Plaques and nodules overlying joints of extremities (especially hands), "EED-like" clinically	• Dense neutrophilic infiltrate (upper half); plasma cells and macrophages with neutrophilic debris; no vasculitis; may form microabscess in papillary dermis or intraepidermal blisters (similar to dermatitis herpetiformis)

Behçet's disease	• Usually Young, adult males
	• Middle East and Japan
	
	• Multisystem disorder with presence of recurrent, painful aphthous ulcers (heal 7–14 days)
	• Diagnostic criteria:
	Three episodes in 1 year and two of the following:
	  • Skin findings (erythema-nodosum-like nodules on legs, cutaneous pustules)
	  • Eye findings (uveitis, retinal vasculitis)
	  • Recurrent genital ulcerations
	  • Positive "pathergy" test (self-healing pustule forms at site of trauma)
	• Associated with HLA-Bw51 and B12
	• Disease activity marker = IL-8
	• MAGIC syndrome (mouth and genital ulcers with inflamed cartilage) = Behçet's disease + relapsing polychondritis (antibodies to collagen II)
		• *Note:* Behçet's is usually diagnosed clinically
		• Epidermis with ulceration or pustule; variable mixed infiltrate (especially neutrophils); vasculitis

Name	Predilection and Clinical Key Features	Histopathology
Chronic lymphocytic vasculitis		
Toxic erythema	<ul><li>Also known as "morbilliform eruption"</li><li>Trunk/proximal extremities</li><li>Associated with viral infections and drugs (antibiotics, OCP, aspirin)</li><li>Macular or blotchy erythema</li></ul>	<ul><li>Superficial perivascular infiltrate (lymphocytes); small amount of nuclear dust, no fibrin extravasation usually</li></ul>
Collagen vascular disease	<ul><li>Group with skin, soft tissue, muscle, joint, organ involvement</li></ul>	<ul><li>Superficial and deep lymphocytic vasculitis; mild fibrin</li></ul>
PUPPP	<ul><li>PUPPP = Pruritic urticarial papules and plaques of pregnancy</li><li>Third trimester (typically does not recur)</li><li>In and around abdominal striae; spares periumbilical region (unlike pemphigoid gestationis)</li><li>Resolves with delivery or spontaneously (no adverse effects to fetus)</li></ul><ul><li>Intensely pruritic papules and urticarial plaques</li></ul>	<ul><li>Lymphocytic vasculitis with eosinophils and edema of dermis</li></ul><ul><li>Negative DIF (differs from pemphigoid gestationis) and NO fibrin deposition</li></ul>
Prurigo of pregnancy	<ul><li>Controversial entity</li><li>Occurs in early pregnancy (second trimester); earlier than PUPPP</li><li>Acral areas</li><li>Scattered, pruritic, acral papules; may continue after pregnancy</li></ul>	<ul><li>Varies histologically; possible lymphocytic vasculitis; parakeratosis, acanthosis</li><li>Infiltrate may be loosely arranged around vessels with no vasculitis</li></ul>

Name	Predilection and Clinical Key Features	Histopathology

Erythema annulare centrifugum	• Adults
	• Trunk/proximal extremities
	
	• Annular, erythematous lesions; fine scale on advancing edge; may be pruritic
	• Firm pink papules that expand centrifugally and then clear centrally
	• Often idiopathic, may be associated with infection (tinea pedis, rickettsia, viruses), drugs (penicillin, cimetidine, antimalarials)
	• Two forms:
	  1. Superficial = trailing white scale
	    • favors thighs and hips
	  2. Deep = infiltrated borders (cord-like, no scale)
		• Superficial and deep dense infiltrate, well demarcated, "coat-sleeve" distribution; no fibrin extravasation
		• Reminder: "EA sleeve in EAC"
		
		• Advancing edge has spongiosis, mounds of parakeratosis
		• Possible differential for "PEGS" of parakeratosis:
		P = pityriasis rosea
		E = EAC
		G = guttate psoriasis
		S = small plaque parapsoriasis

Erythema gyratum repens (Gammel's disease)	• Figurate erythema that is migratory and composed of concentric rings with "wood-grain" appearance (increase 1 cm/day) • Associated with paraneoplastic phenomenon; most common neoplasm is lung cancer (also breast and esophagus)	• Superficial and deep lymphohistiocytic infiltrate around vessels; eosinophils; edema • DIF = IgG/C3 along BMZ (beneath lamina densa)
Erythema marginatum	• Cutaneous manifestations of acute rheumatic fever (10%) • Group A β-hemolytic streptococcal infection of pharynx • Children • Asymptomatic, transient, migratory annular and polycyclic erythematous eruption; pink/red border and paler center	• Perivascular infiltrate in upper dermis; lymphocytes and lots of neutrophils

Name	Predilection and Clinical Key Features	Histopathology
Erythema chronicum migrans (Lyme disease) [Warthin–Starry]	• Annular erythema develops at site of *Borrelia burgdorferi*-infected *Ixodes* tick • Occurs average of 15 days after tick bite (favors trunk) • Centrifugally spreading erythematous lesion at site of tick bite, may be multiple	• Superficial and deep perivascular infiltrate (including plasma cells, and adjacent to site are eosinophils) • Spirochete organism seen with Warthin–Starry stain
Pityriasis lichenoides et varioliformis acuta (PLEVA)	• "Mucha–Habermann" (acute form of pityriasis lichenoides) • Males • Second to third decades • Anterior trunk and flexor surfaces • Papular eruption becomes hemorrhagic crusts, ulcers, vesicles, pustules then varioliform scars (more CD8)	• Top-heavy, lymphoid infiltrate with extravasated erythrocytes, scale crust and focal epidermal changes (PLEVA has more infiltrate and cell death than PLC) • Histopathology of "PLEVA": P = parakeratosis L = lichenoid E = extravasation of erythrocytes V = vasculitis (lymphocytic) A = apoptotic keratinocytes and "eight" (mostly CD8 T cells)

Name	Predilection and Clinical Key Features	Histopathology
Pityriasis lichenoides chronica (PLC)	• Milder, chronic form of pityriasis lichenoides • Males in 20s and 30s • Anterior trunk and flexor surfaces • Scaly, red–brown maculopapules; central adherent, "mica" scale; heal with hypopigmentation in darker skin (more CD4)	• Similar to PLEVA, but less dense and more superficial
Pigmented purpuric dermatoses [Perls' stain for hemosiderin/iron]	• Purpuric lesions with variable pigmentation from hemosiderin deposition due to RBC extravasation • Young adults • Lower extremities • Multiple clinical variants, see below	• Variable infiltrate (majority CD4) and infiltrate upper dermis (perivascular); lymphocytic vasculitis; hemosiderin in papillary dermis; no fibrosis as in stasis dermatitis; spongiosis (except lichen aureus) • DDx: Stasis dermatitis has deeper involvement, mild spongiosis, fibrosis, loss of follicles, increased vessels

Name	Predilection and Clinical Key Features	Histopathology
Progressive pigmentary dermatosis	• Variant of pigmented purpuric dermatoses (PPD) • "Schamberg's disease" • Pre-tibial area • Symmetric, punctate purpuric, "cayenne pepper" macules	• Upper dermal infiltrate with lymphocytes and histiocytes; RBC extravasation; usually no epidermal involvement
Purpura annularis telangiectodes of Majocchi	• Variant of PPD • Trunk area • Annular patch with perifollicular, red punctate lesions and telangiectasis	• Similar to Schamberg's on HP with spongiosis

Name	Predilection and Clinical Key Features	Histopathology
Pigmented purpuric lichenoid dermatosis of Gourgerot and Blum	• Variant of PPD • Lower legs • Symmetric, lichenoid papules/plaques • Associated with hepatitis C	• Similar to Schamberg's on HP, but more lichenoid and spongiosis
Lichen aureus	• Variant of PPD • Lower legs, trunk • Unilateral, grouped macules/papules with rusty, golden, or purple color	• The most lichenoid-like, superficial, heavy infiltrate; no exocytosis or spongiosis (as in others)
Eczematid-like purpura of Doucas and Kapetanakis	• Variant of PPD • Lower extremities and progress proximally • Pruritic, eczematous-like and orange color • Case reports associated with infliximab	• Spongiosis and similar other variants (hemosiderin, etc.)

Name	Predilection and Clinical Key Features	Histopathology
Miscellaneous pigmented purpura dermatosis	• Purpuric contact dermatitis – associated with allergic contact dermatitis to textile dyes/resins • PPD/mycosis fungoides overlap	

Malignant atrophic papulosis (Degos' disease)
 	
[Colloidal iron/alcian blue for mucin]
	• Rare, progressive arterial occluding disease of small and medium size vessels that results in tissue infarction (especially GI) and initially involves the skin
	• Two variants:
	  1. Benign cutaneous variant
	  2. Malignant systemic variant (involves skin, GI, CNS); often die from fulminant peritonitis (GI perforations)
	• Trunk and arms (spares face)
	• Crops of red papules that slowly evolve to umbilicated papules with a white center and telangiectatic rim, then to a depressed, atrophic, "porcelain-white" scar
		• Epidermal atrophy with hyperkeratosis (older lesion); underlying wedge-shaped cutaneous ischemia (dermal infarct); dermis hypereosinophilic fibrin-thrombi in vessels; abundant mucin and fibrin
		• "Endovasculitis" (primary endothelial defect with secondary thrombosis leading to an infarct)

Perniosis	• "Chilblain"
	• Localized inflammatory lesion that develops in individuals exposed to cold
	• Variants:
	  • Classic perniosis = fingers/toes
	  • Equestrian perniosis = butt and thigh of female horse riders in winter
	  • When exposed to cold temperature, painful, erythematous to purplish swellings; may evolve to ulcers/necrosis
	  • Diagnosis is primarily clinical
	  • DDx: lupus may mimic perniosis (chilblain lupus)
		• Lymphocytic vasculitis; dermal edema; thickening of vessel walls that appear like "fluffy edema" in vessels (lymphocytes in vessel musculature and around sweat ducts)

Rickettsial and viral infections	• Rickettsial infections and viral infections (i.e. herpesvirus) may develop lymphocytic vasculitis	

Name	Predilection and Clinical Key Features	Histopathology
Pyoderma gangrenosum	• Ulcerative cutaneous condition (unknown etiology), may involve other organs as sterile neutrophilic abscesses • Mid-adult life • Lower extremities • Erythematous nodule/pustule that rapidly becomes necrotic ulcer with ragged, undermined, violaceous edge • Associated with Crohn's, RA, IgA monoclonal gammopathy • Primary variants of pyoderma gangrenosum: • Ulcerative (classic): • legs • Atypical or vesiculobullous: • hands, more superficial • associated with AML, IgA monoclonal gammopathy • Pustular: • multiple small pustules • associated with IBD, Behçet's • Superficial granulomatous or vegetative: • following trauma, surgery • PAPA syndrome: • Pyogenic sterile arthritis + pyoderma gangrenosum + acne • Mutation = PSTPIP1 (proline–serine–threonine phosphatase interacting protein-1), also called CD2BP1 (CD2 antigen-binding protein-1)	• Histology depends on variant (ulcerative, pustular, bullous and vegetative) Early lesion = folliculitis • Late lesion = necrosis of superficial dermis and ulcer with base showing mixed inflammatory cells with abscess formation • Advancing edge of lesion = perivascular infiltrate of lymphocytes and plasma cells with endothelial swelling and fibrinoid extravasation

Name	Predilection and Clinical Key Features	Histopathology
Polymorphic light eruption (PMLE)	• Most common form of idiopathic photodermatoses • Develops several hours after sun exposure (UVA > UVB or visible) • Typically occurs in spring • Papules, plaques or "erythema-like" lesions in sun-exposed areas	• Subepidermal edema leading to blister; cobweb-like appearance with collagen fibers separated by edema; superficial and deep perivascular lymphocytic infiltrate
TRAPS	• Tumor necrosis factor Receptor-Associated Periodic Syndrome (TRAPS) • TNFRSF1A gene, encodes tumor necrosis factor receptor • Periodic fever syndrome with migratory macules and patches in first few years of life • DDx: other familial fever syndromes, such as hypergammaglobulinemia D syndrome and familial Mediterranean fever	• Superficial and deep perivascular infiltrate
Sclerosing lymphangitis of the penis	• Sudden appearance of firm, cord-like nodular lesions on coronal sulcus or dorsum shaft of penis	• Dilated vessels, lumen with eosinophilic material or fibrin thrombus; inflammatory cell infiltrate • Possibly lymphatic or vein involvement
Leukemic vasculitis	• Leukocytoclastic vasculitis may develop in leukemia patients secondary to sepsis and medications	

Name	Predilection and Clinical Key Features	Histopathology
Vasculitis with granulomatosis		
Wegener's granulomatosis	<ul><li>Necrotizing vasculitis and granulomas of upper and lower respiratory tracts, usually focal necrotizing glomerulitis</li><li>Skin lesions in 30–50% cases</li><li>Adults (fourth to fifth decades)</li><li>Elbows, knees, buttocks</li></ul><ul><li>Symmetric, papulonecrotic lesions; sinusitis, etc.; "rheumatoid nodule-like" but RF negative</li><li>Classic triad: systemic vasculitis + necrotizing granulomas of respiratory airway + glomerulonephritis</li></ul>	<ul><li>Epidermis necrotic/ulcerated; small-to-medium vessel vasculitis; palisading necrotizing granuloma with neutrophil predominantly infiltrate; thrombi; RBC extravasation; giant cells</li><li>80% anti-neutrophil cytoplasmic antibodies (ANCA)+; mostly cytoplasmic ANCA (c-ANCA, IgG to proteinase 3):<ul><li>ANCA titers reflect disease activity</li><li>Renal-limited disease has myeloperoxidase subtype of p-ANCA</li></ul></li></ul>
Lymphomatoid granulomatosis	<ul><li>Angiocentric lymphoma</li><li>Middle age (median survival 14 months)</li><li>Erythematous or violaceous nodules/plaques on trunk and lower extremities; fever, cough, weight loss</li></ul>	<ul><li>Polymorphous, angiocentric infiltrate of atypical lymphocytes; sweat glands involved; fibrinoid necrosis</li></ul>

Name	Predilection and Clinical Key Features	Histopathology

Churg–Strauss syndrome (CSS)	• "Allergic granulomatosis"
	• Systemic vasculitis with hypereosinophilia + asthma + necrotizing vasculitis with granulomas
	• Young adults with pre-existing asthma and allergic rhinitis
	• Scalp or symmetric on extremities
	• Petechiae, purpura or red nodules; urticarial and tender; weight loss; GI symptoms; arthralgias, peripheral eosinophilia
	• Differentiate from Wegener's by:
	  • CSS affects GI, heart instead of renal
	  • CSS has H/O asthma and extrapulmonary involvement
		• Three major features (may not coexist):
		  1. Palisading granulomas (extravascular)
		  2. Lots of eosinophils (possible "flame figures")
		  3. Necrotizing vasculitis
		• p-ANCA > c-ANCA

Name	Predilection and Clinical Key Features	Histopathology
Giant cell (temporal) arteritis	• Granulomatous vasculitis involving large or medium size elastic arteries • Elderly (>50 years old) • Superficial temporal and ophthalmic arteries • Associated with polymyalgia rheumatica (syndrome with >4 weeks of aching in neck, proximal muscles) • Dx = temporal artery biopsy (3 cm) • Classic symptoms = tender, swollen, pulseless temporal artery • Necrosis of scalp with ulceration; headache; jaw claudication; visual and neurological disturbances; alopecia; tip of tongue necrosis; hyperpigmentation; morning stiffness of neck, pelvis, shoulders; eye blindness risk (rarely returns); elevated ESR	• Granulomatous arteritis involving inner media of artery with prominent giant cells (Langhans and foreign body) • Staining for elastin [VVG stain] shows focal destruction of elastin in inner elastic lamina
Takayasu's arteritis	• "Aortic arch syndrome" or "pulseless disease" • Large vessel granulomatous vasculitis (aortic arch) • Young females • Erythema nodosum, pyodermatous ulcers, rashes, urticaria; necrotizing vasculitis; bruits; asymmetric pulses • Diagnosis with angiogram	• Large vessel granulomatous reaction
Miscellaneous vascular disorders		

Erythromelalgia (or erythermalgia)	• Possibly due to platelet dysfunction and abnormal vascular dynamics
	• Females
	• Recurrent, red, warm extremities with burning pain; exacerbated by exercise, heat, fever, standing, and decreased symptoms by cooling
	• Variants:
	  • Type I = associated with essential thrombocythemia; adult onset; often unilateral; best results if treated with aspirin
	  • Type II = idiopathic primary form; often bilateral; onset in childhood
	  • Type III = associated with underlying disorder (vasculitis, SLE, etc., but not thrombocythemia); adult onset
		• Thickening of capillary basement membrane; moderate endothelial swelling; perivascular edema; scant infiltrate

Disorders of Epidermal Maturation and Keratinization

9

Ichthyosis vulgaris

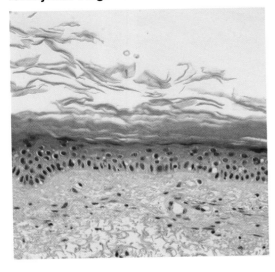

Major keratins and specific locations

- K1–8 (type II) = basic and high molecular weight (chromosome 12)
- K9–20 (type I) = acidic and low molecular weight (chromosome 17)
- Upper spinous and granular layer = K2e and K10
- Stratum spinosum = K1 and K10
- Basal layer = K5 and K14
- Cornea = K3 and K12
- Mucosa = K4 and K13
- Palms/soles = K6 and K16 (also in psoriasis, warts, AK, SCC)

Name	Predilection and Clinical Key Features	Histopathology
Ichthyoses		
Ichthyosis vulgaris	<ul><li>Most common ichthyosis</li><li>Autosomal dominant</li><li>Present in early childhood</li><li>Spares antecubital and popliteal flexural areas (unlike lamellar ichthyosis) and spares preauricular area (unlike X-linked ichthyosis)</li><li>Mutation = profilaggrin (FLG gene), resulting in decreased filaggrin</li><li>Retention hyperkeratosis with normal proliferation</li></ul> <ul><li>Fine, whitish scale, especially extensor areas; keratosis pilaris (KP); hyperlinear palms</li></ul>	<ul><li>Decreased to absent granular layer; hyperkeratosis; involves hair follicles</li></ul>

Name	Predilection and Clinical Key Features	Histopathology
X-linked ichthyosis	• X-linked recessive • Birth to first few months • Retention hyperkeratosis • Mutation = steroid sulfatase (leukocytes and fibroblasts, increased cholesterol sulfate disrupts barrier function and proteases) • Large, dark-brown scale, often involves preauricular area (unlike ichthyosis vulgaris); cryptorchidism; corneal comma-shaped opacities • Spares flexural creases and palms/soles (unlike lamellar ichthyosis) • OB complications = placental sulfatase deficiency may cause mother's labor of child not to begin or progress (may require C-section for delivery) • Contiguous gene deletion may cause Kallmann syndrome (impaired smell + delayed puberty) and X-linked recessive chondrodysplasia punctata • Associated with Goldenhar syndrome (oculo-auriculo-vertebral syndrome, due to first brachial arch developmental abnormality) • *Note:* think of "3-Cs" to include: • C-section often for delivery (failure to progress) • Comma-shaped, corneal opacities • Cryptorchidism risk	• Obvious acanthosis; hyperkeratosis of follicles
Collodion baby differential	• Lamellar ichthyosis/LI (#1 cause) • Congenital ichthyosiform erythroderma (CIE) • Sjögren–Larssen syndrome • Conradi–Hünermann syndrome • Trichothyiodystrophy • Ectodermal dysplasia • Infantile Gaucher disease • Hay–Wells syndrome • Neutral lipid storage disease	

Name	Predilection and Clinical Key Features	Histopathology
Ichthyosis congenita • Types: • Type I = Congenital ichthyosiform erythroderma (CIE), see below • Type II = Lamellar ichthyosis (LI), see below • Type III = lamellar scales; collodion baby • Type IV = variable		
Congenital ichthyosiform erythroderma (CIE)	• Previously called "non-bullous CIE" • Autosomal recessive • Mutation = TGM1 (transglutaminase-1), ALOXE3, ALOX12B and ABCA12 genes • Accelerated epidermal turnover rate • Newborn = collodion baby • Infants = erythroderma and fine, pale scales (high content of n-alkanes); collodion baby; cicatricial alopecia; ectropion	• Hyperkeratosis; focal parakeratosis; keratotic plugging (same as LI)
Lamellar ichthyosis (LI)	• Mutation = TGM1 (transglutaminase-1) gene: also ABCA12 and ALOC3/12 • Autosomal recessive • Causes excessive turnover with hyperkeratosis • Mutation affects crosslinking of loricrin and involucrin • Hyperproliferation hyperkeratosis • Newborn features = collodion baby; risk of hypernatremic dehydration • Child/adult = large plate-like scale, involves palms/soles; scarring alopecia; PPK; erythroderma; risk of skin cancers	• Hyperkeratosis (LI > CIE); keratotic plugging

Name	Predilection and Clinical Key Features	Histopathology
Bullous ichthyosis	• Epidermolytic hyperkeratosis (EHK) • Autosomal dominant • Seen at birth (six subtypes) • Widespread erythema and some blistering; coarse, verrucous scales (especially on flexures), "corrugated cardboard-like" • Risk of bacterial infections; foul odor • Gene mutation = keratin 1 and 10 • Keratin 1 and 10 mutations cause keratinocyte fragility, so friction causes blisters and recurrent shear forces cause accentuated scale • Keratin 1 = severe PPK • Keratin 10 = lacks PPK	• Epidermolytic, hyperproliferative hyperkeratosis, marked hyperkeratosis and vacuolar changes in upper epidermal layers; mild perivascular infiltrate • EM = aggregation of tonofilaments at cell periphery with perinuclear areas free (clumped keratin filaments)
Ichthyosis bullosa of Siemens	• Autosomal dominant • Mutation = keratin 2e • Subsides with age and develops hyperkeratosis • Milder form of EHK (often limited to flexural areas) • Mauserung phenomenon = circumscribed shedding ("molting") of the stratum corneum overlying hyperkeratotic skin	

Name	Predilection and Clinical Key Features	Histopathology

Netherton's syndrome	• Autosomal recessive
	• Birth to first few months
	• Ichthyosis linearis circumflexa or migratory annular and polycyclic erythema with double-edge scale; abnormal hair shafts (especially eyebrows > scalp); abnormal immune system
	• Mutation = SPINK5 (encodes LEKT1, serine protease inhibitor)
	• Netherton's syndrome triad:
	  1. Ichthyosis linearis circumflexa
	  2. Trichorrhexis invaginata (bamboo or ball-and-socket)
	  3. Atopic diathesis
	• *Note:* avoid tacrolimus/pimecrolimus topically due to increased absorption and serum levels possible
		• Hyperkeratosis, well-developed granular layer; parakeratosis
		• Margin of lesions = parakeratosis with psoriasiform hyperplasia, lacks granular layer
		• EM = increased mitochondria and lipoid bodies in stratum corneum; premature secretion of lamellar body contents

Erythrokeratoderma variabilis (EKV)	• Autosomal dominant • Infancy • Mutation = GJB3, GJB4 gene (encode connexin 31, 30.3) • Transient, well-demarcated geographic erythematous patches (change daily); fixed focal hyperkeratotic plaques	• Hyperkeratosis, irregular acanthosis, mild papillomatosis, superficial infiltrate

Name	Predilection and Clinical Key Features	Histopathology
Progressive symmetric erythrokeratoderma	• May be a variant of ichthyotic variant of Vohwinkel's syndrome • Symmetric erythematous plaques, PPK (lacks migratory erythematous lesions as in EKV) • Mutation = loricrin gene • One of most responsive genodermatoses to oral retinoids	• Non-specific findings: hyperkeratosis, irregular acanthosis, mild papillomatosis, possible dyskeratotic, grain-like cells
Harlequin fetus	• Autosomal recessive • Usually incompatible with life, but may survive • Mutation = multiple genes including ABCA12 gene (ATP-binding cassette gene, involved in transport of lipids to stratum corneum and formation of lamellar granules) • Thick, plate-like scales with deep fissures; severe ectropion, eclabium, absent ears	• Massive hyperkeratosis • EM = absent lamellar bodies/granules
Follicular ichthyosis	• Birth to early childhood • Abnormal epidermal differentiation in hair follicles; hyperkeratosis (especially head/neck); photophobia; alopecia	• Compact hyperkeratosis in follicle; prominent granular layer
Acquired ichthyosis	• Adults • Similar to ichthyosis vulgaris • Associated with malignancy (especially lymphoma), malnutrition, hypothyroidism, drugs (clofazimine, nafoxidine)	• Compact orthokeratosis and/or parakeratosis without spongiosis
Pityriasis rotunda	• Possible variant of acquired ichthyosis • Black adults (especially South Africa) • Trunk, buttocks, extremities • Sharply demarcated, nearly perfectly round, asymptomatic, scaly patch • Possibly associated with systemic illnesses (especially hepatocellular carcinoma)	• Similar ichthyosis with mild hyperkeratosis and an absent or reduced granular layer

Name	Predilection and Clinical Key Features	Histopathology
Refsum's syndrome	• Autosomal recessive • Mutation = phytanic acid storage disease due to deficiency of peroxisomal enzyme phytanoyl-CoA hydroxylase (PAHX gene) or peroxin-7 (PEX7 gene) • Characterized by ichthyosis, cerebellar ataxia, peripheral neuropathy and retinitis pigmentosa ("salt and pepper" pigment); deafness; cardiac arrhythmias • Required diet = chlorophyll-free diet (avoid phytanic acid by not eating green vegetables or dairy products)	• Hyperkeratosis, acanthosis, vacuolated basal keratinocytes with lipids • EM = non-membrane-bound vacuoles in basal and suprabasal keratinocytes
Other ichthyosis-related syndromes		
Sjögren–Larsson syndrome	• Autosomal recessive • Infancy (ichthyosis) and 2–3 years old (CNS symptoms) • Often seen in Sweden • Mutation = FALDH (fatty aldehyde dehydrogenase gene) • Dark scales (similar to lamellar ichthyosis); retinal degeneration (glistening white dots in perimacular area); intense pruritus (due to leukotrienes) • Clinical triad = "SIR Sjögren": S = spastic paralysis (scissor-type gait) I = ichthyosis (congenital) R = retardation (mental)	• Acanthosis, mild papillomatosis, mild thick granular layer, basket-weave hyperkeratosis
"KID" syndrome	• Autosomal dominant and autosomal recessive • Birth • Mutation = GJB2 (encodes connexin 26 in skin and cochlea), same gene as Vohwinkel's syndrome • K = keratitis; I = ichthyosis; D = deafness • Recurrent infections; SCC of skin, tongue; alopecia; possible blindness; stippled PPK • Beware: oral retinoids may worsen corneal neovascularization	• Generalized hyperkeratosis with follicular plugging

Name	Predilection and Clinical Key Features	Histopathology
Conradi–Hünermann–Happle syndrome	• Form of chondrodysplasia punctata • X-linked dominant • Mutation = cholesterol biosynthesis (emopamil-binding protein, EBP gene, Smith–Lemli–Opitz syndrome involved in same pathway) • Chondrodysplasia with ichthyosis and palmar/plantar hyperkeratosis; stippled epiphyses (punctate calcifications); asymmetric limb shortening; follicular atrophoderma hyperpigmentation; frontal bossing; "cheesy-scale" on skin	• Hyperkeratosis; prominent granular layer (parakeratosis with a diminished granular layer possible); dilated ostia of pilosebaceous follicles; intracorneal calcification localized to keratotic follicular plugs (diagnostic for this condition)
"CHILD" syndrome	• X-linked recessive (lethal to males) • Congenital hemidysplasia, ichthyosiform erythroderma limb defects ("CHILD") • Mutation = cholesterol biosynthesis (NSDHL gene) • Unilateral ichthyosiform erythroderma with sharp midline cutoff; alopecia; stippled epiphyses; agenesis of organs below ichthyosis	• Psoriasiform epidermal hyperplasia; possible verruciform xanthoma changes
Tay's syndrome	• Photosensitivity + trichothiodystrophy (IBIDS, see below) • Close-set eyes, beaked nose, and sunken cheeks	
IBIDS	• IBIDS = Ichthyosis with Brittle hair, Impaired intelligence, Decreased fertility, and Short stature • PIBIDS if photosensitivity present • Most common mutation = ERCC2 gene (DNA excision repair gene)	
Multiple sulfatase deficiency	• Disorder affecting activity of several sulfatases resulting in severe neurodegenerative disease, ichthyosis and signs of mucopolysaccharidosis	
"MAUIE" syndrome	• "MAUIE" = Micro-pinnae, Alopecia Universalis, Congenital Ichthyosis. and Ectropion	
Neutral lipid storage disease (Dorfman–Chanarin syndrome)	• Autosomal recessive • Mutation = acylglycerol recycling (triacylglycerol to phospholipid in fibroblasts), resulting in lipid accumulation • Combines fatty liver with muscular dystrophy and ichthyosis	• Hyperkeratosis; mild acanthosis; discrete vacuolation with lipids in basal keratinocytes; lipid droplets in circulating granulocytes and monocytes (not lymphocytes or RBCs)
Shwachman syndrome	• "Swachman–Diamond syndrome" • Pancreatic insufficiency and bone marrow dysfunction with xerosis and/or ichthyosis	

Name	Predilection and Clinical Key Features	Histopathology
Palmoplantar keratoderma and related conditions		
Palmoplantar keratoderma (overall)	• Group of inherited conditions with thick hyperkeratotic palms/soles • Autosomal recessive types usually most severe (i.e. mal de Meleda, Papillon–Lefèvre) • Transgrediens = hyperkeratosis that crosses palm/sole edge (Greither's, Olmsted's, Vohwinkel's, mal de Meleda)	• Diffuse forms = prominent orthokeratotic hyperkeratosis, thick granular layer, acanthosis • Punctate forms = dense, homogeneous keratin plug with usually a slight depression in epidermis below plug
Unna–Thost syndrome	• "Non-epidermolytic PPK" • Autosomal dominant • Appears in first few months of life • Mutation = keratin 1 • Diffuse palmoplantar keratoderma form; bilateral, symmetric hyperkeratosis palms/soles; hyperhidrosis, bromhidrosis, deafness	• Orthokeratosis (Vorner's PPK variant has epidermolytic hyperkeratosis)
Greither's syndrome	• Autosomal dominant • Mutation = keratin 1 • Hyperhidrosis + diffuse non-epidermolytic keratoderma: • characteristic feature = transgrediens lesions extend to ventral aspect of wrist and Achilles tendon	
Olmsted's syndrome	• Diffuse mutilating keratoderma with periorificial plaques, oral leukokeratosis; transgrediens • Mutation = keratin 5 and 14	

Vohwinkel's syndrome	• Autosomal dominant disorder
	• Autoamputation of digits, starfish-shaped keratoses on dorsal digits; linear keratosis on knees and elbows; honeycomb PPK; scarring alopecia; transgrediens PPK
	• Mutation variations:
	  • loricrin gene = no deafness
	  • GJB2 gene (connexin 26 in gap junctions) = classic Vohwinkel + deafness – same gene as "KID" syndrome	

Name	Predilection and Clinical Key Features	Histopathology
Vorner's syndrome	• "Epidermolytic PPK" • Autosomal dominant • Birth to 1 year • Mutation = keratin 9 (most common) and keratin 1 • Bilateral, symmetric, thick, yellowish hyperkeratosis on palms/soles; hyperhidrosis, bromhidrosis (same as Unna–Thost clinically)	• Epidermolytic hyperkeratosis, papillomatosis, cytoplasmic vacuolation and conspicuous intracytoplasmic inclusions • Unna–Thost PPK variant has orthokeratosis only and without epidermolysis

Howel–Evans syndrome	• Autosomal dominant disorder
	• Second decade to adulthood
	• "Pressure-point" keratoderma, esophageal cancer risk (SCC type)
	• Two types:
	  • type A = late-onset PPK and high risk of esophageal cancer (fifth decade)
	  • type B = early onset and benign course
	• Mutation = TOC gene (tylosis esophageal cancer gene)	

Papillon–Lefèvre syndrome	• Autosomal recessive
	• "PPK + periodontitis":
	  • sharply demarcated PPK (glove-and-stocking); destructive periodontitis and premature loss of teeth; pyoderma; hyperhidrosis, fetid odor; dural calcifications in CNS; pyogenic infections
	• Mutation = cathepsin C (CTSC) gene:
	  • cathepsin C is a lysosomal protease, important in innate immunity and neutrophil function
	  • same gene defect seen in Haim–Munk syndrome (autosomal recessive): PPK + periodontitis + arachnodactyly (long, thin, curved fingers) + acro-osteolysis (bone loss in digits) + pes planus + onychogryphosis	

Mal de Meleda	• "Keratosis palmoplantaris transgrediens of Siemens" • Autosomal recessive • Birth to first few months • Mutation =ARS B gene: encodes SLURP-1 (secreted Ly-6/uPAR related protein-1); a cell-signaling and adhesion protein • Diffuse transgrediens keratoderma (glove-and-stocking distribution; i.e. sharp cut-off at wrist/ankle); hyperhidrosis; fetid odors; koilonychia nails	

Name	Predilection and Clinical Key Features	Histopathology

PPK + woolly hair conditions	• Woolly hair = unruly, kinky, curly hair on the scalp of a Caucasian
	  • develops as a child when hair initially grows
	• Two variants:
	  1. Naxos disease
	    • mutation = plakoglobin (JUP gene)
	    • autosomal recessive disorder
	    • diffuse PPK, right ventricular cardiomyopathy, woolly hair
	  2. Carvajal syndrome
	    • mutation = desmoplakin (DSP gene)
	    • autosomal recessive disorder
	    • epidermolytic PPK, dilated cardiomyopathy, woolly hair	

Punctate palmoplantar keratoderma	• "Spiny keratoderma" • Autosomal dominant • Childhood to early adult • Small foci of discrete, hard hyperkeratotic papules • Different variations and types	• Keratin plug with slight depression of epidermis

Striate palmoplantar keratoderma	• Rare form of PPK with linear hyperkeratotic streaks along the volar surface of fingers and focal keratoderma over the soles
	• Three types:
	  • Type I (desmoglein 1 gene mutation)
	  • Type II (desmoplakin gene mutation)
	  • Type III (keratin 1 gene mutation)	

Circumscribed keratoderma	• Heterogeneous group of focal areas of thickening on palms/soles • Includes hereditary painful callosities, keratoderma palmoplantaris striata, etc. • Corneal dystrophy possible	
Acquired keratoderma	• Palms and soles • Discrete, asymptomatic keratotic papules • May occur in myxedema, MF, lymphoma, cancers, exposure to arsenic	• Hyperkeratotic papules

Name	Predilection and Clinical Key Features	Histopathology
Arsenic keratosis	<ul><li>Type of acquired keratoderma</li><li>Palms and soles</li><li>Discrete, asymptomatic keratotic papules; Mee's lines on nail plates (transverse white lines on multiple nail plates)</li><li>Arsenic source may be due to poisoning or contaminated drinking water</li></ul> <ul><li>Mees' lines (photo above)</li></ul>	<ul><li>Compact hyperkeratosis, atypical keratinocytes</li></ul>

Name	Predilection and Clinical Key Features	Histopathology
Aquagenic acrokeratoderma	• "Transient reactive papulotranslucent acrokeratoderma" or "aquagenic syringeal acrokeratoderma" • Palms and soles • Rapid development of transient whitish, symmetric, hypopigmented flat-topped papules after sweating or exposure to water • Dermoscopy photo, above, showing dilated eccrine ostia along the palmar ridges	• Spongy appearance to cornified layer; dilation of intraepidermal eccrine ducts and some hyperkeratosis around dilated ducts; "crenulated" (wavy or serrated) eccrine coils • Dilated eccrine ducts • Distinctive crenulated appearance in the eccrine coils

Name	Predilection and Clinical Key Features	Histopathology
Oculocutaneous tyrosinosis	• "Richner–Hanhart syndrome" • Autosomal recessive • First few months life • Painful weight-bearing PPK + pseudoherpetic keratitis + blindness; possible mental retardation • Mutation = tyrosine aminotransferase gene (causes deficiency of hepatic enzyme and accumulation of tyrosine) • Treatment includes a diet avoiding tyrosine and phenylalanine	
Acrokeratoelastoidosis	• Variant of PPK, occurs sporadic and autosomal dominant • Early childhood to early adult • Female predominance • Side of palms/feet and dorsum of hands/feet, especially the inner side of the thumb and adjoining index finger. May coalescence to form large plaques • Multiple, 2–5-mm, firm, translucent papules, especially along junction of dorsum and palmar/plantar surface • Genodermatosis in which dermal elastic fibers are usually fragmented and decreased in number • Clinically, lesions between thumb and adjacent index finger may appear similar to collagenous and elastotic plaques of the hands (see p. 259)	• Prominent hyperkeratosis with shallow depression of epidermis, hypergranulosis and acanthosis; sparse perivascular infiltrate (lymphocytes); decreased and fractured elastic fibers Trichrome stain (above)

Name	Predilection and Clinical Key Features	Histopathology
Pachyonychia congenita	• Rare form of PPK • Usually autosomal dominant  • Symmetrical, hard thickening of nails with: • Type I (Jadassohn–Lewandowsky): • oral leukokeratosis, PPK, keratosis pilaris, blisters • mutation = keratin 6a and 16 • Type II (Jackson–Lawler): • similar to type I but natal teeth prior to birth, multiple cysts (but no oral leukokeratosis) • associated with steatocystoma multiplex • mutation = keratin 6b and 17	• Extremely thick subungual hyperkeratosis, intercellular edema, thickened epidermis

Cornoid lamellation

- Cornoid lamella = thin column of parakeratotic cells with absent or decreased underlying granular layer and vacuolated or dyskeratotic spinous cells
- Caused by a localized area of faulty keratinization and clinically appears as raised thin, thread-like border around lesion

Name	Predilection and Clinical Key Features	Histopathology
Porokeratosis of Mibelli	• Limbs  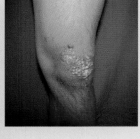 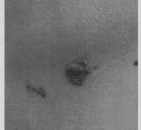 • Solitary (round, oval, or gyrate) plaques with atrophic center and thin, elevated, keratotic rim • Risk of malignant transformation, especially to SCC	• Cornoid lamellae, invagination of epidermis at site of cornoid lamella with adjacent mild papillomatosis; absent granular layer below lamellae 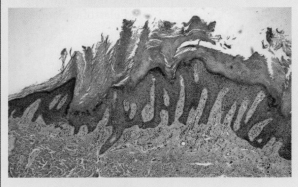 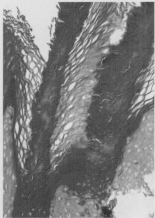 • PAS stain (above) shows purple granules in the cornoid lamellae due to intracellular glycogen and glycoprotein

Name	Predilection and Clinical Key Features	Histopathology
Disseminated superficial actinic porokeratosis (DSAP)	• 30s–40s • Sun-exposed areas • Multiple, annular, keratotic lesions with hyperkeratotic, thread-like border (especially on extremities) • UV light exacerbates	 • Cornoid lamellae; epidermis between lamellae often atrophic with hyperkeratosis, possible superficial band-like lichenoid infiltrate; solar elastosis
Linear porokeratosis	• Rare variant with linear appearance • Risk of SCC transformation 	• Same as DSAP

Name	Predilection and Clinical Key Features	Histopathology
Punctate porokeratotic keratoderma	• Palms and soles • Spiny papules	• Cornoid lamellae on acral skin with parakeratotic plug 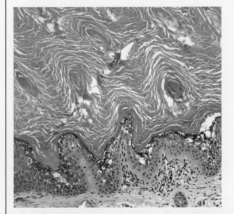
Epidermolytic hyperkeratosis		

Epidermolytic hyperkeratosis (EHK)	• Abnormal epidermal maturation
	• May be seen in various clinical settings:
	  • generalized (bullous ichthyosis)
	  • systematized or localized (epidermal nevus variant)
	  • palmoplantar (PPK variant)
	  • solitary (epidermolytic acanthoma)
	  • multiple discrete (disseminated epidermolytic acanthoma)
	  • incidental (focal EHK, seborrheic keratosis)
	  • solar keratosis related (variant of actinic keratosis)
	  • follicular (nevoid follicular EHK)
	  • mucosal (epidermolytic leukoplakia)
		• Cells appear to "drop-out"
		• Compact hyperkeratosis, granular and vacuolar degeneration of spinous and granular layer cells
		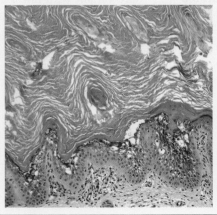

Name	Predilection and Clinical Key Features	Histopathology
Epidermolytic acanthoma	• All ages • Solitary, verrucous-like papule ("wart-like")	• Epidermolytic hyperkeratosis (i.e. hyperkeratosis, vacuolar degeneration); bluish, "moth-eaten" keratinocytes with hazy borders, vacuoles, and cytoplasmic eosinophilic inclusions • EM = clumping of tonofilaments 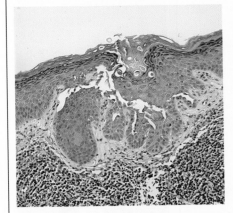

Acantholytic dyskeratosis

(Histological reaction pattern with suprabasilar clefting with acantholytic and dyskeratotic cells at all levels)

Name	Predilection and Clinical Key Features	Histopathology
Focal acantholytic dyskeratosis	• Often clinically inapparent and an incidental foci in a solitary papule	• Focal area of acantholytic dyskeratosis 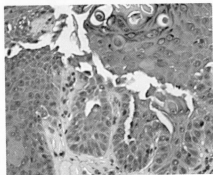

Name	Predilection and Clinical Key Features	Histopathology
Acantholytic acanthoma	• Elderly men • Trunk area • Solitary, asymptomatic keratotic papule/nodule	• Hyperkeratosis, papillomatosis, and acantholysis
Darier's disease	• "Keratosis follicularis" • Autosomal dominant • Onset adolescence (teenagers) • Greasy, crusted papules and papulovesicles; cobblestone oral papules; mental retardation; odor; skin-colored or brownish papules on dorsum of hands, feet; red and white bands on nails with "V-shape" defects distally • Mutation = ATP2A2 gene, endoplasmic reticulum (ER) Ca^{2+} pump in keratinocyte, encodes SERCA2 • Depletion of ER's Ca^{2+} stores causes acantholysis due to loss of cell adhesion and dyskeratosis due to apoptosis • *Note:* worsens with lithium intake, sweat, heat, UVB	• Acantholytic dermatosis; suprabasilar clefts with acantholysis and dyskeratotic cells forming corps ronds and grains; keratin plug with orthokeratosis and parakeratosis • Grains = small cells with elongated, "cigar-shaped" nuclei in stratum corneum • Corp ronds = pyknotic nucleus, clear perinuclear halo, eosinophilic cytoplasm in upper epidermis • Differs from Grover's which likely has several HP features (i.e. spongiosis, pemphigus, etc.), and lacks eosinophils

Name	Predilection and Clinical Key Features	Histopathology
Galli–Galli disease	• Acantholytic variant of Dowling–Degos • Autosomal dominant • Progressive pigmented lesions involving large body folds and flexural areas • Mutation = KRT 5 (keratin 5)	• Multiple foci of acanthosis with overlying parakeratosis; elongated finger-like strands of keratinocytes extending into the papillary dermis similar Dowling–Degos see p. 231

Grover's disease	• "Transient acantholytic dermatosis"
	• Elderly men
	• Upper trunk
	
	• Pathogenesis = unknown
	• Sudden onset of small, crusted, erythematous papules and papulovesicles ("heat rash"-like); Intensely pruritic
	• Usually transient course
		• Four pattern types:
		  1. Darier-like
		  2. Hailey–Hailey-like
		  3. Pemphigus vulgaris-like
		  4. Spongiotic
		• May contain >1 type of pattern histologically
		
		• Often contains eosinophils (which are often lacking in Darier's disease)

Name	Predilection and Clinical Key Features	Histopathology
Persistent acantholytic dermatosis	• Variant of Grover's disease with persistent course • Upper trunk • Pruritic, crusted papules	• Same pathology as Grover's disease
Hailey–Hailey disease	• "Familial benign chronic pemphigus" • Autosomal dominant • Onset in 20s to 30s • Neck, axillae, groin, and intertriginous areas • Recurrent, erythematous, vesicular plaques that progress to small flaccid bullae that rupture/crust; malodor, burning sensation • Mutation = ATP2C1 gene, Golgi Ca^{2+} pump; depletion of Golgi's Ca^{2+} causes a broader area of acantholysis only (due to loss of cell adhesion)	 • Broad, suprabasilar clefting with acantholytic cells lining clefts; epidermal hyperplasia; "dilapidated brick wall" appearance (partial acantholysis at different epidermal levels); dyskeratosis not a prominent feature • DIF = negative

Name	Predilection and Clinical Key Features	Histopathology
Warty dyskeratoma	• Middle age to elderly • Head and neck 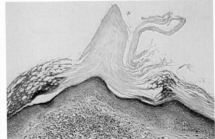 • Solitary papule with an umbilicated/pore-like center on sun-damaged skin	• Cup-shaped or comedo-like invagination of epidermis with down growths; hyperkeratosis, parakeratosis, dyskeratotic keratinocytes (including corps ronds and grains)

Discrete keratotic lesions

Name	Predilection and Clinical Key Features	Histopathology
Flegel's disease	• "Hyperkeratosis lenticularis perstans" • Sporadic; autosomal dominant • 40–50 years of age • Defect = Odland or lamellar bodies (membrane-coating granules in the stratum corneum) • Dorsum of feet; anterior lower legs; thighs; pinnae of ear • Persistent, multiple, red–brown, discrete 1–5-mm keratoses (papules with scale) • Pin-point bleeding, if remove scale (unlike stucco keratosis) • Reported in association with diabetes or hyperthyroidism	• Focal area of compact, deeply eosinophilic orthokeratotic hyperkeratosis and only patchy parakeratosis; dense band-like infiltrate (lymphocytes); acanthosis at margins of lesions; absent granular layer 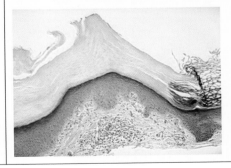

Name	Predilection and Clinical Key Features	Histopathology
Kyrle's disease	• Females; 40s • Lower limbs • Hyperkeratotic papules with a central, cone-shaped plug • Associated with chronic renal failure, liver dysfunction and diabetes	• Keratotic plug overlying an invaginated atrophic epidermis; focal parakeratosis; basophilic cellular debris present; inflammatory infiltrate
Multiple minute digitate keratoses	• Adults • Upper part of trunk; proximal limbs • Hundreds of minute keratotic spikes	• Spicules with densely compact, thin stacks of orthokeratotic material (not related to hair follicles); mild epidermal hyperplasia (normal dermis)
Waxy keratoses	• Childhood • Trunk area • Shiny, yellowish, "waxy", hyperkeratotic papules	• Marked orthokeratotic hyperkeratosis, tenting/papillomatosis of epidermis and some acanthosis

Miscellaneous epidermal genodermatoses

Acrokeratosis verruciformis of Hopf	• Autosomal dominant • Present around puberty • Males • Often seen in Darier's patients • Dorsum of hands and fingers • Multiple, skin-colored, warty papules (resemble plane warts)	 • Hyperkeratosis, regular acanthosis, regular undulating appearance ("church spires") • No parakeratosis and no dermal infiltrate

Name	Predilection and Clinical Key Features	Histopathology
Xeroderma pigmentosum (XP)	<ul><li>Means "dry pigmented" skin</li><li>Autosomal recessive</li><li>Photophobia, solar sensitivity, pigmentary changes (lentigines at an early age), xerosis, Possible neurologic abnormalities</li><li>Risk of all skin cancers at an early age; risk of internal malignancies</li><li>XP mutation = DNA nucleotide excision repair</li><li>Various sites of mutation, XPA through XPG</li><li>XP variant mutation = DNA polymerase</li><li>Usually no neurological abnormalities</li></ul> *Note:* <ul><li>Cockayne syndrome may have mutations involving XPB, XPD, and XPG</li><li>Trichothiodystrophy may have mutations in XPB and XPD genes</li></ul>	
Ectodermal dysplasias	<ul><li>Large group of inherited disorders with a primary defect of two or more tissues of embryonic ectoderm origin (i.e. skin, hair, nails, eccrine glands, teeth)</li></ul> 1. Anhidrotic ectodermal dysplasia (Christ–Siemens–Touraine):<ul><li>X-linked disorder</li><li>EDA gene mutation</li><li>anhidrosis + anodontia + hypotrichosis, characteristic facies, nail dystrophy</li></ul>2. Hidrotic ectodermal dysplasia (Clouston's syndrome):<ul><li>autosomal dominant</li><li>GJB6 gene mutation (gap junction protein connexin 30)</li><li>normal perspiration + prominent PPK + alopecia (and eyebrow/eyelash) + nail dystrophy</li></ul>3. Orofaciodigital syndrome:<ul><li>X-linked dominant disorder (lethal to males)</li><li>marked reduction of sebaceous glands, dental dysplasia, milia, cleft lip, digit malformations</li></ul>4. Ectodermal dysplasias with clefting:<ul><li>several syndromes</li><li>ectodermal dysplasia with cleft lip/palate; due to mutation in p63 gene</li></ul>	

Name	Predilection and Clinical Key Features	Histopathology
Nevoid hyperkeratosis of the nipple	• Areola and nipple (may be bilateral) • Hyperpigmentation of the areola with accompanying verrucous thickening; may be unilateral or bilateral • Associated with acanthosis nigricans	• Hyperkeratosis, papillomatosis, and acanthosis with marked elongation of the rete ridges (often filiform interconnecting pattern); keratin-filled spaces and ostia
Peeling skin syndrome	• Autosomal recessive • Variants may be localized to the palm, face, or acral regions • Spontaneous, continual skin peeling of the stratum corneum • Mutation in acral variant = transglutaminase-5	• Hyperkeratosis, parakeratosis, reduced granular layer, acanthosis; separation of stratum corneum from the underlying granular layer

Name	Predilection and Clinical Key Features	Histopathology
Miscellaneous disorders		
Granular parakeratosis	• Acquired abnormality of keratinization • Middle-aged women • Axilla, intertriginous areas, abdomen • Pruritic, erythematous, hyperkeratotic, and hyperpigmented patches or plaques (spontaneous resolution and recurrence) • Apparent defect in processing profilaggrin to filaggrin (filaggrin absent in affected keratinocytes); results in a failure to degrade keratohyaline granules	• Thick parakeratotic stratum corneum layer with retention of keratohyaline granules
White sponge nevus	• Autosomal dominant • Early childhood • Buccal mucosa • Thickened, spongy mucosa with a white opalescent tint • Mutation = KRT4 and KRT13	• Epithelial thickening, parakeratosis, and extensive vacuolization of the suprabasal keratinocytes

Disorders of Pigmentation

Dowling–Degos disease
"Reticulate pigmented anomaly of the flexures"

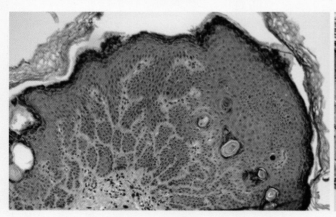
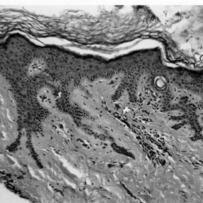

Name	Predilection and Clinical Key Features	Histopathology
Disorders characterized by hypopigmentation		

Phenylketonuria	• Autosomal recessive disorder (screened for disorder at birth)
	• Neurological abnormalities + oculocutaneous pigmentary dilution
	• Mutation = enzyme L-phenylalanine hydroxylase deficiency
	• Increased phenylalanine causes:
	  • toxicity to the CNS
	  • generalized hypopigmentation of the skin (inhibits tyrosine and melanogenesis); also affects eyes (blue) and hair (blonde)	

Piebaldism	• "Partial albinism" • Autosomal dominant • Present at birth • Defective proliferation and migration of melanocytes during fetal development • Non-progressive hypopigmentation of the scalp, central anterior trunk, upper arms, and legs, especially mid-forehead, central eyebrows (normal pigmentation on hands/feet); white forelock (80–90%) • Possible association with neurofibromatosis-1 • Mutation = *c-kit*; proto-oncogene (results in abnormal tyrosine kinase receptors, abnormal melanocyte embryogenesis, defective melanoblast proliferation; *c-kit* mutation in mastocytosis also) • Woolf's syndrome = piebaldism + deafness	• No melanocytes and melanin in leukodermic areas
Waardenburg syndrome (WS)	WS I = Pax3 gene mutation (autosomal dominant) • Pax3 is a transcription factor controlling neural creast differentiation, and regulates other genes such as those responsible for melanoblast activation/migration • White forelock + hypopigmented patches + cleft palate + heterochromia irides + deafness + dystopia canthorum of the eyes (increased distance between inner canthi with normal distance to pupil and outer canthi)	
	WS II = MITF gene mutation (autosomal dominant) • MITF is a melanocyte transcription factor • WS I + hearing loss but no dystopia canthorum of the eyes	
	WS III (Klein–Waardenburg syndrome) = Pax3 gene mutation (autosomal dominant) • WS I + pectoral and limb abnormalities	
	WS IV (Shah–Waardenburg syndrome) = SOX10, endothelin-3 signaling gene and endothelin receptor gene mutations (autosomal recessive) • WS I + Hirschsprung disease + deafness + possible dystopia canthorum of the eyes (uncommon)	

Name	Predilection and Clinical Key Features	Histopathology
Vitiligo	• Acquired (genetic predisposition) and idiopathic • Onset 10–30 years old; associated with HLA-DR4 • Three types = localized, generalized, and universal • Defect = loss of melanocytes • Depigmented macules that enlarge and coalesce to form leukodermic areas; predilection to face, back of hands, axillae, groin, genitalia, knees/elbows • 20–30% have associated autoimmune/endocrine disorder (Hashimoto's, hyperthyroidism, ID-diabetes, etc.) • Tx = activate/migrate hair melanocyte to repigment areas (narrow-band UVB > PUVA, excimer laser) • Vogt–Koyanagi–Harada syndrome: vitiligo, granulomatous uveitis, poliosis (premature graying of hair), dysacusis, alopecia, meningeal irritation • Alezzandrini syndrome = white scalp, eyebrows, eyelashes, and depigmented skin on face, all on same side as unilateral vision changes	• Absent melanocytes; possible lymphocytic infiltrate (if active); complete loss of melanin pigment from epidermis • Fontana–Masson stain (above)
Oculocutaneous albinism (OCA)	• Numerous variants • Due to generalized decrease or absence of melanin pigment in eyes, hair and skin; normal number of melanocytes	
OCA1A	• Autosomal recessive (40% cases) • Birth • Mutation = TYR gene (absent tyrosinase activity or transport, mutation in both genes) • Snow-white hair; blue to gray–blue irides; severe nystagmus; prominent red reflex in eye; pink–white color; increased risk of SCC > BCC > MM	
OCA1B	• Birth • Mutation = partially active TYR gene • Hypopigmentation at birth (develop yellow or blond hair) • Minimal pigment (more pheomelanin), clinical variants including a temperature-sensitive albinism variant (no synthesis in warm body areas)	
OCA2	• Tyrosine-positive albinism • Most common variant (50%) • Autosomal recessive • Birth • Mutation = *P* gene, membrane transporter (decreased eumelanin, possibly regulates pH in melanosomes) • Cream to yellow–brown hair; blue to yellow–brown irides; nystagmus; increased risk of skin cancers • *Note:* associated with deletions in *P* gene as seen in Prader–Willi (obesity, hypogonadism, retardation) and Angelman syndromes (retardation, microcephaly, ataxia, inappropriate laughter)	
OCA3	• "Rufous OCA" • Tyrosine-related protein-1 (TYRP1) gene mutation • Red–bronze skin color, ginger–red hair and blue or brown irides	
OCA4	• MATP gene mutation (membrane-associated transporter protein)	

Name	Predilection and Clinical Key Features	Histopathology

Hermansky–Pudlak syndrome	• Clinical variant of OCA with platelet dysfunction
	• Common death = respiratory failure
	• Mutations affect Golgi apparatus trafficking (affects platelets and melanocytes)
	• Cream to red–brown hair; epistaxis; bleeding diathesis (platelet storage defect); ceroid deposition in macrophages (lysosomal membrane defect); pulmonary fibrosis; granulomatous colitis
	• Numerous variants, such as:
	  • Type I = HPS1 gene (16-base pair duplication gene/intracellular trafficking)
	    • Puerto Rico, Swiss Alps
	  • Type II = HSP2 gene (AP3B1 mutation which controls protein packaging and vesicle formation)
	  • Type III = HSP3 gene
		• Complete or partial loss in melanin pigment in skin/hair bulbs; melanocytes normal
		• EM = absent granules in platelets and immature melanosomes
		• Six "P"s clinically:
		  • Pigment dilution
		  • Petechiae
		  • Pigmented nevi
		  • Photophobia
		  • Pulmonary fibrosis
		  • PT/PTT increased
		• Or, "HP" = Hispanic race (usually) and Pulmonary/platelet issues

Chediak–Higashi syndrome	• Autosomal recessive disorder • Birth to first few months • Partial OCA + immunodeficiency disorder (pyogenic infections) + bleeding diathesis • Mutation = LYST gene (tracking protein regulating microtubules), resulting in bad transport of lysosomes in melanocytes, leukocytes, and platelets • Silvery sheen on hair; partial or incomplete albinism; recurrent bacterial infections (cellular metabolism/chemotaxis abnormalities), bleeding	• EM = giant lysosomal granules in neutrophils/melanocytes and giant melanosomes • Think of: a boat called "The Chediak–Higashi" that LYSTs to one side due to giant melanosomes and the crew is ill, bleeding and white in color

Griscelli syndrome (GS)	• First year of life (autosomal recessive)
	• Pigment clumping in melanocytes causes pigmentary dilution and silver–gray hair; neutropenia; fevers; hypotonia
	• *Variants:* organelle trafficking affected, unable to ligate actin, thus bad transport in cells:
	  • GS1 = myosin Va:
	    • neurologic impairment
	    • no immune defects
	  • GS2 = RAB27A:
	    • immune abnormalities (hemophagocytic syndrome possible)
	    • neurologic condition is secondary
	    • possible Tx: hematopoeitic stem cell transplant
	  • GS3 = MLPH (melanophilin links myosin Va and RAB27A)
		• Clusters of melanin seen in hair's medulla
		• EM = no inclusion bodies in neutrophils and large melanosomes (Differs from Chediak–Higashi syndrome which has abnormally large granules)

Elejalde syndrome	• "Neuroectodermal melano-lysosomal disease" • First month to childhood • Triad = silvery hair, hypopigmented skin, CNS dysfunction • Silvery hair, intense tan after sun exposure and CNS dysfunction (seizures, retardation); no immunodeficiency	• EM = hair shaft with irregular, large granules of melanin (Differentiation: Chediak–Higashi has hypopigmentation/infections and Griscelli syndrome has immune defects)
Progressive macular hypomelanosis	• Acquired form of hypopigmentation • Young, adult females (Caribbean origin) • Back	• Decrease in melanin pigment in epidermis; normal melanocytes

Name	Predilection and Clinical Key Features	Histopathology
Ash leaf spot of tuberous sclerosis complex (TSC)	• "Bourneville's disease" • Autosomal dominant • "Ash leaf spot" (above) is a hypopigmented macule in lance-ovate shape with a round end and pointed end "Shagreen patch" Koenen's periungual tumor • TSC may have multiple hamartomas in organs; infantile spasms; facial angiofibromas ("adenoma sebaceum"); hypermelanotic macules; "Shagreen patch" (collagenoma); Koenen's tumor (periungual fibromas) • Triad: epilepsy, mental retardation, angiofibromas ("adenoma sebaceum") • Think of "SHAMED": S = Shagreen patch H = hyperpigmentation A = angiofibromas M = mental retardation E = epilepsy D = dental pits ("TS is the pits") • TSC mutation = TSC1 (encodes hamartin) or TSC2 gene (encodes tuberin)	• Melanin reduced, but not absent; decreased size of melanosomes
Idiopathic guttate hypomelanosis	• Middle-aged to elderly, light-skinned women • Extremities • Acquired, benign leukoderma, especially on anterior aspects of legs, made up of discrete, white macules	• Atrophy and flattened rete ridges; decrease in melanin pigment and reduced number of dopa-positive melanocytes

Name	Predilection and Clinical Key Features	Histopathology
Hypomelanosis of Ito	• "Incontinentia pigmenti achromians" (looks like a negative image of incontinentia pigmenti) • Mosaicism, or sporadic mutations not inherited • Birth to first year • Females • Whorled marble cake hypopigmentation along Blaschko's lines, may be unilateral; alopecia; seizures; anodontia of teeth; scoliosis	• Reduced melanocytes and melanin in basal layer
Nevus depigmentosus	• "Achromic nevus" • Congenital hypopigmented macule/patch (stable size) • Birth to early childhood • Trunk and proximal extremities • Isolated, hypopigmented macule	• Normal melanocytes, but reduced dopa activity (e.g., melanin)
Pityriasis alba	• Dark-skinned atopic patients; usually children/young adults • Face (especially malar area), neck, shoulders • Etiology = possible hypopigmentation due to eczema • Ill-defined, slightly scaly, faintly erythematous patches that resolve to areas of hypopigmentation	 • Focal parakeratosis and focal mild spongiosis reduced basal pigmentation; normal melanocyte number; exocytosis of lymphocytes and mild superficial perivascular infiltrate; possible focal spongiosis and keratotic follicular plugging
Postinflammatory leukoderma	• Hypopigmentation following an inflammatory skin disease (psoriasis, DLE, pityriasis rosea, viral, lichen sclerosus et atrophicus, syphilis) 	• Reduction in melanin pigment in basal layer; typically a normal number of melanocytes; usually variable melanin incontinence

Name	Predilection and Clinical Key Features	Histopathology

Nevus anemicus	• Upper trunk
	• Congenital localized, solitary, vascular constriction anomaly with a hypopigmented patch
	
	• Clinical exam = to help confirm diagnosis:
	  • Use ice (causes redness only around lesion), or
	  • Apply pressure (disappears as surrounding skin blanches)
		• No abnormalities on light or electron microscopy
		• Cause = localized vascular hypersensitivity to catecholamines by local vessels

Disorders characterized by hyperpigmentation		
Generalized hyperpigmentary disorders	• Hyperpigmentation possible in number of metabolic, endocrine, hepatic, and nutrition disorders, as well as topical and oral drugs and heavy metals	
Universal acquired melanosis	• "Carbon baby syndrome" • Progressive pigmentation of skin during childhood	• Hyperpigmentation of epidermis and increase in melanosomes
Acromelanosis	• Newborn to first year of life • Dark-skinned patients • Dorsal surface of phalanges • Increased skin pigmentation, usually located on the dorsal surface of the phalanges	• Basal hyperpigmentation
Familial progressive hyperpigmentation	• Birth • Patches of hyperpigmentation that increase in size/number	• Increase in melanin pigment within epidermis, especially basal layer
Idiopathic eruptive macular pigmentation	• Children to adolescents • Neck, trunk, and proximal extremities • Asymptomatic, pigmented macules on neck/trunk	• Increased basal pigmentation, pigmentary incontinence, sparse infiltrate
Dyschromatosis symmetrica hereditaria	• "Reticulate acropigmentation of Dohi" • Autosomal dominant hereditary skin condition • Develops by age 6; Japan • Dorsum of hands, distal extremities (spares palms, soles and mucosa), face • Symmetrical, hypo- and hyperpigmented macules (freckle-like) • Darken in summer and may spontaneously clear • Mutation = DSRAD (encodes adenosine deaminase)	• Increased basal pigmentation in hyperpigmented areas; and reduced pigment in hypopigmented areas

Name	Predilection and Clinical Key Features	Histopathology
Dyschromatosis universalis hereditaria	• Autosomal dominant hereditary skin condition • Appear birth to age 6; Japan • All over body, including palms and soles (not mucosa) • Asymptomatic, hypo- and hyperpigmented macules in a generalized pattern (no atrophy and telangiectasia) • Areas do not darken in summer or spontaneously clear	• Variable epidermal pigmentation and pigment incontinence
Patterned hypermelanosis	• Rare dermatoses with overlapping features of linear, whorled, or reticulate areas of hyperpigmentation (usually follow Blaschko's lines)	• Whorls of hypermelanosis
Chimerism	• Double fertilization of an ovum, producing individual with differing sets of chromosomes	• Increased melanin in basal layers of epidermis in hyperpigmented lesions
Melasma	• "Chloasma" • Women (especially pregnant, OCPs, Hispanic, hormone replacement) • Face • Tan or dark, irregular facial patches • "Epidermal-only" involvement responds better to treatment (Wood's lamp enhances color contrast)	• Increased melanin in epidermis with mild pigment incontinence
Acquired brachial dyschromatosis	• Middle age, especially women on ACE inhibitors • Dorsum of forearms (usually bilateral) • Asymptomatic, gray–brown patches of pigmentation with interspersed hypopigmented macules	• Epidermal atrophy, increased basal pigmentation, superficial telangiectases and actinic elastosis (no pigment incontinence or amyloid)

Name	Predilection and Clinical Key Features	Histopathology
Ephelis	• "Freckles" • Appear in first 3 years of life • Fair skin (especially if red hair) • Face and shoulders • Related to sun exposure (especially bursts of high intensity) • Multiple, small (1–3-mm), well-circumscribed, red–brown macules • Darken easily with sun exposure	• Increased basal melanin • No elongation of rete ridges and no nests
Café-au-lait spots	• Means "coffee-with-milk" • Hyperpigmented macules that develop in early infancy • Associated with early manifestation of neurofibromatosis (95% of NF1 patients, axillary freckling often present) • McCune–Albright syndrome, tuberous sclerosis, Fanconi anemia, Bloom syndrome, Russell–Silver syndrome, etc. • Cause = increased melanin and giant melanosomes	• Basal hyperpigmentation; no increase in melanocytes; possible giant melanin granules seen

Name	Predilection and Clinical Key Features	Histopathology

Macules of McCune–Albright's syndrome	• Sporadic
	• Females
	
	• Mutation = GNAS1 gene activation (encodes part of G proteins that regulate adenylate cyclase/cAMP), found in endocrine and non-endocrine tissue
	• Triad:
	  1. Polyostotic fibrous dysplasia
	  2. Endocrine dysfunction: i.e. sexual precocity, hyperthyroidism
	  3. Pigmented macules
	• Large café-au-lait macules (irregular "coast of Maine" border and do not cross the midline); recurrent fractures
		• Resemble freckles histologically

Laugier–Hunziker syndrome	• Acquired, benign condition • 20–50 years of age • Macular hyperpigmentation of lips, buccal mucosa, and longitudinal melanonychia of nails (possible pseudo-Hutchinson sign = pigment on proximal nail fold); but no intestinal polyps • Remember "LH" = lips and hands	• Acanthosis, basal hypermelanosis, some melanin incontinence

Peutz–Jeghers syndrome	• "Hereditary intestinal polyposis syndrome"
	• Autosomal dominant
	• Average age at diagnosis = 20s
	• Common mutation = STK11/LKB1 (serine/threonine kinase 11)
	• Polyps + macules + mucosal macules
	• Intussusception (possible first sign); intestinal hamartomatous polyps; mucocutaneous melanocytic macules
	• Slight risk of colon malignancy transformation
	• Increased risk of cancers, especially GI, pancreas, liver
	• DDx:
	  • Cronkhite–Canada syndrome = intestinal polyposis + lentigo-like macules on face, palms, soles (no mucosal macules and no increase in melanocytes)
	  • Laugier–Hunziker = macules + mucosal macules (no intestinal polyps)
		• Basal hyperpigmentation; possible increase in melanocytes

Name	Predilection and Clinical Key Features	Histopathology
Ruvalcaba–Myhre– Smith syndrome	Syndrome with juvenile polyposis coli + macrocephaly (cerebral gigantism) + pigmented (café-au-lait) macules on glans/shaft of the penis	
Becker's nevus	• Young men • Area of shoulder girdle • Unilateral, hyperpigmented area, hypertrichosis • May follow sunburn to area • Associated with connective tissue nevus, accessory scrotum, areolar hypoplasia	• Rete ridges with flat tips; mild papillomatous hyperplasia; acanthosis • *Note:* Areas have increased level of androgen receptors

Name	Predilection and Clinical Key Features	Histopathology
Dowling–Degos disease	• "Reticulate pigmented anomaly of the flexures" • Autosomal dominant • Child to adult onset • Back, neck, axillae • Pigmented, reticulate macule/papule of flexures; pruritus; pitted perioral or facial scars • Mutation = keratin 5 (KRT5) • Galli–Galli disease = acantholytic variant of Dowling–Degos disease • DDx = Reticulate acropigmentation of Kitamura (see p. 232)	• Elongated, pigmented rete ridges (filiform, "antler-like" down growths); thinning of suprapapillary epithelium; perivascular infiltrate; dermal melanosis

(see p. 232)

Name	Predilection and Clinical Key Features	Histopathology
Postinflammatory melanosis	• "Postinflammatory hyperpigmentation" (PIH) • Acquired pigment excess due to preceding conditions (lichenoid reaction such as LP, lichenoid drug, fixed drug; or due to trauma, infection, etc.) • Wood's lamp helps differentiate epidermal PIH (accentuates border) and dermal PIH	• Prominent melanin incontinence; perivascular lymphocytic infiltrate; normal or increased amounts of melanin in the basal layer
Prurigo pigmentosa	• Back, neck, chest • Pruritic, recurrent, red rash that heals with a reticular hyperpigmentation in days	• Papular stage = acanthosis, mild spongiosis, exocytosis of lymphocytes, lichenoid reaction pattern; few eosinophils • Late stage = prominent melanin incontinence
Kitamura	• "Reticulate acropigmentation of Kitamura" • Autosomal dominant • Japanese individuals • Dorsal hands and feet • Reticulate, slightly depressed, pigmented macules; palmar pits • Sunlight may aggravate • Possible variant of Dowling–Dagos (see p. 231)	• "Solar lentigo-like" with club-shaped elongation of the rete ridges, but with intervening epidermal atrophy; melanocytes are increased in number
Generalized melanosis in malignant melanoma	• Melanoma patients • Patients with disseminated malignant melanoma who develop slate-gray or bluish-black pigmentation, especially in light-exposed areas	• Melanin pigment throughout dermis in perivascular and interstitial melanophages and as free granules; no individual melanoma cells present typically

Dermatopathia pigmentosa reticularis (DPR)	• Autosomal dominant form of ectodermal dysplasia
	• By age 2 years
	• Triad:
	  1. Generalized reticulate hyperpigmentation (trunk); does not fade with time
	  2. Alopecia (non-scarring)
	  3. Onychodystrophy: lack of dermatoglyphics (no fingerprints)
	• Also possible acral, non-scarring blisters
	• Mutation = keratin 14 (non-helical head domain)
		• Significant melanin incontinence in areas of hyperpigmentation; normal epidermis

Name	Predilection and Clinical Key Features	Histopathology

Naegeli– Franceschetti– Jadassohn syndrome (NFJ)	• Autosomal dominant form of ectodermal dysplasia that affects the skin, sweat glands, nails, and teeth
	• By age 2 years
	• Dark brown, reticulate pigmentation of trunk/limbs + PPK, also hypohidrosis, enamel hypoplasia, nail dystrophy; heat intolerance, skin blisters
	• Absent dermatoglyphics (i.e. lack of fingerprints)
	• *Note:* pigment often fades after puberty (differs from hyperpigmentation in DPR)
	• Mutation = keratin 14 (defect in non-helical head domain of KRT14 which causes an early translation termination)
	• Clinical DDx:
	  • Dyskeratosis congenita but NFJ lacks leukoplakia, bone marrow involvement, and risk of malignancy (see Ch. 3, Lichenoid Reaction Pattern)
	  • Dermatopathia pigmentosa reticularis but NFJ pigment fades after puberty and does not have alopecia
		• Extensive melanin incontinence in areas of hyperpigmentation; normal epidermis

Incontinentia pigmenti	• "Bloch–Sulzberger syndrome"
	• X-linked dominant
	• Young females (lethal to males)
	• Skin stages:
	  I = Vesicular (birth to 2 weeks): lower extremities
	  II = Verrucous (2–6 weeks)
	  III = Hyperpigmented whorls and swirls (3–6 months)
	  IV = Hypopigmented whorls and swirls (20s–30s)
	
	• Whorls of hyper- and hypopigmentation; scarring alopecia; anodontia and peg-shape/conical teeth; seizures
	• Possible extracutaneous involvement includes:
	  • dental ("peg teeth")
	  • ocular
	  • neurologic
	  • musculoskeletal
	• Mutation = NEMO (results in defective NF-κB activation, a transcription factor in immune, inflammatory, and apoptotic pathways)
		• First stage (vesicular) = spongiosis, eosinophils
		• Second stage (verrucous) = papillomatosis, dyskeratotic cells, hyperkeratosis
		• Third stage (hyperpigmented) = melanin incontinence
		• Fourth stage (hypopigmentation) = atrophic, hypopigmented, thin streaks
		
		• Vesicular stage (pictured above)

Name	Predilection and Clinical Key Features	Histopathology
Frictional melanosis	• Hyperpigmentation develops at sites of chronic friction	• Presence of melanin in upper dermis, mostly in macrophages
Notalgia paresthetica	• Cause = sensory neuropathy (T2–T6 nerves) • Upper back pruritus, burning pain (close to medial scapula)	• Melanin pigment in macrophages in upper dermis
"Ripple" pigmentation of the neck	• Feature of macular amyloidosis, or long-standing atopic dermatitis patients	• Presence of melanin in upper dermis (free and in macrophages)
"Terra firma-forme" dermatosis	• Cutaneous discoloration resembling "dirt" that cannot be washed off with soap, but removes with alcohol • Neck area of children • Possible cause = disordered keratinization	• Mild acanthosis and orthokeratosis with numerous keratin globules in stratum corneum

Disorders of Collagen

Morphea

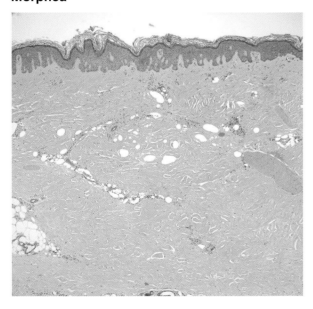

Collagen "basics"

- Major constituent of connective tissue (70% of dry weight)
- Repeating triplet of amino acids glycine–X–Y (X is usually proline)

Transcription step = produces collagen mRNA, regulator of collagen production:

- Stimulated by TGF-β, retinoids, IL-4
- Decreased production by TNF-α, IFN-γ

Translation step = occurs in rough endoplasmic reticulum:

- Hydroxylation of lysine and proline amino acids (stabilizes helix)
  – requires vitamin C and iron
  – scurvy = ascorbic acid deficiency reduces hydroxylation of proline
  – helix unstable and breakdown before excretion
- Glycosylation = add glucose and galactose residues (role in protein folding and assembly in ER)
- Synthesis of interchain disulfide bond (lines up chains so triple helix can form)
- Triple helix procollagen molecule ("the zipper" forms from C-terminus to N-terminus)
- Secretion of procollagen

Extracellular step:

- Cleavage of C- and N-terminal extensions
- Crosslinking of covalent bonds between triple helices (lysyl oxidase enzyme and others)
  – lysyl oxidase requires copper and oxygen
- Assembly into helix . . . then fibril . . . then fibers . . . then bundles

Major types of collagen = location (associated disorders):

- Type I (80%) = skin, bone, tendon; has two identical chains (osteogenesis imperfecta)
- Type II = cartilage (relapsing polychondritis)
- Type III (10%) = GI and vascular, first deposited in wound, contains three identical chains (Ehlers–Danlos, vascular type)
- Type IV = basement membrane
- Type V = skin (classic type of Ehlers–Danlos syndrome, previously type 1 & 2)
- Type VI = beaded filament collagen; increased in keloids and morphea
- Type VII = anchoring fibrils in basement membrane (EBA, bullous SLE, linear IgA)
- Type VIII = endothelium

Name	Predilection and Clinical Key Features	Histopathology
Scleroderma		
Localized scleroderma overall	• Cutaneous scleroderma variant, includes morphea and linear morphea • Usually negative antinuclear antibodies, except linear variant • No visceral involvement or Raynaud's noted • Increased IL-4 and TGF-β in the involved skin areas	
Morphea	• Most common variant of scleroderma • Trunk and extremities • Indurated plaques with ivory center and violaceous border ("lilac ring") • May coincide with lichen sclerosus et atrophicus • Various forms, such as: • guttate morphea • generalized morphea (often ssDNA+) • disabling pansclerotic morphea • subcutaneous morphea (see p. 351)	• Three classic features: 1. Collagen deposition (trichrome stains blue): • broad sclerotic collagen bundles; thick dermis • increased fibroblasts; normal elastic fibers 2. Vascular changes • thickened walls with narrow lumen 3. Inflammatory infiltrate (perivascular/deep): • mainly lymphocytes, some plasma/macrophages
Linear morphea	• Variant with sclerotic areas in a linear pattern • Often ANA+ • Head, trunk, extremities (may lead to joint contractures) • May be associated with Romberg's disease (facial hemiatrophy) if face involved • Coup de sabre-type (above left)	• One of square-looking biopsies (think "Square-O-derma")

Name	Predilection and Clinical Key Features	Histopathology
Diffuse systemic scleroderma	• 20–40% systemic cases • Trunk and acral skin • Symmetrical thickening and induration on trunk/acral with abrupt onset; Raynaud's; synovitis; esophageal involvement; renal failure; ventral pterygium of nails (from adhesion to hyponychium) • Multiple antibodies possibly involved, including: • SCL-70 (60%) = DNA topoisomerase I, unwinds DNA • Centromere (30%)	• Compressed eccrine glands • Similar to localized scleroderma, but systemic scleroderma contains: • less inflammatory changes • subtle collagen deposition early • more prominent vascular changes
Limited systemic scleroderma	• Older women • Usually digits only • Raynaud's often precedes thickening of skin (usually limited to digits); hair loss; anhidrosis; telangiectasia; pulmonary hypertension; ventral pterygium of nails • Antibodies: anti-centromere (80%); anti-Fc receptor (50%); anti-Scl-70 or antitopoisomerase (30%) • "CREST" syndrome: calcinosis; Raynaud's phenomenon; esophageal dysfunction; sclerodactyly; telangiectasia	
Mixed connective tissue disease	• Clinical features of SLE, scleroderma and polymyositis • Antibody to ribonucleoprotein, especially U1RNP (100%), but anti-Sm and DNA negative • Triad ("SRA"): • Swollen/sclerotic fingers • Raynaud's phenomenon and ribonucleoprotein Ab • Arthritis • Also muscle tenderness, proximal weakness, esophageal involvement	• Early lesion = marked dermal edema with collagen separation • Scleroderma-like lesion = dermal sclerosis, thick vessel walls • DIF = speckled IgG epidermal nuclear staining

Name	Predilection and Clinical Key Features	Histopathology

Eosinophilic fasciitis	• "Shulman syndrome"
	• Variant of scleroderma
	• Mid-adult ages
	• Limbs (spares fingers, unlike scleroderma)
	
	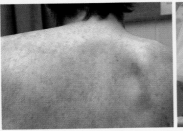
	
	• Sudden onset symmetrical induration of skin and subcutaneous tissue of limbs; usually after strenuous exercise; peripheral eosinophilia; hypergammaglobulinemia
		• Looks like "morphea profunda + eosinophils";
		• Involves deep fascia mainly
		• Early:
		  • Interlobular fibrous septa and deep fascia with edema and mixed infiltrate with eosinophils
		• Later:
		  • Thickening of deep fascia and septa of subcutis; fibrosis and hyalinization of collagen
		
		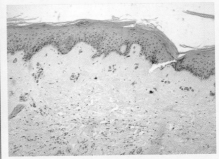

Sclerodermoid disorders

Name	Predilection and Clinical Key Features	Histopathology
Sclerodermoid GVHD	• Rare complication of chronic GVHD • Trunk and proximal extremities 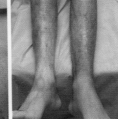 • Develop scleroderma-like lesions usually in a disseminated pattern • Negative antibodies (i.e. ANA, anti-centromere, anti-SCL-70)	• Scleroderma-like lesion, but may extend fibrosis into subcutis; possible GVHD lichenoid changes present 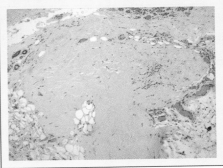

Name	Predilection and Clinical Key Features	Histopathology
Stiff-skin syndrome	• "Congenital fascial dystrophy" • Buttocks, thighs (spares inguinal folds) • Stony-hard skin and limited joint mobility (possible abnormality of dermal/fascial collagen)	• Mild fibrosis of dermis/subcutis with no inflammation

Winchester syndrome	• Inherited osteolysis syndrome
	• Mutation in matrix metalloproteinase-2 (MMP2)
	• Syndrome:
	  • Dwarfism
	  • Carpal–tarsal osteolysis
	  • Thick, leathery skin and coarsened facial features
	  • Hypertrichosis and hyperpigmentation
	  • Corneal opacities
		• Increased basal pigmentation and some dermal thickening; fibroblasts significantly increased; perivascular lymphocytic infiltrate; no increased dermal mucin
		• Memory reminder: think of a short person shooting a Winchester rifle, but difficulty due to eyes (opacities) and hand (osteolysis) problems

"GEMSS" syndrome	• Autosomal dominant • GEMSS = glaucoma, lens ectopia, microspherophakia, stiffness of joints, shortness • Mutation = enhanced TGF-β1 expression	• HP = resembles systemic scleroderma

Pachydermo-periostosis	• Autosomal dominant condition
	• Males
	• Syndrome clinical features:
	  • Digital clubbing
	  • Thick legs and forearms: due to periosteal new bone formation on distal ends of long bones
	  • Coarse facial features with deep furrowed, thick skin on cheeks, forehead, and scalp (cutis verticis gyrata)
		• Diffuse dermal thickening with close, packed collagen; some hyalinization of collagen; increased fibroblasts

Pachyder-modactyly	• Fibrous thickening of the lateral aspects of proximal interphalangeal joints of fingers • Differs from knuckle pads which involve the dorsal aspect of finger joints	
Acro-osteolysis	• Lytic changes in distal phalanges • Sclerodermoid plaques + Raynaud's • Various forms (familial, idiopathic and occupational due to vinyl chloride exposure)	• Thickened dermis, swollen collagen bundles, decreased cellularity, fragmented elastic fibers

Chemical- and drug-related disorders	• Sclerodermoid lesions developing after occupational exposure to polyvinyl chloride, vinyl chloride, herbicides, silica
	  • Texier's disease = pseudoscleroderma lesions following injections of vitamin K1 (phytomenadione)
	    • causes sclerotic lesions with iliac border on buttocks and thighs ("cowboy holster pattern")
		• Resembles systemic sclerosis

Paraneoplastic pseudos-cleroderma	• Sclerotic skin lesions a rare paraneoplastic complication (lung cancer, plasmacytoma, carcinoids)	• Resembles systemic sclerosis

Name	Predilection and Clinical Key Features	Histopathology
Nephrogenic fibrosing dermopathy [CD34+]	• "Nephrogenic systemic fibrosis" • Renal dialysis patients • Thick and hard skin on the trunk and limbs; rippled pigmentation • Associated with gadolinium CT-contrast	• "Sclerodermoid-like but more cellular" • Thick dermis with haphazard collagen arrangement, increased fibrocytes
Lichen sclerosus et atrophicus (LSetA)	• Middle-aged to elderly women • Anogenital region usually • Flat, ivory papules that coalesce to plaques; develop follicular plugging and atrophy; then to parchment-like, depressed scar ("cigarette paper atrophy"); pruritus • Rarely, SCC may develop (in anogenital areas) • Balanitis xerotica obliterans: LSetA involving glans, prepuce and meatus of penis	• Subepidermal edema with homogenized collagen; atrophy; follicular plugging; decreased elastic fibers (unlike morphea) • Early lesions = vacuolar change with lichenoid-like infiltrate • Later lesions show more sclerosis and eosinophils

Name	Predilection and Clinical Key Features	Histopathology
Post-stripping cutaneous sclerosis	• Stripped saphenous vein patients • Multiple hypopigmented and indurated plaques in a linear arrangement along the path of the previously stripped saphenous vein	
Other hypertrophic collagenoses		
Connective tissue nevi	• Cutaneous hamartomas in which one component of extracellular connective tissue (collagen, elastin fibers, glycosaminoglycans) is abundant; subclassification depends on predominant component. • Collagen type: • Collagenoma = asymptomatic, firm, flesh-colored plaque on trunk/upper arms: • associated with cardiomyopathy and Down syndrome • Shagreen patch: • tuberous sclerosis patients (lower part of trunk); slight elevated, flesh-colored plaque on lower trunk with "goose flesh" papules as satellite lesions • HP = dense, sclerotic bundles of collagen with hypertrophied appearing fibroblast • Elastin type = elastoma • Proteoglycan type = nodules in Hunter's syndrome (increased mucopolysaccharides, X-linked recessive)	• Collagenoma connective tissue nevus (photos below): • Thick dermis with broad, haphazard collagen

Name	Predilection and Clinical Key Features	Histopathology
White fibrous papulosis of the neck	• Elderly individuals • Lateral and posterior neck • Multiple, pale, discrete, non-follicular papules	• Circumscribed area of thick collagen bundles similar to connective tissue nevus; elastic fibers usually reduced

Hypertrophic scars and keloids	• Thickened, from papules/plaques
	• Hypertrophic scars:
	  • do not extend beyond original wound
	• Keloids:
	  • sternum (most common area); ears
	  • extend beyond confines of original wound
	  • more common in black races and <30 years old
	  • increased TGF-β
	  • increased type III and VI collagen
	
		• Hypertrophic scar = parallel-oriented collagen and fibroblasts; capillaries oriented perpendicular to skin surface; compressed vessels; often regresses
		• Keloid = broad, homogeneous, brightly eosinophilic, glassy, haphazard collagen; fibroblasts increased in haphazard way; elevated above skin; decreased vascularity; do not regress
		
		• Hypertrophic scar (above)
		
		• Keloid scar (above)

Name	Predilection and Clinical Key Features	Histopathology
Striae distensae	• Females • Abdomen, back, thighs, breasts • Flat, pink, linear lesions that broaden and lengthen with a violaceous color; gradually fade to white, depressed scar • Associated with pregnancy; heavy lifting; Cushing's disease (excess corticosteroid); protease inhibitors	• "Scar-like" with flat epidermis with loss of rete ridges; parallel-arranged collagen; reduced elastic fibers; elastin and fibrillin fibers realign parallel to skin surface in deep dermis
Fibroblastic rheumatism	• Hands • Sudden onset of symmetrical polyarthritis, Raynaud's, and cutaneous 0.2–2-cm nodules	• Proliferation of plump, spindle myofibroblast cells; increased fibroblasts; thick collagen bundles in a whorled pattern
Collagenosis nuchae	• "Nuchal fibroma" • Males • Associated with scleredema, diabetes, Gardner's syndrome • Diffuse induration and swelling on back of neck	• Thick, disorganized collagen bundles replace part of subcutaneous fat; no inflammatory cells; few fibroblasts

Name	Predilection and Clinical Key Features	Histopathology
Lipodermato-sclerosis	• "Sclerosing panniculitis" • Scleroderma-like hardening of the legs in patients with venous insufficiency • Lower extremities • Induration, hyperpigmentation, and depression of the skin ("woody stasis")	• Septal and lobular panniculitis with septal fibrosis and sclerosis; dermal thickening; necrosis; fatty microcysts with foci of membranocystic changes
Weathering nodules of the ear	• Ears • Asymptomatic, white or skin-colored nodules (2-3mm) with gritty texture; usually bilateral and form chain of lesions in ear	• Spur of fibrous tissue with a focus of metaplastic cartilage

Name	Predilection and Clinical Key Features	Histopathology
Atrophic collagenoses		

Aplasia cutis congenita (ACC)	• Group of disorders with areas of absent skin at birth
	• Autosomal dominant, autosomal recessive, and sporadic
	• Often on the vertex of the scalp, but may occur on trunk and limbs
	• Absence of epidermis, dermis, subcutis, and possibly underlying bone
	
	• Solitary (70%), superficial erosions with alopecia on scalp; heal with scar; "hair collar sign"
	• Increased risk of meningitis, sagittal sinus hemorrhage
	• Possible drug cause = methimazole (hyperthyroid drug)
	• Associated syndromes:
	  • Adams–Oliver Syndrome = ACC + transverse limb defects
	  • MIDAS (microphthalmia, dermal aplasia sclerocornea) = aplasia cutis congenita presents as a linear facial skin defect on face/neck
	  • Bart's syndrome = epidermolysis bullosa + congenital absence of skin on lower extremities; inherited autosomal dominant
	  • Opitz syndrome = MID1 gene; ACC + midline defect (palate, cardiac)
		• Epidermis absent/thin; underlying dermis thin with loosely arranged connective tissue

Name	Predilection and Clinical Key Features	Histopathology

Focal dermal hypoplasia	• "Goltz syndrome"
	• X-linked dominant
	• 90% female (lethal in males)
	• Trunk, extremities
	• Linear telangiectasia (Blaschko's lines); pigmentation changes with fat herniations in streaks, perioral/perianal areas with raspberry-like papillomas; lobster claw deformity; osteopathic striata; brittle alopecia; eye coloboma
	• Mutation = PORCN (membrane-bound acyltransferase on endoplasmic reticulum, aids secretion of WNT-gene product)
	• "FOCAL" acronym:
	  F = females only
	  O = osteopathia striata
	  C = coloboma (hole in eye)
	  A = absent dermis, alopecia
	  L = lobster claw deformity
		• Dermal hypoplasia, herniation of fat

Focal facial dermal dysplasia	• Temple area • Congenital • Symmetrical, scar-like lesions	• Thin epidermis (usually depressed); thin dermis; decreased elastic tissue; absence of adnexal structures
Pseudoainhum constricting bands	• Congenital constriction bands resulting in gross deformity or amputation of limb or digit	• Thinning of dermis with finger-like projection of fibrous tissue into underlying subcutis

Keratosis pilaris atrophicans	• Keratosis pilaris associated with mild perifollicular inflammation and subsequent atrophy
	• Congenital follicular dystrophy with abnormal keratinization in upper part of follicle
	
	• Three disorders (based on location and degree of atrophy):
	  1. Keratosis pilaris atrophicans faciei
	  2. Keratosis follicularis spinulosa decalvans
	  3. Atrophoderma vermiculata
		• Follicular hyperkeratosis (below) with atrophy of underlying follicle and sebaceous gland

Name	Predilection and Clinical Key Features	Histopathology
Corticosteroid atrophy	• Atrophy due to long-term topical steroids, especially with occlusion or fluorinated 	• Epidermal thinning with loss of rete ridges, telangiectasias, thin reticular dermis, focal crowding of elastic fibers
Atrophoderma of Pasini and Pierini	• Trunk, especially back • Sharply demarcated, depressed, and pigmented patches; color varies from bluish to slate-gray or brown	• "Morphea + atrophy" • Dermal atrophy; collagen bundles edematous or slightly homogenized in appearance; perivascular lymphocytic infiltrate

Name	Predilection and Clinical Key Features	Histopathology
Linear atrophoderma of Moulin	• Hyperpigmented atrophoderma that follows Blaschko's lines	• Similar to atrophoderma
Acrodermatitis chronica atrophicans	• Third stage of European lyme disease • Spirochete-induced disease (mainly *Borrelia afzelii*) • Hands • May coexist with juxta-articular nodules	• Atrophy of dermis to about half normal thickness; atrophy of pilosebaceous follicles and subcutis
Restrictive dermopathy	• Lethal • Autosomal recessive disorder • Taut and shiny skin with facial dysmorphism, arthrogryposis multiplex, and bone dysplasia	• Hyperkeratosis with hyperplastic epidermis; thin dermis with parallel-arranged collagen; rudimentary hair follicles

Name	Predilection and Clinical Key Features	Histopathology
Perforating collagenoses		

Reactive perforating collagenosis	• Often follows trauma
	• Two clinical variants:
	  1. Common form:
	     • childhood onset
	     • usually on dorsum of hands/feet
	     • recurrent, umbilicated papules that disappear in 6–8 weeks leaving hypopigmented area
	  2. Acquired adult form:
	     • usually in diabetics with renal failure
	     • Kyrle's disease (dialysis) patients
	
		• Cup-shaped depression of epidermis with plug containing parakeratosis, collagen, and inflammatory debris; basophilic, "perforating" collagen fibers vertically oriented through the underlying epidermis to the plug
		
		• Trichrome stain (above)

Name	Predilection and Clinical Key Features	Histopathology
Perforating verruciform "collagenoma"	• Traumatically altered collagen is eliminated in a single, self-limited occurrence with a more verrucous look	• Prominent hyperplasia with some acanthotic down growths encompassing necrobiotic collagen and debris; elastic fibers partly preserved in central plug
Chondrodermatitis nodularis helicis	• Males >50 years old • Upper part of helix (especially right ear of men); or antihelix (more common for women) • Chronic, intermittently crusted, painful nodule	• Central area of ulceration with epidermal hyperplasia; between ulcer and cartilage is granulation tissue, fibrosis, mixed inflammatory infiltrate; degeneration of cartilage
Variable collagen changes		

Ehlers–Danlos syndrome	• Type (defect/inheritance):
	  • Classic (COL5A1, COL5A2/autosomal dominant and Tenascin-X/autosomal recessive):
	    • hypermobility, atrophic scars, bruise easily; "fish-mouth" scars
	  • Hypermobility (unknown/autosomal dominant):
	    • hypermobility of joints, dislocation of joints
	  • Vascular (COL3A1/autosomal dominant):
	    • arterial ruptures, GI and uterine ruptures, bruising, thin skin
	  • Kyphoscoliosis (lysyl hydroxylase deficiency/autosomal recessive):
	    • hypotonia, congenital scoliosis, ocular fragility, laxity of joints
	  • Arthrochalasia (COL1A1, COL1A2/autosomal dominant):
	    • severe joint hypermobility, hip dislocations, scoliosis, bruising
	  • Dermatosparaxis (procollagen N-peptidase/autosomal recessive):
	    • severe skin fragility, cutis laxa-like, bruising	

Name	Predilection and Clinical Key Features	Histopathology

Osteogenesis imperfecta (OI)	• Collagen I production defect (triple helix formation of COL1A1 or COL1A2) so reduced collagen production
	• Bone fragility; decreased skin elasticity; short stature; joint laxity; blue sclerae; otosclerosis
	• Types of OI:
	  • Type I = most common, autosomal dominant, blue sclera, bowed legs, hearing loss
	  • Type II = autosomal dominant/recessive, blue sclera, in utero fractures, die young (resp. failure)
	  • Type III = autosomal dominant/recessive, blue sclera as infants, fractures at birth/in utero
	  • Type IV = autosomal dominant, normal sclera, fractures decrease with age	

Marfan's syndrome	• Fibrillin 1 gene mutation: elastic fiber dysfunction, not collagen • Hyperextensible skin, striae distensae; tall stature; dolichostenomelia (limbs > trunk); ectopia lentis (displace upwards)	
Syndromes of premature aging		
Werner's syndrome (adult progeria)	• Adult form of progeria (autosomal recessive) • Present at 15–30 years of age • Mutation = RECQL2/WRN gene (DNA helicase enzyme) • Bird-like facies; short stature; leg ulcers; diabetes; high-pitch voice; neoplasms (10%, especially fibrosarcoma, osteosarcoma) • Lab: increased urinary hyaluronic acid	• Epidermal atrophy; variable collagen from hyalinization to decreased size; atrophic pilosebaceous units and sweat glands
Progeria (Hutchinson–Gilford syndrome)	• Autosomal dominant; first to second year of life • Mutation = lamin A (nuclear envelope protein) • Thin, atrophic skin; sparse/absent hair; short stature; large cranium:face ratio; CHF; high-pitch voice; "plucked-bird" look • Lab: increased urinary hyaluronic acid	• Epidermal atrophy; dermal fibrosis; decreased adnexal structures and fat; atrophic to lost hair follicles
Acrogeria (Gottron type)	• Milder form of progeria • Autosomal recessive; early childhood • Atrophy, dryness, and wrinkling of skin (esp. face and extremities) • Associated with elastosis perforans serpiginosa and perforating elastomas	• Atrophy of dermis; connective tissue replaces subcutaneous fat; disrupted and irregular elastin fibers
Poikiloderma congenitale	• "Rothmund-Thomson" syndrome • Autosomal recessive • Mutation = *RecQL4* helicase gene • Multisystem disorder of principally skin, eyes, skeletal system • Reticular erythematous eruptions in first year of life followed by hyperpigmentation; poikiloderma; short stature; cataracts; hypogonadism; mental retardation; alopecia; absent thumbs; risk of osteosarcoma/fibrosarcoma	
Cockayne syndrome	• Autosomal recessive • Mutation = DNA helicase (*ERCC8*, *ERCC6* mutations) • Sensitivity to UV and progressive neurologic degeneration • Cachectic dwarf appearance; large ears ("Mickey Mouse" appearance); "salt-and-pepper" retinal pigment; photosensitive eruption in "butterfly" distribution	

Disorders of Elastic Tissue

Elastosis perforans serpiginosa

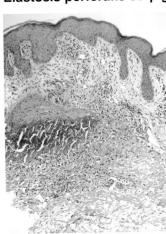 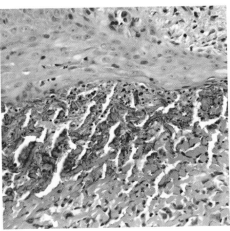

Elastic tissue basics

- Responsible for elasticity and resilience of skin
- Verhoeff-van Gieson (black) or Pinkus acid orcein (dark brown) stains identify elastic fibers
- Major amino acids = desmosine and isodesmosine which crosslink between two tropoelastin polypeptides (need copper)
- Elastic fibers = 90% elastin (produced by fibroblasts/smooth muscle) and 10% fibrillin:
  - three types of elastic fibers = oxytalan fibers (immature, not crosslinked, run perpendicular to basement membrane); elaunin fibers (more mature, crosslinked, run parallel to basement membrane like in "E"); and mature elastic fibers (majority crosslinked)
- Retinoic acid, TNF-α, and vitamin D can decrease elastin

Name	Predilection and Clinical Key Features	Histopathology
Increased elastic tissue		
Elastoma (elastic nevus)	• Variant of connective tissue nevus (increased elastic tissue) • Early age • Lower trunk and extremities • Flesh-colored or yellow papules/plaques • Associated with Buschke–Ollendorf syndrome: • Autosomal dominant disorder (LEMD3 or MAN1 mutations) of connective tissue with multiple elastic nevi symmetrically on trunk (dermatofibrosis lenticularis disseminata) and osteopoikilosis (foci sclerosis or thickening of bone)	• Wavy patterned epidermis; increased, thick, branching elastic fibers in dermis
Linear focal elastosis	• Acquired lesion • Males • Lumbosacral area • Palpable stria-like yellow lines ("keloid of elastic tissue")	• Numerous elongated wavy elastic fibers with "paintbrush" ends
Focal dermal elastosis	• Late onset • PXE-like eruption (see p. 256)	• Increase in normal-appearing elastic fibers (no PXE changes, see p. 256)
Elastoderma	Acquired, localized lax, wrinkled skin (resembles cutis laxa)	• Increased, pleomorphic elastic tissue in upper dermis
Elastofibroma	• Japan • Adults, particularly women • Subscapular fascia • Gray–white or tan nodule • Slow growing proliferation of collagen and abnormal elastic fibers	• Deep mass of proliferation of collagen and elastic fibers, non-encapsulated; "globs" of elastic fibers ("dumbbell-like")

Name	Predilection and Clinical Key Features	Histopathology
Elastosis perforans serpiginosa (EPS)	• Neck, extremities 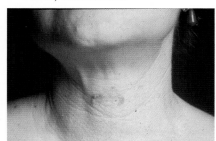 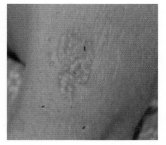 • Grouped, hyperkeratotic, deep-red conical papules in circinate or serpiginous arrangement • Associated with "DERM A POPS" acronym: D = Down syndrome (most common) E = Ehlers–Danlos syndrome R = Rothmund–Thompson M = Marfan's syndrome A = Acrogeria P = Pseudoxanthoma elasticum (PXE) O = Osteogenesis imperfecta P = Penicillamine therapy for Wilson's disease (disrupts desmosine crosslinks in elastin) S = Scleroderma	• Papillary accumulation and transepidermal elimination of elastic tissue (creates channel); keratinous plug overlying channel 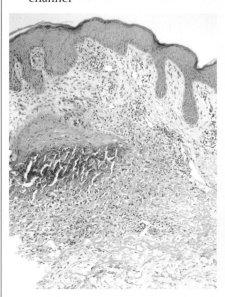 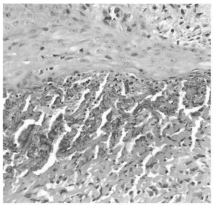 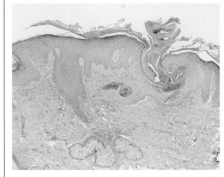 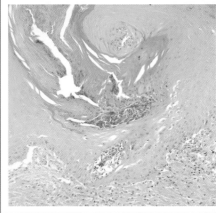

Name	Predilection and Clinical Key Features	Histopathology

Pseudoxanthoma elasticum (PXE)
 	
[von Kossa method stains calcified elastic fibers black; PTAH stains blue and VVG stains elastic fibers]
	• Inherited disorder of connective tissue with calcification and fragmentation of elastic fibers (affects skin, eyes, cardiovascular)
	• In second decade, skin symptoms present
	• Lateral neck (often first location); axillae; flexural creases
	• Mutation = ABCC6 gene (multi-drug resistant protein)
	• Avoid aspirin since increased bleeding risk in PXE
	
	• Skin changes:
	  • Flat, yellowish papules and plaques: "plucked-chicken" look
	• Eye changes:
	  • Angioid streaks are due to calcification and breaking of Bruch's membrane in retina
	    • angioid streaks DDx = PXE, sickle cell anemia, thalassemia, Paget's disease, hyperphosphatemia
	  • "Peau d'orange" or mottling of retinal epithelium
	  • Degenerative choroidoretinitis
	Cardiovascular changes:
	  • Hypertension, CVA, GI hemorrhage
		• "Purple-squiggles" or "bramble-bush" disease
		• Fragmented, short, basophilic, calcified elastic tissue fibers in mid-dermis (only elastic disorder you can see with only H & E stain)
		• Possible calcifications (do not confuse with calcinosis cutis)

Name	Predilection and Clinical Key Features	Histopathology
Acquired pseudoxanthoma elasticum [von Kossa]	• Acquired PXE with late-onset disease • No family history and absence of vascular and retinal stigmata • Possibly seen with exposure to calcium salts (farmers using Norwegian saltpeter), renal failure dialysis patients • May perforate ("perforating calcific elastosis"); often seen in obese, multiparous black women	• Same histology as PXE • von Kossa stain (photo above) • In perforating PXE, a focal central erosion or tunnel surrounding prominent acanthosis; basophilic elastic fibers extrude through defect (photos below)

Name	Predilection and Clinical Key Features	Histopathology
Pseudo-pseudoxanthoma elasticum	• Patients on long-term penicillamine therapy for Wilson's disease (excess copper disorder) • Penicillamine interferes with desmosine crosslinks in elastin	• Appears same as PXE histologically, except von Kossa stain negative (indicating no calcified elastic fibers)
Elastic globes	• Asymptomatic nodules	• Basophilic cytoid, elastic bodies in upper dermis
Solar elastotic syndromes (Accumulation of abnormal elastic tissue due to long-term sun exposure)		
Solar elastosis (actinic elastosis) [Verhoeff stains elastic fibers black]	• Thick, dry, coarse, wrinkled skin with loss of skin tone due to sun exposure 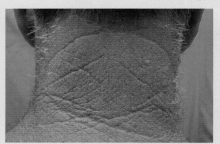 • Clinical variant on the neck = cutis rhomboidalis (photo above)	• Accumulation of curled basophilic elastic fibers and elastic masses in upper dermis; grenz zone of normal-appearing collagen 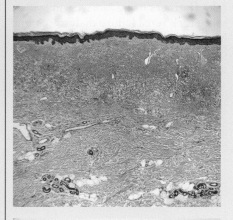 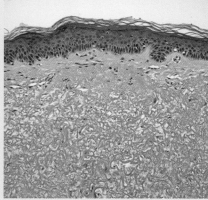
Nodular elastosis with cysts and comedones	• "Favre–Racouchot syndrome" • Males • Periorbital area; head and neck 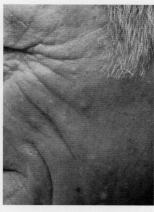 • Thick, yellow plaques with cysts and open comedones	• Solar elastosis; dilated follicles and comedones with keratin debris in lumen; sebaceous glands atrophic 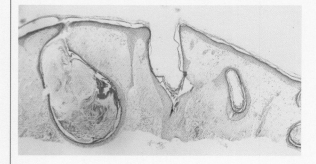

Name	Predilection and Clinical Key Features	Histopathology
Elastotic nodules of the ears	• Anterior crus of antihelix (often bilateral) • Small, asymptomatic, pale papules on ear	• Clumped masses of elastotic material [Verhoeff elastic stain]; elastotic degeneration in dermis; orthokeratosis
Collagenous and elastotic plaques of the hands	• "Keratoelastoidosis marginalis" "digital papular calcific elastosis," or "digital papular calcific elastosis" • Slow, progressive, degenerative condition • Elderly males usually over the age of 50 • Junction of palmar and dorsal skin (especially thumb and adjacent index finger) • Waxy, linear plaques • Related likely to repetitive trauma and sun damage • Clinically, lesions between thumb and adjacent index finger may appear similar to the genodermatosis acrokeratoelastoidosis (see pp. 207 and 262)	• Thick collagen, haphazard but often a proportion of the collagen bundles are running perpendicular to the surface; admixed granular, elastotic material; basophilic elastotic masses found in upper dermis; possible focal deposits of calcification in the dermis

Name	Predilection and Clinical Key Features	Histopathology
Erythema ab igne	• Lower legs, lower back • Reticulated, hyperpigmented patch • Due to repeated heat exposure • Possible risk of keratoses or SCC	• Thinning of epidermis with effacement of rete ridges; some basal vacuolar changes; small amount of hemosiderin; usually prominent elastotic material in mid-dermis; sometimes areas of epithelial atypia resembling actinic keratosis
Decreased elastic tissue		
Nevus anelasticus	• Early onset • Lower trunk • Papular lesions (absence or decrease of elastic fibers)	• Localized reduction in elastic fibers; normal collagen; no inflammation
Perifollicular elastolysis	• Face and back • Associated with acne vulgaris • Gray/white, finely wrinkled lesion with central hair follicle	• Complete loss of elastic tissue around follicles; no inflammation
Anetoderma	• Localized "relaxed skin" with herniation • Late teens to adults • Trunk and upper arms • Well-circumscribed, small, "bag-like" outpouching of shiny wrinkled skin; usually herniates inward with finger-tip pressure • Primary anetoderma: • Jadassohn–Pellizzari type: inflammatory lesions present • Schweninger–Buzzi type: no precursor inflammatory lesions • Secondary anetoderma: • Develops at site of prior lesions such as: syphilis, leprosy, sarcoidosis, GA, TB, HIV, lupus erythematosus, lymphoma	• Loss of elastic fibers, particularly in dermis

Name	Predilection and Clinical Key Features	Histopathology
Cutis laxa	• Congenital variant = defect in elastic synthesis or assembly • *Acquired (Marshall's syndrome)* = associated with penicillin, penicillamine, INH, SLE, celiac disease • Classic facies are hooked nose and long upper lip ("bloodhound" face) • Widespread, large folds of pendulous skin • Often involves internal organs • Mutations: • Autosomal recessive form = fibulin-5: calcium-dependent, elastin-binding protien • Autosomal dominant form = elastin gene (ELN) mutation • X-linked recessive form = ATP7A: • same mutation as Menkes' syndrome (see below) • emphysema and occipital horn exostoses	• Fragmentation and loss of elastic fibers; mixed infiltrate • Differential diagnosis includes Costello syndrome: • Genetic disorder with loose skin localized to hands, feet, neck + retardation + short stature + heart problems + growths around nose/mouth • Short and ruptured elastic fibers also
Williams' syndrome	• Multisystem, congenital disorder • "Elfin" facial features; low nasal bridge; full lips; cheerful demeanor (negative outbursts); retardation; love for music • Mutation = chromosome 7 (elastin gene and other genes)	• Skin appears normal histologically
Papillary-dermal elastolysis	• Neck and upper trunk • Papules and cobblestone plaques similar to PXE	• Complete loss of elastic tissue in papillary dermis; no calcification of remaining fibers; does not appear like PXE histologically
Mid-dermal elastolysis	• Women • Upper extremities • Widespread patches of fine wrinkling due to loss of elastic fibers in mid-dermis • 50% preceded by erythema, urticaria, or burning	• Loss of elastic tissue limited to mid-dermis; does not involve papillary or lower reticular dermis
Menkes' syndrome (kinky hair disease)	• X-linked recessive (copper storage disease): sparse, brittle, "steel wool" coarse hair; pili torti (monilethrix and trichorrhexis); growth failure; seizures; hypotonia; hypermelanotic skin • Mutation = ATP7A or MNK gene (do not absorb copper) • *Note:* copper mutation also seen in Occipital Horn syndrome and Ehlers-Danlos type IX • Think of "Pillsbury dough-boy" = male with doughy skin, who wears a hat because of coarse hair	
Fragile X syndrome	• X-linked (#1 cause of inherited mental impairment) • Large testicles (macro-orchidism); hypotonia; autism; long face with large ears, high-arched palate; heart defects • Mutation = FMR1 gene at long arm end of X chromosome (role in normal brain development)	
Wrinkly skin syndrome	• Autosomal recessive disorder • Wrinkling of skin on dorsum of hands, feet, and abdomen; increased number of palmar and plantar creases; hypermobility of joints; poor growth; developmental delay; venous pattern on chest (decreased elastic coil due to decreased elastic fiber number and length)	
Granulomatous diseases	• Anetoderma that develop as a complication of sarcoidosis, leprosy, TB	
"Granulomatous slack skin"	• Cutaneous T-cell lymphoma patient • Pendulous skin in flexural areas	Lymphoid cells; granulomas with multinucleate giant cells; absence of elastic fibers

Name	Predilection and Clinical Key Features	Histopathology
Myxedema	• Associated with prolonged hypothyroidism • Coarse, thickened skin; facial changes, puffiness around eyes; slow speech (see Ch. 13, Cutaneous Mucinoses)	
Acrokerato-elastoidosis	• Variant of PPK, occurs sporadic and autosomal dominant • Early childhood to early adult • Female predominance • Side of palms/feet and dorsum of hands/feet • Multiple, 2–5-mm, firm, translucent papules, especially along junction of dorsum and palmar/plantar surface • Genodermatosis in which dermal elastic fibers are usually fragmented and decreased in number • Clinically, lesions between the thumb and adjacent index finger may appear similar to collagenous and elastotic plaques of the hands (see p. 259)	• Prominent hyperkeratosis with shallow depression of epidermis, hypergranulosis and acanthosis; sparse perivascular infiltrate (lymphocytes); decreased and fractured elastic fibers • Trichrome stain (Photo above)

Name	Predilection and Clinical Key Features	Histopathology
Variable or minor elastic tissue changes		
Leprechaunism	• "Donohue syndrome" • Rare autosomal recessive disorder • Abnormal resistance to insulin • Characteristic facies (thick/wide lips, low-set ears, flaring nostrils), skin abnormalities, enlarged clitoris/penis, endocrine abnormalities	
Wrinkles	• Sun damage and environment (i.e. smoking) contribute	

Scar tissue	• Scar tissue order of repair:
	  1. Fibronectin
	  2. Collagen III
	  3. Collagen I
	• Macrophages are required for proper wound healing	

Marfan's syndrome	• Autosomal dominant disorder of connective tissue • Mutation = fibrillin-1 (FBN 1) • Ocular, skeletal, and CV conditions; striae distensae; elastosis perforans serpiginosa	

13 Cutaneous Mucinoses

Stain	Material Stained and Color
Alcian blue pH 2.5	• Acid mucopolysaccharides (usually hyaluronic acid) • Light blue color
Alcian blue pH 0.5	• Only sulfated acid mucopolysaccharides, i.e. chondroitin sulfate (Hurler's syndrome) and heparin sulfate • Light blue color
Colloidal iron stain	• Acid mucopolysaccharides • Blue-green color • If add hyaluronidase, removes hyaluronic acid
Toluidine blue	• Acid mucopolysaccharides • Purple color
Mucicarmine	• Epithelial mucin (not dermal mucin); use in Paget's disease, adenocarcinoma • Red color

Name	Predilection and Clinical Key Features	Histopathology
Dermal mucinoses		
Generalized myxedema [Colloidal iron]	• Hypothyroid patient (increased mucin due to impaired degradation of glycosaminoglycans by low thyroxine level) • Eyelids, nose, cheeks • May deposit in other organs • Thickened, waxy, non-pitting, edematous skin; macroglossia; hypothermia; PPK	• Subtle changes; mucin deposition (especially hyaluronic acid) often perivascular or perifollicular; no fibroblast changes • Colloidal iron stain (photo above)

Name	Predilection and Clinical Key Features	Histopathology
Pretibial myxedema	• Graves' disease (1–4%), hyperthyroidism, or may develop after hyperthyroidism treated • Associated with autoimmune thyroiditis (possibly increased mucin due to elevated circulating factors that increase synthesis in fibroblasts) • Anterolateral aspect of lower legs and dorsum of feet • "Elephantiasis-like" skin thickening; sharply circumscribed nodular lesions or diffuse non-pitting edema	• Increased mucin in mid-dermis (mostly hyaluronic acid); mild infiltrate; hyperkeratosis; no increase in number of fibroblasts (stellate appearance) • Colloidal iron stain (above)
Lichen myxedematosus or papular mucinosis	• Hands, forearms, face • Rare association with hepatitis C, HIV • Multiple, asymptomatic, pale/waxy, 2–3-mm papules • Associated with paraproteinemia (especially IgG lambda type) • Not associated with thyroid disease	• Papular mucinosis resembles focal mucinosis

Name	Predilection and Clinical Key Features	Histopathology
Scleromyxedema	• Generalized variant of lichen myxedematosus • Involves entire body • Associated with paraproteinemia (especially IgG lambda type), multiple myeloma, Waldenström's macroglobulinemia • "Papules + skin thickening" • Lichenoid papules/plaques with skin thickening • No associated thyroid disease	• Mucin + increased fibroblasts + whorled collagen appearance; atrophy of follicles; flattened epidermis

Name	Predilection and Clinical Key Features	Histopathology
Acral persistent papular mucinosis	• Variant of lichen myxedematosus • Women • Back of hands, forearms, calf • Discrete, flesh-colored papules; usually no associated disease	• Resembles papular mucinosis (mucin deposition and fibroblast proliferation less pronounced and more in upper dermis)
Cutaneous mucinosis of infancy	• Variant of lichen myxedematosus • Possible connective tissue nevi of proteoglycan-type (i.e. nevus mucinosis) • Infants • Upper extremities, trunk • Multiple, small papular lesions	• Abundant mucin; no significant fibroblast increase
Self-healing juvenile cutaneous mucinosis	• Variant of lichen myxedematosus • Childhood • Head and trunk • Infiltrated plaques with spontaneous resolution; rapid onset, but resolves over months	• Normal epidermis over edematous dermis (mucin separating collagen)
Nephrogenic fibrosing dermopathy [CD34+]	• "Nephrogenic systemic fibrosis" • Renal dialysis patients • Thick and hard skin on the trunk and limbs; rippled pigmentation • Association with gadolinium CT-contrast	• "Sclerodermoid-like but more cellular"; thick dermis with haphazard collagen arrangement, increased fibrocytes

Name	Predilection and Clinical Key Features	Histopathology
Reticular erythematous mucinosis (REM) [Colloidal iron better than alcian blue]	• Young to middle-aged females • Midline chest and back • Erythematous macules, papules, or infiltrated plaques in a reticulated, or net-like, pattern • Sunlight and hormones may exacerbate • May progress to tumid lupus (dermal variant of lupus)	• "Tumid-lupus" like; superficial and deep perivascular lymphocytic infiltrate; prominent mucin; epidermis normal • DIF = IgM along BMZ (granular) • Colloidal iron staining mucin (photo above)

Name	Predilection and Clinical Key Features	Histopathology

Scleredema
 	
[Alcian blue, toluidine blue (pH 5.0 or 7.0), or colloidal iron]
	• All ages; female
	• Symmetric involvement of posterior neck, shoulders, upper trunk
	
	• Non-pitting induration of the skin; systemic manifestations (EKG, ocular, tongue muscle)
	• May be associated with gammopathy (especially IgG)
	• Clinical setting variants:
	  • Follows acute febrile illness (*Strep*.); child
	  • Associated with insulin-dependent diabetes; obese male
	  • Associated with monoclonal gammopathy
	  • Insidious onset, protracted course
		• "Dermal sclerosis + mucin"
		• Thickening of reticular dermis with swelling and separation of collagen; variable mucin; epidermis normal but flattening of rete ridges and basal hyperpigmentation; swelling of collagen with separation (unlike scleroderma)
		• No increase in fibroblasts (unlike scleromyxedema)
		• No deep inflammatory infiltrate (unlike morphea)
		
		• Colloidal iron stains mucin between the collagen (picture below)

Name	Predilection and Clinical Key Features	Histopathology
Focal mucinosis [Alcian blue (pH 2.5), toluidine blue (pH 3.0), colloidal iron]	• Adults • Face, trunk, proximal extremities • Dome-shaped solitary, flesh-colored nodule (1 cm)	• Nodule with prominent mucin in upper dermis; variable collagen; spindle-shaped fibroblasts

Name	Predilection and Clinical Key Features	Histopathology
Digital mucous (myxoid) cyst [Alcian blue (pH 2.5), colloidal iron]	• "Focal mucinosis on the hands" • Middle age to elderly female • Digits • Solitary, dome-shaped, shiny, tense cystic nodule • Variants: • Base of nail • If over DIP joint, then possible ganglion cyst variant	• "Acral skin + deep focal mucinosis" • Ganglion cyst variant has cystic space with fibrous wall and possibly synovial lining; connects to joint (pictured below)

Name	Predilection and Clinical Key Features	Histopathology

Mucocele of the lip
 	
[Alcian blue (pH 2.5), colloidal iron]
	• May result from rupture of a minor salivary duct
	• Lower lip
	
	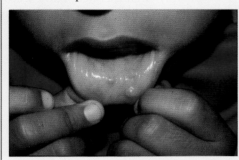
	
	• Translucent, white, or blue nodule with firm cystic consistency; may rupture
		• "Mucosa + cystic space"
		• Possibly sebaceous gland adjacent
		• Numerous neutrophils and eosinophils in cystic space (not true cyst since it lacks epithelial lining)
		
		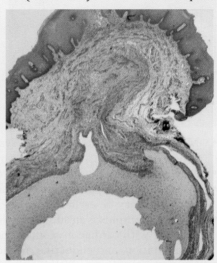
		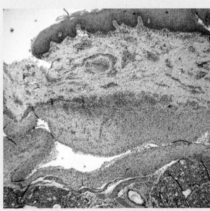
		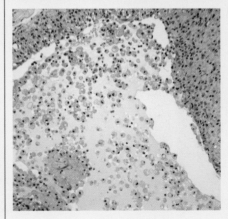
		
		• Two types histologically:
		  1. Pseudocystic space with surrounding macrophages and vascular loose fibrous tissue
		  2. Granulation tissue with mucin, muciphages, and inflammatory cells

Name	Predilection and Clinical Key Features	Histopathology
Cutaneous myxoma	• Benign cutaneous mass • Eyelids, nipples, buttocks • May not be associated with any systemic abnormalities • May be associated with Carney's complex • 50% of Carney's patients have cutaneous myxoma (may be earliest sign) • Carney's complex is an autosomal dominant disorder with cardiac myxomas, spotty pigmentation, and endocrine overactivity • Carney's mutation = PRKAR1A; tumor-suppressor gene	• Similar to focal mucinosis but prominent capillaries and deep in dermis • Sharply circumscribed, non-encapsulated lesion; prominent mucin; variable fibroblasts • Colloidal iron stain (above)

Name	Predilection and Clinical Key Features	Histopathology
Nevus mucinosus	• Variant of connective tissue nevus with deposition of acid mucopolysaccharides (proteoglycans) • Birth to early adult age • Extremities and trunk • Grouped, zosteriform, or linear papules	• Mucin in expanded papillary dermis; increased fibroblasts present, acanthosis
Progressive mucinous histiocytosis	• Rare autosomal dominant histiocytosis of childhood • Multiple small papules composed of epithelioid and spindle-shaped histiocytes in abundant stromal mucin	
Secondary dermal mucinoses	• Mucin and changes caused by underlying disease such as: • SLE, DM, Degos' disease, granuloma annulare, Jessner's lymphocytic infiltrate, neurofibroma, BCC, chondroid syringomas	
Follicular mucinoses		

Follicular mucinosis
 	
[Colloidal iron]
	• "Alopecia mucinosa"
	• Adults (30–40s)
	
	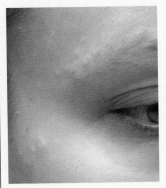
	
	• Follicular papules or plaques with hair loss and follicle degeneration
	• Three types:
	  1. Benign transient form:
	    • face, scalp (alopecia)
	    • resolve in <2 years
	  2. Widely distributed form:
	    • course >2 years
	  3. Widespread lesions:
	    • associated with lymphoma, MF, Hodgkin's, leukemia cutis (15–30%)
		• Mucin in hair follicles and attached sebaceous glands with some cellular attachment dissolution; follicular and perivascular infiltrate
		
		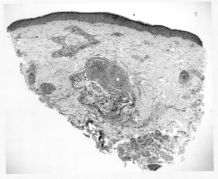
		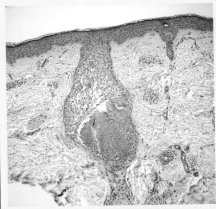
		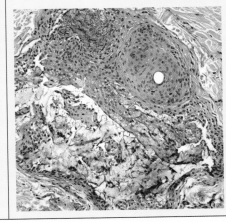

Secondary follicular mucinoses	• Inflammatory process may stimulate fibroblasts to produce excess mucin • Follicular mucinosis may be associated with LSC, arthropod bite, hypertrophic lichen planus, DLE, acne vulgaris	

Mucopolysaccharidoses

- Deposited material is dermatan sulfate, chondroitin sulfate or heparan sulfate
- Stains with alcian blue pH >0.5; not hyaluronic acid like mucinosis disorders

- Group of lysosomal storage diseases resulting from deficient specific lysosomal enzymes
- Major types:
  - Hurler's syndrome (MPS I), autosomal recessive:
    - gigantism, corneal clouding
    - mutation = α-L-iduronidase (deposits dermatan, heparan sulfate)
  - Hunter's syndrome (MPS II), X-linked recessive:
    - white papules between scapulae, no corneal clouding
    - mutation = iduronate 2-sulfatase (deposits dermatan, heparan sulfate)

- Metachromatic granules in fibroblasts, sometimes eccrine glands and keratinocytes
- Hunter's syndrome = extracellular mucin visible in maculopapular lesions

Cutaneous Deposits

Calcinosis cutis

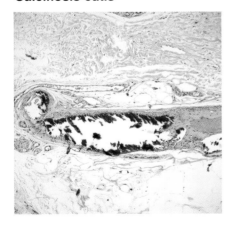

Name	Predilection and Clinical Key Features	Histopathology
Calcium calcinosis cutis • Stains with von Kossa's silver, which stains calcium deposits black; and alizarin red, which stains calcium a red-orange colour		
Subepidermal calcified nodule (idiopathic)	• Infants/children • Often on the ear • Solitary nodule on the head, extremities	• Multiple, small globular subcutaneous calcium deposits (dark, basophilic, fractured deposits)
Idiopathic scrotal calcinosis	• Children and young adults • Single to multiple lesions on the scrotal skin; may discharge chalky material	• Amorphous masses in the scrotal skin with dark, basophilic, fractured deposits
Tumoral calcinosis (idiopathic)	• Healthy, black individuals • Overlying large joints • Subcutaneous mass	• Large, dense, subcutaneous deposits
Auricular calcinosis ("petrified ear")	• One or both ears • Associated with inflammation, frost bite, trauma, Addison's disease, ochronosis	
Infantile calcinosis of the heel (dystrophic)	• Infants (heel pricks) • Present at 10–12 months, disappears at 1 year	• Pseudoepitheliomatous hyperplasia, associated with transepidermal elimination of granules
Milia-like calcinosis	• Pin-size nodules in genital area, thigh, knees • Associated with Down syndrome	

Name	Predilection and Clinical Key Features	Histopathology
Dystrophic calcification	• Calcium deposited in damaged or degenerative tissue • Does not involve internal organs and is without systemic metabolic abnormalities • Associated with trauma, dermatomyositis, LE, scars, keloids, violin pressure points	• Large subcutaneous deposits of dark, basophilic, fractured deposits

Metastatic calcification	• Variant of calcinosis cutis involving a dysfunction of the calcium regulatory system
	• Axillae, abdomen, medial thigh/flexural areas
	
	• #1 cause = renal disease
	• Accompanies hypercalcemia that is associated with primary or secondary hyperparathyroidism, destructive bone lesions, hypervitaminosis D
	• "Calciphylaxis":
	  • Rare disease with progressive cutaneous necrosis and ulceration with widespread calcification and thrombosis
	  • Associated with renal failure and secondary hyperparathyroidism; metastatic breast cancer
		• Large, dense subcutaneous deposits of dark, basophilic, fractured deposits; involve vessels
		
		• Calciphylaxis histology = epidermal ulceration, focal dermal necrosis and vascular calcifications; acute/chronic calcifying panniculitis

Name	Predilection and Clinical Key Features	Histopathology
Bone		

Cutaneous ossification	• Osteoma cutis = "bone in the skin"
	• Types:
	 • Primary (osteoma cutis) = lacks pre-existing lesion
	 • Secondary (metastatic ossification) = associated with inflammatory, traumatic, or neoplastic process
	• Variants:
	 • Multiple osteomas = birth, childhood; multiple foci of cutaneous ossification
	 • Multiple miliary osteomas of the face = history of previous acne or dermabrasion; multiple miliary osteomas of face with hard, flesh-colored papules
	 • Osteomas of distal extremities = rare group of bony tumors of the digits with no cartilage or bony connection
	 • Secondary ossification = majority of cases; bone may be found in nevi, BCC, pilomatricoma (20%), sites of trauma/infection, abdominal wounds
	• Genetic disorder variants:
	 • Fibrodysplasia ossificans progressiva (FOP):
	  • endochondral bone formation; unlike other genetic variants which have intramembranous ossification
	  • involves skin only via extension from the deep tissue
	  • often die at young age due to restricted chest movement
	  • mutation = ACVR1 gene (encodes activin A receptor, a bone morphogenic protein receptor)
	 • Plate-like osteoma cutis (POC) = develops at birth:
	  • thigh, scalp; slow development of large mass of bone in dermis; usually involves only few areas (possible limited for POH)
	  • mutation = inactivation of GNAS1
	 • Progressive osseous heteroplasia (POH) = develops in childhood
	  • idiopathic disorder with cutaneous calcification and ossification; usually asymptomatic papules; progresses rapidly
	  • mutation = inactivation of GNAS1
	 • Albright's hereditary osteodystrophy (AHO) = develops at an early age
	  • pseudohypoparathyroidism or pseudo-pseudohypoparathyroidism, obesity, brachydactyly, short stature; ossification of dermis, round facies, short-thick fingers
	  • mutation = inactivation of GNAS1 (activated in McCune–Albright's syndrome)
	  • mutation also seen in POC and POH
		
		• Small spicules or large masses of bone in deep dermis or subcutaneous tissue; Haversian systems and cement lines present; osteoclasts uncommon

Name	Predilection and Clinical Key Features	Histopathology
Cartilage		
Cartilaginous lesions of the skin	*Presence of cartilage with varying maturity:* • Chondromas: • rare dermal tumor without bony connection • Hamartomas containing cartilage: • accessory tragus, Meckel's cartilage ("wattle"), bronchogenic and dermoid cysts • Soft tissue tumors with cartilaginous differentiation: • extraskeletal tumors usually in finger soft tissue • Skeletal tumors with cartilaginous differentiation: • osteochondromas, synovial chondromatosis, and subungual exostoses • Miscellaneous lesions: • eccrine tumor, chondroid syringoma, nuchal fibrocartilaginous pseudotumor	 Accessory tragus (above) Synovial chondromatosis (below)

Name	Predilection and Clinical Key Features	Histopathology
Hyaline (pink amorphous "blob") deposits		
Gout	• Men, age 40–50 • Tophi = cutaneous manifestation of gout with monosodium urate crystal deposits around joints • Whitish–red nodules over digits and joints; arthritis • Associated with uric acid accumulation and metabolic defect • Gout Tx = may use allopurinol (xanthine oxidase inhibitor, blocks uric acid production); NSAIDs, colchicine 	• Granulomatous reaction with macrophages and foreign body giant cells; acellular bluish material in dermis; negative birefringence with polarized light (unlike pseudogout) • Formalin-fixed = amorphous, eosinophilic deposits in dermis and subcutaneous tissue (crystals dissolved) • Alcohol-fixed = brown, needle-shaped crystals (doubly refractile) • Gout fixed with alcohol (above)

Name	Predilection and Clinical Key Features	Histopathology
Pseudogout ("calcium gout")	• Deposits of calcium pyrophosphate dihydrate crystals • Typically affects elderly and larger joints (knee, shoulder, wrist) • Larger joints (knee, shoulder, wrist) • Possibly associated with hyperparathyroidism and hemochromatosis	• Unlike gout, positive birefringence (while gout is negative), and crystals are shorter, more rhomboid in shape

Amyloidosis overall	*Cutaneous relevant amyloidosis fibril proteins and associations:*
	• AL (amyloid-light proteins of Aλ and Aκ immunoglobulins):
	  • primary systemic amyloidosis; myeloproliferative diseases
	• AA (amyloid-associated protein):
	  • chronic inflammatory disease such as RA (secondary systemic amyloidosis); or heredofamilial amyloidosis (i.e. familial Mediterranean fever and Muckle–Wells syndrome)
	• ATTR (amyloid-transthyretin protein):
	  • familial amyloidosis
	• Aβ2M (amyloid-β2 microglobulin protein, not filtered by dialysis):
	  • predilection to deposits in synovial membranes
	  • associated with long-term hemodialysis
	• AK (amyloid-keratin protein):
	  • cutaneous amyloidosis
	Stains for amyloid:
	• Congo red = apple-green birefringence
	• Crystal violet = metachromatic color on H & E
	• Thioflavin T = bright yellow–green fluorescence
	• Cotton dye Pagoda Red no. 9 = specific to amyloid (does not stain lipoid proteinosis, colloid milium, or solar elastosis)	

Primary systemic amyloidosis [Congo red, crystal violet, thioflavin T]	• Elderly • Eyelids (periorbital), tongue, heart, GI, skin • Associated with 6–15% of multiple myeloma patients • Main amyloid protein = AL (light chains of immunoglobulin) 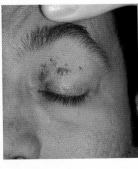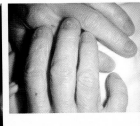 • Shiny, smooth, firm, waxy papules; macroglossia; periorbital purpura after cough/sneeze; purpuric lesions and ecchymoses ("pinch purpura," #1 cutaneous manifestation); purpura due to vessel infiltration by amyloid • Amyloidosis clinical suspicion = carpal tunnel + macroglossia • Tx = often melphalan (risk of marrow suppression, malignancy)	• Amorphous, eosinophilic deposits with fissures; may have deposits in vessel walls 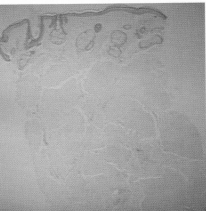 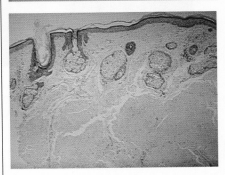 • Biopsy locations = rectal mucosa, abdominal subcutaneous fat aspiration, gingiva, and tongue

Name	Predilection and Clinical Key Features	Histopathology

Secondary systemic amyloidosis	• Rarely cutaneous involvement:
	   • AA (amyloid-associated protein) type of amyloid (produced by liver)
	• Result of underlying chronic inflammatory condition:
	   • non-infectious (5–11% of RA patients, dystrophic EB, inflammatory bowel disease)
	   • infectious (lepromatous leprosy, hidradenitis suppurativa)
	   • often involves adrenal, liver, spleen, kidney (rarely involves skin)
	• Loses birefringence after treatment with potassium permanganate (other types do not)	

Heredofamilial amyloidosis	• Family syndromes associated with amyloidosis; amyloid protein = AA
	   1. *Muckle–Wells syndrome (autosomal dominant):*
	     • Chronic recurrent urticaria from birth, fever, secondary amyloidosis, arthritis, deafness
	     • Mutation = *CIAS1* gene (cryopyrin protein)
	       • same gene as familial cold urticaria
	   2. *Familial Mediterranean fever (autosomal recessive):*
	     • similar to Muckle–Wells (urticarial lesions, recurrent fever, amyloidosis), but also recurrent pleuritis, peritonitis, or synovitis
	     • mutation = *MEFV* gene (pyrin protein)
	   3. *MEN IIA (Sipple's):*
	     • medullary carcinoma of the thyroid; pheochromocytomas; hyperparathyroidism caused by parathyroid hyperplasia
	     • mutation = *RET* gene (putative tyrosine kinase receptor)	

Amyloid elastosis	• Cutaneous lesions and progressive systemic disease	• Elastic fibers in skin and serosae coated with amyloid material; amyloid localized to microfibrils of elastic fibers
Lichen amyloidosus [EAB-903 keratin stain +]	• Cutaneous amyloidosis variants with no systemic disease; often involves friction or rubbing • Protein component is amyloid keratin (AK) • Shins (often bilateral) • Itchy, small, brown, lichenoid papules • Associated with EBV infection and MEN IIA (Sipple's) syndrome (medullary thyroid cancer, pheochromocytoma, hyperparathyroidism)	• Amyloid deposits limited to dermal papillae; melanin incontinence; epidermal hyperkeratosis and acanthosis (resembles lichen simplex chronicus)

Name	Predilection and Clinical Key Features	Histopathology
Macular amyloidosis [EAB-903 keratin stain +]	• Chronic cutaneous amyloidosis variants with no systemic disease; often involves friction or rubbing • Protein component is amyloid keratin (AK) • Interscapular region of back • Pruritic, brown, rippled macules ("salt-and-pepper" look) • Clinically similar to notalgia paresthetica • Associated with MEN IIA	• Subtle amyloid blobs in papillary dermis; melanin incontinence • *Clue:* widened papillae due to amyloid
Biphasic amyloidosis	• Presence of concurrent lesions of macular and lichen amyloidosus	
Auricular amyloidosis	• "Collagenous papule of the ear" • Possibly variant of lichen amyloidosus • Auricular concha of the ear • Papule or plaque	• Amyloid deposits localized to widened dermal papillae

Name	Predilection and Clinical Key Features	Histopathology
Nodular amyloidosis	• Rarest cutaneous amyloidosis variant • Amyloid protein = AL (likely produced by plasma cells) • Lower extremities, face • Multiple, large, waxy nodules • Risk of developing multiple myeloma later • Associated with Sjögren's syndrome	• Numerous plasma cells; large masses of amyloid in dermis and subcutis; accentuated deposits around deep vascular channels and adnexal structures; plasma cells; Russell bodies at margins and in amyloid islands (below) • [Negative staining for anti-keratin antibodies unlike other cutaneous amyloidosis] • Differentiate from colloid milium since VVG stains milium black
Poikilodermatous amyloidosis	• Poikilodermatous cutaneous amyloidosis syndrome: • poikilodermatous amyloidosis, short stature, early onset, light sensitivity, PPK	• Resembles primary systemic amyloidosis
Anosacral amyloidosis	• Rare form of primary cutaneous amyloidosis in Chinese • Light-brown lichenified plaques in perianal region and extending to lower sacrum	• Amyloid deposits in papillary dermis; hyperkeratosis, acanthosis, melanin incontinence
Familial primary cutaneous amyloidosis	• Rare, autosomal dominant genodermatosis • Keratotic papules, swirled hyper- and hypopigmentation on extremities/trunk	• Transepidermal elimination of papillary dermal deposits characteristic
Secondary localized cutaneous amyloidosis	• Amyloid found in stroma of cutaneous tumors (BCC, SCC, cylindromas, pilomatricoma, etc.)	

Name	Predilection and Clinical Key Features	Histopathology
Porphyria	• Metabolic disorder with cutaneous manifestations (see p. 109 and pp. 378–381 for more information) • In PCT (possibly associated with hemochromatosis), blisters form in light-exposed areas, especially dorsa of hands	• Subepidermal blister with deposition of lightly eosinophilic, hyaline material in and around small vessels in upper dermis • PCT (pictured below) • In erythropoietic protoporphyria (EPP; pictured below), hyaline material forms irregular cuffs around vessels and does not encroach adjacent dermis, unlike lipoid proteinosis

Lipoid proteinosis (Urbach–Wiethe disease)
 	
[Alcian blue, colloidal iron, Sudan black, PAS with or without diastase]
	• Autosomal recessive genodermatosis with deposits of amorphous, hyalin-like material in skin, mucosa, and viscera
	  • By age 2 = vesicles and crusts with "ice-pick" scars
	  • Second stage = papules, verrucous lesions
	• Inner lips, tongue, face, vulva, dorsal aspect of extremities, eyelid margin
	• Mutation = loss of function with extracellular matrix protein-1 (ECM1 gene)
	• Hoarse cry at birth
	• Hyperkeratotic wart-like lesions on dorsal aspect hands, elbows; yellow, transparent, beaded papules on eyelid margins; recurrent skin infections
	• Bilateral sickle-shaped temporal calcifications on X-ray (pathognomonic finding); possible epilepsy
		• Hyperkeratosis; papillomatosis; diffuse amorphous, eosinophilic deposits in dermis with tendency to be perpendicular to epidermis and arranged around vessels/adnexal structures (unlike erythropoietic protoporphyria, which is PERIVASCULAR ONLY)
		• May form "onion-skin" appearance around vessels

Name	Predilection and Clinical Key Features	Histopathology
Waldenström's macroglobulinemia	• Translucent papules may form by deposits of monoclonal IgM in Waldenström's macroglobulinemia	• Hyaline deposits in papillary and upper reticular dermis [PAS+]; deposits encase vessels and hair follicles

Name	Predilection and Clinical Key Features	Histopathology
Colloid milium and colloid degeneration [Verhoeff-van Gieson stains elastic black which will differ from amyloidosis yellow color; also stains with crystal violet, thioflavin T; colloid is PAS positive]	• Deposition of colloid likely due to elastic fiber degeneration from sun exposure or exposure to petroleum, etc. • Four variants: 1. Colloid milium (classic adult type) = grouped yellow–brown, semitranslucent dome-shaped papules: • cheeks, ears, dorsa of hands • H/O exposure to petroleum products or excessive sunlight (associated with solar elastosis) • Congo red positive 2. Juvenile colloid milium = rare, papules/plaques on face, neck prior to puberty: • Congo red negative 3. Pigmented colloid milium (hydroquinone related) = follows excessive use of hydroquinone bleaching creams 4. Colloid degeneration (paracolloid) = nodular, plaque-like areas on the face	• Epidermal atrophy; nodular, fissured masses of homogeneous, eosinophilic material in dermis; fissures and clefts divide material into smaller islands; solar elastosis (especially adult variant) • "Cracked-and-fissured" colloid material • Looks similar to nodular amyloidosis, but VVG stains colloid milium black • PAS stain of colloid (above)
Massive cutaneous hyalinosis	• Massive amorphous deposits of hyaline material in deep dermis and subcutis of face and upper trunk	
Corticosteroid injection sites	• Due to local injection of steroids into keloids and subsequent biopsy	• Well-defined, irregularly contoured lakes of lightly staining material in dermis/deeper tissue; variable histiocytic response; fine granular/amorphous material present and surrounded by variable histiocytic response, crystal-shaped empty spaces may be seen within material.
Hyaline angiopathy	• Pulse granuloma • Associated with chronic inflammation • Oral cavity and skin near GI tract openings • Possible unusual foreign body reaction to implanted material	• Amorphous, eosinophilic material within and around vessels; acute or chronic inflammation

Name	Predilection and Clinical Key Features	Histopathology
Infantile systemic hyalinosis and juvenile hyaline fibromatosis	• Infancy to childhood • Autosomal recessive disorder • Scalp, ears, face • White, firm, cutaneous nodules • Characterized by large tumors (especially on scalp); white cutaneous nodules; hypertrophy of gingiva; flexural contractures; osteolytic bone erosion • Recurrent infections may lead to death • Mutation = CMG2 (capillary morphogenesis protein 2)	• Thickened dermis with a "chondroid appearance" • Fibroblast-like cells with abundant granular cytoplasm embedded in an amorphous, hyaline-like, eosinophilic ground substance • [PAS+]

Name	Predilection and Clinical Key Features	Histopathology
Cytoid bodies	• Derived from degenerating keratinocytes, usually associated with lichenoid reaction pattern • Ovoid, round discrete deposits (including amyloid, colloid bodies, Russell bodies and elastic globes)	

Pigment and related deposits

Ochronosis [Methylene blue, cresyl violet stains black color]	• Forehead, temples, nose, lower jaw 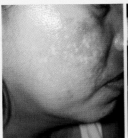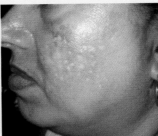 • Yellow–brown or ocher pigment deposited in collagen-containing tissues due to either: 　• Endogenous: alkaptonuria (autosomal recessive disorder, homogentisic acid oxidase deficiency, so tyrosine and phenylalanine increase and there is an increase in melanin precursors which float around the body) 　• Exogenous: hydroquinone derivatives (inhibit homogentisic acid) • Possible clinical differences: 　• Alkaptonuria: 　　• bluish and bluish–black pigment of face, neck, dorsa of hands 　　• blue color in sclerae, cartilage (ear) 　　• black-colored urine 　• Hydroquinone induced: 　　• hyperpigmentation in malar area of face, neck, ears 　　• due to application of hydroquinone cream, phenol, or antimalarial drugs	• "Brown banana-shaped" fibers; yellow–brown pigment granules in endothelial cells; rare foreign body giant cells 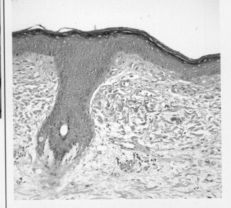 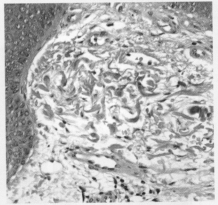 • "Bananas-in-the-dermis" (above) 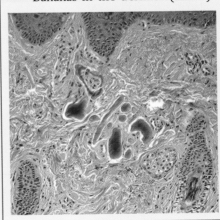

Name	Predilection and Clinical Key Features	Histopathology

Tattoos	• Mechanical introduction of insoluble pigments into the dermis
	• *Note:*
	  • Titanium dioxide ink responds poorly to laser therapy
	  • Cadmium sulfide (yellow pigment) may cause photoallergic or phototoxic reaction
		
		• Pigment localized around vessels in upper/mid-dermis in macrophages and fibroblasts

Hemochromatosis [Perls' stain]	• Most common autosomal recessive disorder • "Bronze diabetes" • Adult onset • Generalized skin bronzing (especially on face) or hypopigmentation; diabetes; cirrhosis; fatigue; impotence • Risk of hepatocellular carcinoma • Possibly associated with PCT • Mutation = *HFE* gene (disrupts transferrin receptor function) • Too much iron builds up in parenchymal organs causing damage (liver, heart, pancreas, skin)	• Thinning of epidermis; increased melanin in basal layer; increased yellow–brown granules of hemosiderin in dermis, especially around vessels and sweat glands basement membrane

Name	Predilection and Clinical Key Features	Histopathology
Hemosiderin from other sources	• Hemosiderin may be noted in the skin after the following: • Application of Monsel's solution; venous stasis of lower legs; pigmented purpuric dermatoses; Zoon's balanitis; granuloma faciale	
"Bronze baby" syndrome	• Dark grayish–brown discoloration of the skin caused by unusual complication of phototherapy treatment of hyperbilirubinemia of the newborn	
Argyria	• "Silver deposition" • Ingestion of silver-containing compounds or application to mucous membranes • Permanent blue–gray pigmentation in sun-exposed areas; blue lunulae on nails 	• Multiple, minute, brown–black granules deposit in band-like fashion to basement membrane of sweat glands (especially eccrine glands); granules not in dermal macrophages • Dark-field examination = "stars in heaven" pattern
Gold deposition (chrysiasis)	• Gold salt deposits in dermis following gold injections for RA and pemphigus • Permanent blue–gray pigmentation of skin in sun-exposed areas	• Small, round/oval, black granules in dermal macrophages; localized around vessels in upper/mid dermis • Dark-field examination = visualize gold • Polarized light = orange–red birefringence

Mercury	• Slate-gray pigmentation related to topical application of mercury salts
	• Possibly results in "pink disease" or acrodynia (painful extremities):
	  • rarely seen now, but noted in early childhood due to chronic mercury ingestion in teething powders
	  • dusky pink color of acral areas with extreme pain	

Arsenic	• Ingestion of arsenic results in diffuse, macular, bronze pigmentation • Pronounced on trunk with "raindrop" areas of normal or depigmented skin	
Lead	• May result in blue line at gingival margin due to subepithelial deposits of lead sulfide granules	

Aluminum	• Rare complication of:
	  • aluminum-absorbed vaccines (nodular lesion), or
	  • tattoo due to aluminum salts or topical aluminum chloride in cauterization of biopsy sites
		• Nodule variant = heavy lymphoid infiltrate; confirm aluminum by X-ray
		• Aluminum tattoos/cautery = macrophages with stippled cytoplasm

Bismuth	• Generalized pigmentation resembling argyria following systemic use of bismuth	
Titanium	• Exposure to titanium dioxide	

Name	Predilection and Clinical Key Features	Histopathology
Drug deposits and pigmentation		

Antimalarial drugs	• Various pigmentations possible:
	  • Ochronosis-like deposits (see p. 291)
	  • Pretibial pigment with slate-gray to blue–black	

Phenothiazines	• Progressive gray–blue pigment in sun-exposed areas • Stain with Fontana–Masson (melanin) but not Perls' (hemosiderin)	
Tetracycline	• Bluish pigmentation of cutaneous osteomas and bluish-green pigmentation in areas of trauma following tetracycline use	
Methacycline	Antibiotic which may produce gray–black pigmentation in light-exposed areas and conjunctival pigmentation	
Minocycline	Three different patterns possible: 1. Blue–black pigment in scars, related to hemosiderin or an iron chelate of minocycline 2. Blue–gray pigment of lower legs and arms (hemosiderin and melanin) 3. Generalized "muddy brown" pigmentation due to increased melanin in basal layer 	• Pigment in macrophages, dermal dendrocytes, and eccrine myoepithelial cells (localized patterns) • Extremity pigmentation stains with Perls' (hemosiderin) and Fontana–Masson (melanin), not PAS • Scar pigmentation stains with Perls' only and not Fontana
Amiodarone [Fontana–Masson, Sudan black and PAS, acid-fast]	• Dermal lipofuscin causes blue–gray pigment in light-exposed skin with long-term use 	• Yellow–brown granules of lipofuscin found in macrophages (around vessels at papillary and reticular junction)
Clofazimine	• Used in treatment of leprosy, DLE • Cutaneous and conjunctival pigmentation with reddish–blue hue	

Chemotherapeutic agents	• Pigmentation of skin may occur following bleomycin, fluorouracil, busulfan, doxorubicin, etc.
	  • Bleomycin (cytotoxic antibiotic used in Hodgkin's disease and testicular cancer) may cause "flagellate pigmentation" (linear hyperpigmented streaks often on chest and back)
	  • Similar pigmentation ("flagellate mushroom dermatitis") may be seen with ingestion of raw shiitake mushrooms	

Name	Predilection and Clinical Key Features	Histopathology
Cutaneous implants		
Silicone implants	• Often for cosmetic reasons • Breasts, penis, calves • Painful, indurated areas	• Various reactions dependent mainly on silicone form (liquid, gel, or solid) • Liquid silicone = vacuoles of varying size surrounded by macrophages and foreign body giant cells (silicone removed in processing)
Collagen implants	• Bovine collagen (Zyderm) used to correct acne scars, aging	• Mild lymphocytic and histiocytic infiltrate around vessels in vicinity; not birefringent under polarized light (unlike native collagen)

Name	Predilection and Clinical Key Features	Histopathology
Miscellaneous deposits		
Oxalate crystals	• Usually in primary oxalosis (inherited liver disorder with overproduction of oxalate) > secondary oxalosis (i.e. chronic renal failure on dialysis) • Occurs when kidneys stop excreting calcium oxalate (i.e. kidney stones)	• Light yellow to brown, rhomboid-shaped crystals that are birefringent
Fiberglass	• Rare today; may be seen in stratum corneum and dermis after contact with fiberglass	
Myospherulosis	• Incidental finding • Nose • Iatrogenic reactive process due to the interaction of RBCs with petrolatum, lanolin, or traumatized human adipose tissue	• "Sac-like structures with endobodies" • Type of lipogranuloma formation • Spherules derived from erythrocytes altered by foreign lipids and human fat
Miscellaneous cutaneous implants	• Suture • Suture material under polarized light 	• Gelfoam • Splinter

Diseases of Cutaneous Appendages

15

Endothrix infection

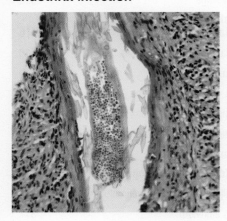

Hair basics

Hair follicle formation:

- Nine weeks's gestation, follicles seen
- By 18th week, hair on entire body (except palms/soles/genitalia)
- Growth rate = 1 mm every 3 days (or 0.35–0.37 mm/day), or 1 cm per month
- Lose an average of 50–100 hairs per day

Pigment predominantly in cortex layer:

- Eumelanin = brown/black hair
- Pheomelanin = red/blonde hair: red hair often has variant to MC1R gene (melanocortin receptor)

Three stages of hair cycle (discussed further under "Alopecia" on p. 315):

1. Anagen (growth phase; years; 85% of hair follicles)
2. Catagen (degenerative/transition from growth-to-resting phase, weeks)
3. Telogen (resting, months)
   - Sonic Hedgehog (Shh), a signaling molecule, appears to mediate the transition from telogen to anagen

Three zones of hair follicle (superficial-to-deep):

1. Infundibulum = ostium to sebaceous duct opening
2. Isthmus = sebaceous duct to insertion of arrector pili muscle
3. Inferior segment = below insertion of muscle:
   - contains bulb (or matrix) and stem
   - Adamson's fringe = level where hair cornification starts; below area, the hair bulb is mitotically active

Hair layers (in order of "inner-to-outer"):

- Medulla (central part of hair fiber) = contains citrulline:
  - vellus hairs have no medulla
- Hair cuticle = outer layer of hair shaft
- Inner root sheath (IRS) = function is to mold hair by hardening filaments and decomposes around sebaceous gland duct level; contains trichohyalin granules:
  - three components of IRS = cuticle of IRS (innermost), Huxley's layer, and Henle's layer (outermost, keratinizes first)
- Outer root sheath (ORS) = characterized by trichilemmal keratinization; forms outer cylinder of hair follicle (merges into epidermis and hair bulb at each end):
  - bulge = segment of ORS near arrector pili insertion; major area of epithelial stem cells of the hair follicle; cells below bulge degenerate in catagen and telogen stages

Name	Predilection and Clinical Key Features	Histopathology
INFLAMMATORY DISEASES OF THE PILOSEBACEOUS APPARATUS **Acneiform lesions**		
Acne vulgaris	• Inflammatory disease of sebaceous follicles and presence of comedones (dilated/plugged hair follicle) • Teenagers • Face and upper trunk • Closed comedones ("whiteheads"); open comedones ("blackheads"); red papules; pustules, cysts, scars • Multifactorial, but four pathogenetic events occur: 　1. Abnormal follicular keratinization with keratinous material retention in follicle 　2. Increased sebum production 　3. Gram+ anaerobic diphtheroid *Propionibacterium acnes* (bacteria not essential for comedone formation) 　4. Inflammation: due to activation of Toll-like receptor 2 (TLR2) • *Note:* may develop "Morbihan's disease": 　• solid, persistent, non-pitting facial edema without inflammation or pustules 　• also called "rosacea lymphedema"	• Comedones (pictured below) • Follicular plugging; often ruptured pilosebaceous apparatus with perifollicular mixed infiltrate; possible intraepidermal pustule over follicle or abscess/sinus tract formation • Gram stain (above right)

Name	Predilection and Clinical Key Features	Histopathology
Neonatal cephalic pustulosis	<ul><li>"Neonatal acne"</li><li>Onset at 2–3 weeks of age (3% neonates)</li><li>Cheeks</li><li>Resolves over weeks to months</li><li>Possibly associated with yeast *Malassezia sympodialis*</li><li>Papulopustules (no comedones)</li></ul>	<ul><li>Histopathology demonstrates a superficial pustule</li><li>Giemsa stain of pustule may show yeast forms, since often associated with *Malassezia* spp</li></ul>
Acne fulminans	<ul><li>Rare, acute form of acne</li><li>Young adult males</li><li>Sudden, painful, ulcerated, and crusted lesions with fever, muscle pain, leukocytosis, lytic bone lesions (especially sternoclavicular bone and chest wall area)</li><li>Associated with Crohn's disease, erythema nodosum, testosterone use, SAPHO syndrome (synovitis, acne, pustulosis, hyperostosis, and osteitis)</li></ul>	<ul><li>Extensive inflammatory lesions in dermis with necrosis of follicles and overlying epidermis; follicles distended with neutrophils (comedones uncommon); severe dermal scarring usually follows</li></ul>
Chloracne	<ul><li>Due to systemic poisoning by halogenated aromatic compounds (chlorinated or brominated), such as dioxin and agent orange</li><li>Malar crescents, retroauricular, scrotum, penis</li></ul> <ul><li>Mostly comedones with small cysts intermingled</li></ul>	<ul><li>Follicular hyperkeratosis with infundibular dilation forming bottle-shaped and columnar funnels containing keratin debris; comedones and keratinous cysts; small inflammatory component</li></ul>

Name	Predilection and Clinical Key Features	Histopathology
Superficial folliculitides		
Acute superficial folliculitis	• "Impetigo of Bockhart" • Small pustules around follicular ostia and often piercing hair • Possible cause = *Staph. aureus*	• Subcorneal pustule overlying follicular infundibulum; mixed infiltrate (neutrophils, lymphocytes, macrophages)
Actinic folliculitis	• Pustular folliculitis of face and upper trunk after exposure to sunlight; resembles superficial folliculitis	
Acne necrotica	• Adults • Forehead, frontal hairline • Crops of erythematous, follicle-based papules that become necrotic, umbilicated, crusted and heal with varioliform scar	• *Early lesions:* intense perivascular and perifollicular lymphocytic infiltrate to mid dermis; edema; spongiosis • *Older lesions:* necrosis of upper follicle, epidermis, dermis with neutrophils
Acne necrotica miliaris	• Pruritic, non-scarring variant of acne necrotica • Possible neurotic excoriations with a bacterial folliculitis	• Follicular vesiculopustules on scalp with superficially inflamed excoriations centered on the follicle
Necrotizing folliculitis of AIDS	• Rare cutaneous manifestation of AIDS	• Necrosis confined to upper part of follicle and adjacent epidermis/dermis, usually in wedge-shaped area; fibrinoid vessel necrosis at wedge apex

Name	Predilection and Clinical Key Features	Histopathology

Eosinophilic folliculitis	• Form of folliculitis with papulopustules with numerous eosinophils in or around follicles with lymphocytes
	
	Clinical subsets:
	• Classic form (Ofuji's disease):
	  • adult males
	  • chronic, recurrent, sterile, follicular papules/pustules; often form circinate plaques with central clearing and hyperpigmentation; involve "seborrheic areas" (face) and non-hair-bearing palms/soles (20%)
	
	• HIV associated (most common):
	  • severe pruritus with papules, but do not form circinate lesions, palmoplantar lesions, or involve face
	• Pediatric:
	  • usually confined to scalp on children; variant called "eosinophilic pustular folliculitis of infancy"
	  • birth to first few days; recurrent crops of pruritic pustules on scalp and face
	  • best prognosis
	• Fungal:
	  • localized with erosive and pustular plaques
	• Miscellaneous group:
	  • *Pseudomonas* bacteria or patient with myeloproliferative/hematologic disorders
		• Eosinophilic spongiosis and pustulosis involving especially the infundibular region of follicle; infiltrate extends to attached sebaceous duct/gland; numerous eosinophils; perivascular and perifollicular infiltrate of mainly lymphocytes

Name	Predilection and Clinical Key Features	Histopathology
Infundibulo-folliculitis	• Black patients (almost exclusively) • Trunk and proximal extremities • Follicular, pruritic papular eruption	• Follicular spongiosis; few neutrophils; mononuclear infiltrate usually surrounds upper dermal portion of hair follicle; keratin plug
Deep infectious folliculitides		
Furuncle	• "Boil" • Deep-seated infection centered on pilosebaceous unit ("abscess involving follicle") • Sites of friction (back of neck, buttocks, inner thighs) • Painful, follicular papules with surrounding erythema and induration with the center becoming yellow and discharging pus • Usually *Staph. Aureus*	• Deep dermal abscess centered on hair follicle; hair follicle usually destroyed but may see residual hair shaft in abscess center; inflammation of subcutis; overlying epidermis destroyed and surface covered by crust
Pseudomonas folliculitis	• Develop 8–48 hours after exposure to organism (*Pseudomonas aeruginosa*), found in sponges, whirlpools and hot tubs • Trunk, axillae, proximal extremities • Erythematous follicular eruption • Self-limited condition (no treatment usually required)	• Acute suppurative folliculitis (both superficial and deep)
Gram-negative folliculitis	• Gram–negative bacterial folliculitis after prolonged antibiotic therapy for acne vulgaris • Usually due to *Klebsiella*, *Enterobacter* or *Proteus* • Possible Tx = oral isotretinoin (possibly antibiotics also)	• Superficial and deep folliculitis; variable perifollicular dermis involvement

Name	Predilection and Clinical Key Features	Histopathology
Viral folliculitis	• Folliculitis usually due to HSV I infection (especially resolving outbreak); vesicles may not be obvious • Follicular pustules/papules	• Partial or complete follicle necrosis with exocytosis of lymphoctyes; epidermis may show typical herpetic infection features (inclusion bodies, multinucleate cells) or a "bottom-heavy" perivascular/interstitial infiltrate
Dermatophyte folliculitis [PAS stain]	• Folliculitis due to fungal organisms (*Trichophyton tonsurans*, *Microsporum canis* and *M. audouinii*) • Possibly forms a kerion (inflamed boggy mass); see p. 442	• Variable inflammation of follicle and perifollicular dermis; hyphae and arthrospores within hair shaft • If kerion, abscess formation with partial or complete destruction of hair follicle occurs
Pityrosporum folliculitis [PAS stain]	• Folliculitis due to *Malassezia* spp (*Pityrosporum*) • Follicular pustules	• Dilated infundibulum with abscess formation; small, oval yeasts seen on PAS within inflamed follicle and adjacent dermis if ruptured PAS stains (above)

Name	Predilection and Clinical Key Features	Histopathology
Deep scarring folliculitides		
Folliculitis decalvans	• Chronic form of deep folliculitis with scarring • Scalp • Oval patches of scarring alopecia at margins which have follicular pustules • Folliculitis barbae (lupoid sycosis) is a related condition confined to the beard area	• Initially folliculitis, followed by disruption of follicle wall and release of contents into dermis; mixed inflammatory infiltrate, including plasma cells
Folliculitis keloidalis nuchae (acne keloidalis)	• Idiopathic inflammatory condition • Adult males, common in black patients • Nape of neck • Follicular papules/pustules that form confluent, thick plaques; scarring results	• Rupture and destruction of follicle and release of hair shaft into dermis ("naked hair shaft"); chronic inflammatory infiltrate, including plasma cells; hair shafts with surrounding microabscesses; fibrosis of dermis; loss of sebaceous glands and follicle "Naked hair shafts"

Name	Predilection and Clinical Key Features	Histopathology
Follicular occlusion triad = Hidradenitis suppurativa, dissecting cellulitis of the scalp and acne conglobata (Pilonidal cyst often added to triad)		
Hidradenitis suppurativa	• "Acne inversa" or "apocrine acne" • Chronic, relapsing, inflammatory follicular disorder and involves apocrine gland-bearing areas • Multifactorial (genetics, hormones, endocrine, cigarettes) • Females • Axillae, groin, perineum • Recurrent, deep-seated inflammatory nodules, complicated by draining sinuses, scarring and pain • May develop SCC later • Associated with lithium, Dowling-Degos, Crohn's disease • Hurley's staging criteria: I. Abscess without sinus tracts/scarring II. Recurrent abscesses with sinus tracts and scars III. Diffuse abscesses and tracts throughout an area	• Heavy, mixed inflammatory infiltrate in lower half; abscesses; sinuses lined by stratified squamous epithelium and may lead to surface; granulation tissue

Name	Predilection and Clinical Key Features	Histopathology
Dissecting cellulitis of the scalp	• "Perifolliculitis capitis abscedens et suffodiens" or "Hoffman's disease" • Severe form of scalp folliculitis • Vertex and occipital scalp • Tender, suppurative nodules with interconnecting draining sinuses and subsequent scarring; patchy alopecia • May develop SCC later	• Similar to folliculitis decalvans + sinus tracts (does not have epithelial lining) • Folliculitis and perifolliculitis with a heavy infiltrate of neutrophils leading to abscess formation in the dermis; draining sinuses; destruction of hair follicle
Acne conglobata	• Males (after puberty); may occur after pregnancy • Hair-bearing areas, especially trunk, buttocks, and proximal extremities • Tender, inflamed nodules/cysts/sinuses that heal leaving disfiguring scars • Does not have systemic manifestations as in acne fulminans • Possible Tx = isotretinoin + prednisone	• Similar to hidradenitis suppurativa; comedones present

Name	Predilection and Clinical Key Features	Histopathology
Miscellaneous folliculitides		
Pseudofolliculitis barbae (PFB)	• Inflammatory response to an ingrown hair • Adult black males (face); females (legs) • Beard area of face, neck, and legs • Male pattern (photo above) • Female pattern (photo above) • Papules and pustules close to hair follicles; scarring and keloids may result • Dermoscopy image (photo above) showing hair shaft piercing skin	• Parafollicular inflammatory foci; small foreign body granulomas; mixed infiltrate
Pruritic folliculitis of pregnancy	• Later half of pregnancy • Pruritic, erythematous papules • Clear spontaneously at delivery or post-partum • No adverse effects on fetus	• Acute folliculitis with possible destruction of follicular wall and forms abscess • In later lesions, possible perifollicular granulomas

Name	Predilection and Clinical Key Features	Histopathology
Perforating folliculitis	• Type of perforating disorder • Buttocks, extensor extremities • Discrete, keratotic, scaly follicular papules on buttocks, thighs • Associated with psoriasis, juvenile acanthosis nigricans, HIV, renal failure, etc.	• Dilated follicular infundibulum filled with keratinous and cellular debris; curled hair shaft possible; degenerative changes of adjacent dermis involving connective tissue, collagen, and elastic fibers
Follicular toxic pustuloderma	• Acute pustular eruption with follicular localization, but not always follicular based • Associated with drugs (antibiotics) and enterovirus	
Sterile neutrophilic folliculitis with perifollicular vasculopathy	• Cutaneous reaction pattern accompanying systemic disease (i.e. IBD, Reiter's, Behçet's, hepatitis B, etc.) • May present as folliculitis, vasculitis, vesiculopustular, or acneiform lesions; often arthritis, fever, malaise	• Neutrophilic or suppurative/granulomatous folliculitis with follicular central neutrophilic vascular reaction (Sweet's-like)
Pseudolympho-matous folliculitis	• Subset of cutaneous lymphoid hyperplasia • Solitary lesion on face (1 cm)	• Dense dermal lymphocytic infiltrate simulating cutaneous lymphoma; atypical lymphocytes; enlarged walls of hair follicles

Name	Predilection and Clinical Key Features	Histopathology
HAIR SHAFT ABNORMALITIES **Fractures of the hair shaft**		

Trichorrhexis nodosa
(Most common structural hair abnormality)
	• Acquired or congenital
	• Caused by trauma (mechanical or chemical)
	• Weakness in hair may make susceptible and may be due to:
	• Pilar dystrophy (pili torti, monilethrix, Menkes), or
	• Inborn errors of metabolism, such as:
	  • arginosuccinic aciduria = ASL gene mutation causes deficiency of arginosuccinate lyase ammonia accumulates in blood/urine), hair will fluoresce red color. Present few days after birth as ammonia increases
	  • trichothiodystrophy (see below)
		• "Broom-like" hair cuticle (two brooms pushed together) appearing as small, beaded swellings along hair shaft (fracture easily)

Trichoschisis	• Seen in trichothiodystrophy due to brittle hair (see below)	• Clean transverse fracture of hair shaft • Under polarized light have "tiger-tail" appearance
Trichothio-dystrophy	• Group of autosomal recessive disorders (IBIDS/Tay's, BIDS, PIBIDS) with short brittle hair with low sulfur and cysteine content; also impaired nucleotide excision repair • No increased risk of skin cancer • May also see trichorrhexis nodosa and trichoschisis • PIBIDS = photosensitivity, ichthyosis, brittle hair, intellectual impairment, decreased fertility, short stature	• Ribbon-like appearance • If polarized, a "tiger-tail" appearance • Low sulfur amino acids (i.e. cysteine and methionine) seen in hair/nails
Trichoclasis	May follow trauma or associated with hair abnormalities (i.e. pili torti, monilethrix, etc.)	• Oblique fracture of the hair shaft with irregular borders and a cuticle partly intact (resembles a "greenstick fracture")
Trichorrhexis invaginata	• Present in infancy (short, sparse hair) • Eyebrows • Associated with Netherton's disease (SPINK5 gene encoding LEKT1, serine protease inhibitor, and migratory double-edge scale called ichthyosis linearis circumflexa); or possibly due to trauma, hair shaft abnormalities	• "Bamboo" hair (develops small nodules along shaft); appears as cup-like expansion of proximal part of hair shaft surrounding club-shaped distal segment (like a "ball and socket") • Abnormal keratinization results in soft hair cortex and invagination
Tapered fractures	• Progressive narrowing of emerging hair shaft due to inhibition of protein synthesis in the hair root • "Pencil-pointing" hair, associated with anagen effluvium caused by cytotoxic drugs	
Trichoptilosis	• "Split-ends" • Persistent trauma • Results from separation of longitudinal cortical fibers following the loss of the cuticle from wear and tear	• Longitudinal distal fracture ("split-ends")
Trichoteiromania	• Self-inflicted damage to hair resulting from rubbing of hair • Discrete patches of alopecia with split or broken hairs	
Trichotemnomania	• Factitious disorder with hair loss resulting from an obsessive-compulsive habit of cutting the hair with scissors or razor • Alopecia, but all infundibula have hair shafts	

Name	Predilection and Clinical Key Features	Histopathology
Irregularities/abnormalities of hair shafts		
Pili canaliculi et trianguli	• Uncombable hair syndrome (or "spun-glass" hair syndrome) • Hair appears dryer, glossier, and lighter and does not lie flat; to see clinically, at least 50% of hairs affected	• Longitudinal groove in hair seen as a homogeneous band on one edge under polarized light; hair appears normal under light microscopy • Possibly due to abnormal keratinization of internal root sheath causing irregular shaped hair shaft
Pili bifurcati	• Intermittent bifurcations of the shaft that subsequently rejoin further along the shaft to form a normal structure	• Bifurcation of single hair at multiple, irregular intervals along the shaft (i.e. single hair splits then rejoins) • Each ramus has its own cuticle
Pili multigemini	• "Multi-hairs" from one canal • Beard area, face • Associated with cleidocranial dysostosis (hereditary condition resulting in skull and clavicle bone abnormalities)	• Multiple hair shafts within a single follicular canal (each fiber has its own inner root sheath, but a common outer root sheath)
Trichostasis spinulosa	• Retention of vellus hairs that protrude from a single dilated ostium 	• Multiple hairs enveloped in a keratinous sheath within a dilated hair follicle
Pili annulati	• Autosomal dominant disorder • Associated with alopecia areata • Sparkly hair due to alternating light and dark bands along hair shaft, no increase in fragility	• "Tiger-tail hair" = alternating light and dark bands along hair shaft when viewed by reflected light (due to "air-bubbles" in the hair shaft); bands about every 0.5 mm • *Note:* trichothiodystrophy also has "tiger-tail" hair but under polarized light

Name	Predilection and Clinical Key Features	Histopathology
Monilethrix	• Inherited autosomal dominant • Means "necklace hair" • Present after birth to the first few months of life • Occipital region and spreads (short, fragile, broken hair) • Patchy alopecia and associated with keratosis pilaris • Mutation = KRT hHB1 and hHB6 (part of KRT86/KRT81 gene family) human hair basic keratins	• "Beaded" hair = elliptical nodes along shaft causing beaded appearance; fractures easily due to narrow portions; elliptical nodes every 0.7–1 mm; tapered nodes lack a medulla
Tapered hairs	• Hairs progressively taper to "pencil pointing" appearance similar to tapered fractures; associated with any process suddenly inhibiting cellular division in matrix (i.e. cytotoxic agents), or following a surgical operation/trauma (Pohl–Pinkus mark)	
Bubble hair	• Results from heat-induced gas accumulation in hair shaft (i.e. excessive hair dryer heat on wet hair) • Presents as localized area of brittle, easily broken hairs on scalp	• Large cavity forms in the shaft, especially medullary region with a "bubble" appearance on light microscopy
Trichomegaly	• Enlargement and hypertrichosis of the eyelashes • May be associated with congenital or acquired form, such as interferon-α 2, ciclosporin, latanoprost, and epidermal growth factor receptor (EGFR)	
Coiling and twisting abnormalities		

Pili torti	• Hair shaft flattened and twisted with >180° twist
	• Associated with :
	  • Menkes' kinky hair syndrome (MKN or ATP7A gene defect = copper-binding enzyme resulting in defective copper transport and metabolism); often die in infancy
	  • Bazex's syndrome (follicular atrophoderma, multiple BCC, hypotrichosis, pili torti)
	  • Bjornstad syndrome (hearing loss + pili torti): mutation = BCS1L gene
	  • Crandall syndrome (Bjornstad + hypogonadism, due to deficiency in luteinizing and growth hormones)
	• *Note:* Test child with pili torti for hearing loss due to associated syndromes
		• Structural defect causing hair shaft to coil and twist on its axis with flattening of the hair at sites of twisting (seen on light microscopy)

Woolly hair	• Curly, kinky hair occuring in Caucasian patients (normal in black patients) • Various clinical settings: autosomal dominant (affects entire scalp); autosomal recessive (familial type); and diffuse partial variant with curly and normal hair mixed (wooly hair nevus variant, 50% also with linear epidermal nevi) • Associated with Naxos disease (plakoglobin defect) and Carvajal syndrome (desmoplakin defect); both have PPK + Woolly hair + cardiomyopathy (Naxos has right sided and Carvajal has left sided)	• Prominent curly or coiled hair involving the scalp in focal or diffuse manner • Hair varies from normal appearance to more oval on cross-section to triangular

Name	Predilection and Clinical Key Features	Histopathology
Acquired progressive kinking	• "Pubic scalp hair" • Occurs in young males, who then develop male pattern alopecia with fairly rapid onset • Onset at puberty or after puberty • Affects regions of scalp (not entire scalp) • Hair resembles pubic hair in texture and color	• Hairs show some flattening of hair shaft with partial twisting at irregular intervals
Circle hair, rolled hair and trichonodosis	• Circle hair = shaft coiled into circle under a thin transparent roof of stratum corneum (appears as black circle); forms on abdomen, thigh, back of middle-aged men • Rolled hair = hairs are irregularly coiled but do not form a perfect circle; often associated with keratosis pilaris • Trichonodosis = "knotted hair"; often incidental finding in scalp hair, especially curly African hair; may lead to fracturing and breaking when combed	
Extraneous matter on hair shafts		
Tinea capitis	• Usually *T. tonsurans*, *T. violaceum* 	• Hairs fragile and break near skin surface Endothrix
Black piedra	• Ascomycete which forms minute concretions on hair • Tropics • Usually due to *Piedraia hortae* • Gritty black nodules on hair (firmer, darker, and more adherent than white piedra)	• Brown hyphae with ovoid ascii
White piedra	• Yeast-like fungus which forms minute concretions on hair • Face, scalp, scrotum • South America • Usually due to *Trichosporon ovoides* (old name: *T. beigelii*) • Numerous cream-colored nodules that form sleeve-like concretions (slide, and not as adherent as black piedra)	• KOH shows fungal arthrospores in mass encasing hair shaft

Name	Predilection and Clinical Key Features	Histopathology
Trichomycosis axillaris	• Most commonly caused by *Corynebacterium tenuis:* Gram positive diphtheroid bacterium • Tiny, cream–yellow nodules attached to axillary or pubic hair • Treatment = shave hair or topical antibiotic	
Pediculosis capitis	• Small white–brown ovoid nits attached to the hair shaft • Nits are the eggs of the lice 	• Eggs lie to one side of hair shaft and do not slide (hair casts can slide); attached to hair by a sheath that envelops shaft and egg base

Hair casts	• Two types:
	  1. Parakeratotic hair casts:
	    • most common variant
	    • associated with inflammatory diseases (such as psoriasis, seborrheic dermatitis)
	    • due to outer root sheath pulled out of follicle
	  2. Peripilar keratin cast = normal finding in young girls
	• Firm, yellow–white concretions (3–7 mm) ensheathing and able to move along hair ("pseudo-nits" and able to slide)
		• Follicular opening with parakeratotic keratinous material which breaks off to form hair casts

Deposits	• Substances may become adherent to hair, such as paint, hair spray, lacquer, and glue	

Name	Predilection and Clinical Key Features	Histopathology
ALOPECIAS **Basic hair stages**		
Anagen stage	• 85–90% of hair • Stage lasts years (actual time varies by location on body)	 • "Ribbon-shaped" and fully pigmented
Catagen stage	• 1% of hair • Stage lasts 2–3 weeks	 • Scattered apoptotic cells develop in outer root sheath; inner root sheath disappears

Name	Predilection and Clinical Key Features	Histopathology
Telogen stage	• 10–15% of hair • Stage Lasts 3–4 months	 • "Club-shaped" and depigmented end
Congenital and hereditary alopecias		
Alopecia universalis congenita	• Congenital alopecia group without associated defects • May be autosomal recessive (human hairless gene mutation) or autosomal dominant • Follicles hypoplastic and reduced in number • Does not form papules as in atrichia (below)	
Hereditary hypotrichosis	• "Marie–Unna type" • Autosomal dominant • Present at birth • Short, sparse hair; childhood hair growth coarse and wiry; progressive loss of hair at adolescence	• No specific features; mild to moderate perifollicular reaction; reduced follicles; milia and fibrosis may form
Atrichia with papular lesions	• Autosomal recessive • Mutation = HR gene (human hairless gene) • Begins in first few months of life • Progressive shedding of scalp/body hair (spares eyelashes); milia-like cysts on face, neck, scalp in childhood/early adult • Forms papules (differs from alopecia congenitalis)	• Small follicular cysts with keratinous material with no vellus hairs in lumen; lack of development of germinal end of follicle with no shaft formation
Keratosis pilaris atrophicans	• Group of clinically related syndromes with inflammatory keratosis pilaris that lead to atrophic scarring (see p. 322)	
Hallermann–Streiff syndrome	• "Mandibulo-oculofacial dyscephaly" • Branchial arch syndrome with characteristic facies, ocular abnormalities, and alopecia	• Atrophic areas composed of loosely woven collagen

Name	Predilection and Clinical Key Features	Histopathology
Short anagen syndrome	• "Hair that never needs cutting" • Short, fine scalp hair with normal body hair and eyelashes • Possibly due to persistent synchronized scalp hair growth with associated short anagen duration	• Unremarkable biopsy
Premature catagen/telogen		
Trichotillomania and traumatic alopecia (traction)	• "Trichotillosis" • Deliberate avulsion of hair • Primarily affects crown and occipital scalp • In adults, women are more common; in children, no predilection	• Presence of empty hair ducts and increased catagen hairs (associated with anagen hairs); deformed hair shafts; sparse infiltrate; pigmented casts in follicles; perifollicular hemorrhage or fibrosis

Telogen effluvium	• Diffuse hair loss often 2–3 months after a stressful event (e.g. childbirth, surgery, fever)
	• Hair typically grows back
	
	• Various possible subtypes:
	  • Immediate anagen release (post-fever)
	  • Delayed anagen release (post-partum alopecia)
	  • Short anagen (child with hair that "does not grow long")
	  • Delayed telogen release (seasonal hair loss)
	  • Immediate telogen release (topical minoxidil)
	  • Chronic telogen effluvium (hair shedding in middle-aged women)
		• Increased telogen vs. vellus-like ratio; no inflammation

Name	Predilection and Clinical Key Features	Histopathology
Premature telogen with anagen arrest		
Alopecia areata	<ul><li>Immunologic-based hair loss</li><li>Possible family history (10–25%)</li><li>Age 15–40; Down syndrome patients</li></ul> 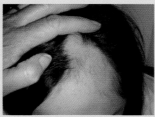 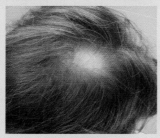 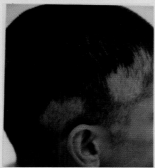 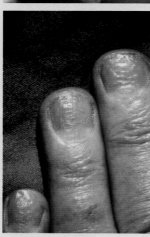 <ul><li>Sudden onset of discrete, asymptomatic patches of non-scarring hair loss; "exclamation mark" hairs (tapered at base) near advancing margin; nail pitting, trachyonychia longitudinal ridging ("sandpaper-like" roughness in lines)</li><li>Variants:<ul><li>Alopecia totalis = complete scalp alopecia</li><li>Alopecia universalis = entire body hair loss</li><li>Ophiasis = involves band from temple to occiput</li><li>Diffuse alopecia areata = general thinning of scalp</li></ul></li></ul>	<ul><li>Lymphocytes around lower follicle (bulb) like a "swarm of bees" (also may be eosinophils, plasma cells, etc.); increased miniature telogen and catagen follicles at expanding edge</li></ul> 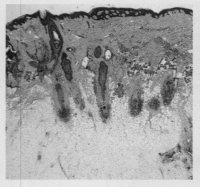 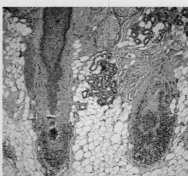 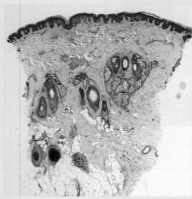 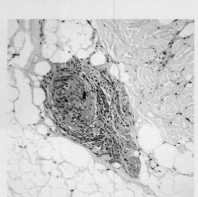 <ul><li>Fibrous tracts extending along site of previous follicles in the subcutis; inversion of anagen:telogen ratio (anagen decrease, telogen increase)</li></ul> 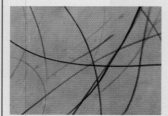 <ul><li>Dermoscopy (photo above) often demonstrates yellow dots in follicular ostium of empty and hair-bearing follicles; exclamation point hairs</li></ul>

Name	Predilection and Clinical Key Features	Histopathology
Vellus follicle formation		

Androgenic alopecia	• "Common baldness"
	• Progressive replacement of terminal hairs with smaller diameter hairs until conversion to fine, virtually unpigmented, vellus hairs
	
	• Patterns:
	  • Male (frontal, central, and temporal)
	  • Female (vertex, frontovertical, and male-like)
	• Possible Tx:
	  • Finasteride (type II 5α-reductase inhibitor), decreases DHT level
	  • Minoxidil (HTN medication originally); possibly due to secondary vasodilation at dermal papilla
		• Early stage: progressive miniaturized telogen follicles; focal basophilic degeneration of connective tissue sheath in lower third of anagen follicles
		• Late stage: miniaturized vellus follicles; increased telogen hairs; enlarged sebaceous glands; decreased anagen:telogen ratio; Arao–Perkins bodies (clusters of elastic tissue at neck of follicular papilla); bodies will follow along fibrous tract at successive higher levels (like an Arao–Perkins body "ladder")

Temporal triangular alopecia	• Triangular patch of alopecia extending to the frontotemporal hairline; usually unilateral • Associated with colonic polyposis, eye defects and phakomatosis pigmentovascularis (congenital syndrome with vascular malformations and pigmented nevi)	• Replacement of normal abundant terminal follicles with vellus follicles • Decreased telogen:vellus ratio

Name	Predilection and Clinical Key Features	Histopathology
Anagen effluvium		
Loose anagen syndrome	• Diffuse hair loss in children (short hair that seldom needs cutting) • Fine hair that pulls out easily and painlessly (classically a blonde girl)	• Early keratinization of inner root sheath preventing normal interdigitation of sheath cuticle and hair cuticle; marked cleft formation between hair shafts and regressively altered inner root sheaths • Microscopy of hair = ruffled proximal cuticle and absence of root sheath
Drug-induced alopecia	• Diffuse, non-scarring hair loss that is reversible with drug withdrawal • Such as thallium, excess vitamin A, retinoids, antimitotic drugs, antithyroid drugs, chemicals to straighten hair, etc.	
Scarring alopecias		
Idiopathic scarring alopecia	• "Pseudopelade of Brocq" • Rare, asymptomatic, idiopathic non-inflammatory form of scarring alopecia with patchy loss • Women over age 40 • "Footprints in the snow" due to islands of clumps of terminal hairs persisting in sclerosis background	• Early lesions: lymphocytes around upper two-thirds of follicle Older lesions: absent follicles and sebaceous glands; fibrosis with elastic fibers [orcein, Verhoeff van Gieson (VVG) elastic stains useful] • No interface changes; DIF negative • DDx: lichen planus and SLE have positive DIF and lack elastic fibers [VVG stain]
Traction alopecia with scarring	• Black women • Scarring alopecia on crown, but periphery of scalp spared	• Early stage: lichenoid perifolliculitis; lymphocyte infiltrate around infundibula • Later stage: sparse infiltrate; granulomatous reaction; loss of follicle, and increased fibrosis
Postmenopausal frontal fibrosing alopecia	• Black women • Progressive frontal fibrosing alopecia with perifollicular erythema	• Similar to lichen planopilaris histologically
Fibrosing alopecia in a pattern distribution	• Inflammatory scarring alopecia affecting only the balding central scalp • Possible variant of lichen planopilaris in which an immune reaction is directed against miniaturized follicles of androgenic alopecia	
Folliculitis decalvans	• See "deep scarring folliculitides" section (p. 305)	

Name	Predilection and Clinical Key Features	Histopathology
Central centrifugal cicatricial alopecia	• "Folliculitis decalvans of central scalp" or "hot-comb alopecia" • Black women • Symmetric cicatricial alopecia on crown/vertex of scalp; may form pustules • Possible cause = premature desquamation of inner root sheath	• Loss of inner root sheath early; "onion-skin" fibrosing of follicles; inflammatory infiltrate (possible granulomatous inflammation)
Tufted-hair folliculitis	• Areas of scarring alopecia with tufts of hair emerging from single follicular openings • May be seen in folliculitis decalvans and acne keloidalis	• Classic feature = several closely set, complete follicles with a common follicular opening with multiple hair shafts emerging • Also folliculitis, perifolliculitis, and scarring can be seen
Miscellaneous alopecias		
Lipedematous alopecia	• Adult black females • Acquired condition with a thick, boggy scalp with hair loss and scalp twice as thick (expanded subcutaneous fat layer)	• Thickening of the subcutis (appears to encroach dermis); no inflammation; mild hyperkeratosis, acanthosis, and keratinous follicular plugging

Name	Predilection and Clinical Key Features	Histopathology
MISCELLANEOUS DISORDERS **Pilosebaceous disorders**		

Sebaceous gland basics:

- Develops as a bud from primordial hair follicle in 13th–15th fetal week
- Distributed throughout body except palms and soles
- Largest distribution in the skin of the face and upper trunk ("seborrheic areas")
- Hormonal control (increase in size at puberty)

"Named" sebaceous glands:

- Meibomian gland = tarsal plate of upper/lower eyelids (chalazion, blepharitis):
  - produces oil for eyes, and not associated with hair follicle
  - #1 source of sebaceous carcinoma on eyelids
- Glands of Zeis = margin of eyelid with eyelashes
- Ectopic (or "free" glands, not associated with a hair follicle):
  - Fordyce's spot = lips (vermilion border)
  - Montgomery's tubercle = areola
  - Tyson's gland = penis (corona area, secretes smegma)

Name	Predilection and Clinical Key Features	Histopathology
Hypertrichosis	• Hypertrichosis = growth of hair on any part of body in excess of the amount usually present based on age, race, sex • Does not include hirsutism which is androgen-induced hair growth in women	
	• Congenital hypertrichosis lanuginosa: • rare familial disorder (often autosomal dominant) with excessive growth of lanugo hair and possible dental/eye abnormalities	
	• Acquired hypertrichosis lanuginosa: • generalized hypertrichosis (not palms/soles) • associated with underlying cancer, drugs, porphyria, etc.	
	• Congenital circumscribed hypertrichosis: • localized areas of hypertrichosis (congenital pigmented nevi, Becker's nevus, etc.)	
	• Acquired circumscribed hypertrichosis: • hypertrichosis develops at sites of persistent friction (plaster casts) and sites of inflammation (bites)	
Keratosis pilaris (KP)	• Disorder of keratinization involving the infundibulum of the hair follicle with spiny follicular papules • Common in males (5%) and females (30%) • Posterior aspect of arms, lateral thighs • Firm, spiny papules centered around follicles • Associated with atopic dermatitis, obesity, hyperandrogenism, insulin-dependent diabetes	• Follicular plug that protrudes above the surface; sparse perifollicular infiltrate

Name	Predilection and Clinical Key Features	Histopathology
Keratosis pilaris atrophicans	• Group of three related disorders with keratosis pilaris, mild perifollicular inflammation, and subsequent atrophy • HP = follicular hyperkeratosis with atrophy of the underlying follicle and sebaceous gland; comedones/milia present; perifollicular fibrosis	
	• Keratosis pilaris atrophicans faciei (ulerythema ophryogenes): • Develop shortly after birth • follicular papules with an erythematous halo involving the lateral eyebrow, later may involve forehead, cheek • pitted scars; alopecia; KP on extremities, buttocks • associated with woolly hair, Noonan's syndrome, Rubinstein–Taybi syndrome 	
	• Keratosis follicularis spinulosa decalvans: • begins in infancy • "moth-eaten" scarring of the malar area + diffuse KP + scarring alopecia of scalp/eyebrows	
	• Atrophoderma vermiculata: • late childhood • involves preauricular region and cheeks with horny follicular plug formation that is shed and followed by reticulate atrophy with comedones/milia; KP of the limbs • no alopecia as in other variants • associated with Marfan's syndrome and Rombo syndrome (atrophoderma vermiculatum of face, multiple milia, telangiectases, peripheral vasodilation with cyanosis, and risk for BCCs)	
Follicular spicules	• Horny, follicular spicules that develop on face of multiple myeloma and cryoglobulinemia patients • Spicules composed of eosinophilic, compact, homogeneous material (due to the monoclonal protein of the underlying gammopathy)	
Lichen spinulosus	• Adolescence • Extensor surface of arms and legs (symmetrically) • Follicular keratotic papules with horny spines that group into plaques; horny spines protrude 1–2 mm above the surface	• Keratotic plug in follicular infundibulum; heavy perifollicular infiltrate of lymphocytes

Name	Predilection and Clinical Key Features	Histopathology
Rosacea	<ul><li>"Acne rosacea"</li><li>Adults, typically on the face</li><li>Five clinical forms: 1. Erythematous telangiectatic type (70% of cases) 2. Papulopustular type 3. Granulomatous type 4. Hyperplastic glandular type (pymatous rosacea), results in rhinophyma 5. Ocular disease</li></ul>	<ul><li>Granulomatous rosacea (photo below)</li></ul><ol><li>Erythematous, telangiectatic type = telangiectasia; perifollicular and perivascular infiltrate of lymphocytes with plasma cells; no comedones as with acne</li><li>Papulopustular type = more inflammatory cell infiltrate (superficial and mid-dermis); superficial folliculitis; keratotic follicular plugging</li><li>Granulomatous type = non-caseating epithelioid granuloma in vicinity of damaged hair follicles; necrosis (mimicking caseation) may be present</li><li>Hyperplastic glandular type/rhinophyma = hypertrophy of sebaceous glands; scattered follicular plugging; telangiectasias</li></ol>
Pyoderma faciale	<ul><li>"Rosacea fulminans"</li><li>Fulminant variant of rosacea</li><li>Women in 20s</li><li>Face</li><li>Sudden onset of confluent nodules and papulopustules; inflammatory</li><li>Associated with inflammatory bowel disease (IBD)</li></ul>	<ul><li>Heavy dermal infiltrate of neutrophils, lymphocytes with occasional granulomas with multinucleate giant cells; perifollicular abscesses; sinus formation</li></ul>
Squamous metaplasia of sebaceous glands	<ul><li>Squamous metaplasia at sites of pressure following cardiac surgery</li><li>Ischemia likely plays a role in formation</li></ul>	
Neutrophilic sebaceous adenitis	<ul><li>Circinate plaques on the face of teenage males which show a neutrophilic infiltrate of the sebaceous glands</li></ul>	
Follicular sebaceous casts	<ul><li>Multiple spiky lesions forming in the nasolabial region following isotretinoin therapy for acne</li></ul>	

Name	Predilection and Clinical Key Features	Histopathology
Apocrine disorders		

Apocrine basics:

- Derived from primary epithelial germ along with hair follicles and sebaceous glands
- Acetylcholine (sympathetic innervation) and adrenergic stimulation control
- Found in axilla, anogenital region, areola/nipple
- "Decapitation" mode of secretion (apical cap separates from the cell into the lumen)
- Modified apocrine gland = Moll's gland (eyelid); auditory canal (ceruminous gland); breast

Name	Predilection and Clinical Key Features	Histopathology
Fox–Fordyce disease	• "Apocrine miliaria" • Women • Axilla and anogenital area • Extremely pruritic, chronic eruption of papules	• Spongiosis or vesicle in plugged follicle near the point of apocrine duct entry; mild infiltrate with lymphocytes and neutrophils; perifollicular foamy histiocytes (unique feature)
Apocrine chromhidrosis	• Production of colored sweat by the apocrine gland	• Orange–brown cytoplasmic granules in the apocrine sweat glands

Name	Predilection and Clinical Key Features	Histopathology	
Eccrine disorders			
Eccrine basics:			
• Derived from primitive epidermal ridge; most numerous on the sole of the foot; secretion is mostly water • Located on entire body, except lips, external auditory canal, clitoris and labia minora • Most numerous on sole of foot • Secretion is mostly water and aids dissipation of body heat by surface evaporation • Secretory coil composed of glycogen-containing clear cells and dark cells that are surrounded by a layer of myoepithelial cells • Glands active at birth • Secretion by exocytosis • Secretory coil stains with IKH-4, EKH-5, EKH-6 (do not stain apocrine secretory portion) • Innervation is post-ganglionic sympathetic fibers with acetylcholine (not norepinephrine); controlled by hypothalamic sweat center			
Eccrine duct hyperplasia	• Seen in variety of circumstances (keratoacanthomas, overlying intradermal nevus, etc.)		
Syringolymphoid hyperplasia	• Hyperplastic sweat ducts sleeved by a dense lymphocytic infiltrate • Associated with cutaneous T-cell lymphoma		
Eccrine metaplasia	• Various types including clear cell metaplasia (may be incidental finding), squamous syringometaplasia (squamous metaplasia of glandular and ductal epithelium; associated with ischemia, radiation, chemotherapy), mucinous syringometaplasia (verruca-like lesion of foot sole or finger)		
Neutrophilic eccrine hidradenitis	• Complication of induction chemotherapy used to treat underlying cancer (i.e. cytarabine for AML) which is excreted from eccrine glands • 1–2 weeks after starting chemotherapy • Plaques and nodules form (especially on trunk); resolve after 2–3 weeks	• Neutrophils surrounding eccrine secretory coils/glands; vacuolar degeneration and necrosis of secretory epithelium; squamous metaplasia sometimes present	
Palmoplantar eccrine hidradenitis	• "Idiopathic palmoplantar hidradenitis" • Children • Plantar surface of the feet (less often palms) • Sudden onset of tender, erythematous plantar nodules. • Resolves in 2–4 weeks without treatment	• Dense neutrophilic infiltrate localized around the eccrine unit; partial sparing of secretory segment often seen • Lacks squamous metaplasia usually, unlike neutrophilic eccrine hidradenitis	
Sweat gland necrosis	• Associated with vesiculobullous skin lesions in patients with drug-induced and carbon monoxide-induced coma • May be associated with a "coma blister"	• Necrotic secretory cells of the sweat glands; sparse infiltrate in dermis including neutrophils; blisters are predominantly subepidermal; focal necrosis of keratinocytes in and adjacent to acrosyringium 	
Vestibular gland disorders			
Vulvar vestibulitis	• Characterized by dyspareunia, point tenderness localized to vulvar vestibule	• HP = chronic inflammatory infiltrate (mostly lymphocytes); squamous metaplasia of minor vestibular gland	

Cysts, Sinuses, and Pits

16

Steatocystoma

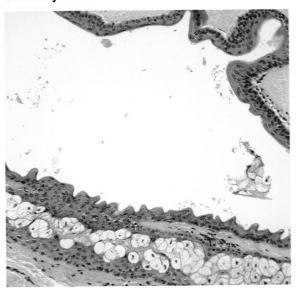

Basic cyst algorithm

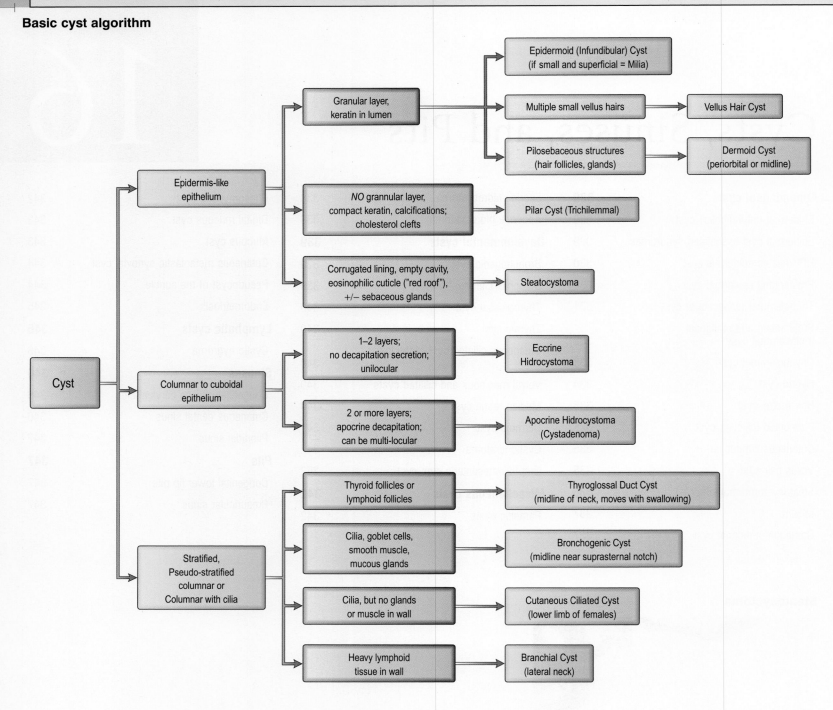

Name	Predilection and Clinical Key Features	Histopathology
Appendageal cysts		
Epidermal (infundibular) cyst	• May be derived from pilosebaceous follicle, traumatic implantation of epidermis, etc. • Young to middle age adults • Trunk, neck, and face; also scrotum and labia majora • Solitary, slowly growing, smooth, dome-shaped cyst often with a surface punctum; does not typically "shell out" easily at removal • Cells express keratin 10	• Epidermal cyst lined with stratified squamous epithelium with a granular layer showing epidermal, "cornflake" keratinization (results in formation of keratohyaline granules and flattened surface epithelium)

Epidermal cyst associated syndromes	• Multiple epidermoid cysts associated with:
	  • Gardner's syndrome:
	    • epidermal cysts (especially head and neck areas), polyposis coli, jaw osteomas, intestinal fibromatoses, and congenital hypertrophy of retinal pigment epithelium (CHEPE)
	    • mutation = APC (Adenomatous Polyposis Coli) gene; tumor suppressor gene regulating β-catenin
	  • Basal cell nevus syndrome (Gorlin syndrome):
	    • epidermal cysts, multiple basal cell carcinomas, odontogenic cysts, bifid ribs, palmoplantar pits
	    • mutation = PTCH1 gene; tumor suppressor gene encoding sonic hedgehog transmembrane receptor protein	

Name	Predilection and Clinical Key Features	Histopathology
HPV-related epidermal cyst (verrucous cyst)	• Variant of epidermal cyst associated with HPV infection • Three types: 1. HPV-60 variant: • involves plantar surface pressure points • usually solitary 2. Verrucous epidermal cyst: • does not usually involve palms/soles • causes verrucous changes in the cyst epithelial lining 3. Cystic structure mimicking molluscum bodies: • big toe • HPV-1 infection	1. HPV-60 type = intracytoplasmic inclusions and vacuolar keratinous changes; eccrine ducts sometimes in cyst wall 2. Verrucous cyst type = epidermal cyst with a papillated and/or digitated lining with prominent hypergranulosis and irregular keratohyaline granules (see photos below) 3. Cystic structure mimicking molluscum bodies
Proliferating epidermal cyst	• Risk of carcinomatous changes (20%) • Variants: 1. Tricholemmal type (p. 332): • female • scalp 2. Epidermal type: • male • widespread distribution including pelvic, anogenital, scalp, upper extremities, and trunk areas	• Multilocular cystic spaces containing keratinous material or proteinaceous fluid; subepidermal cystic tumors with a granular layer, often connecting to epidermis (narrow opening or dilated hair follicle) • Proliferating epithelium extends into adjacent stroma; may show squamous eddies

Name	Predilection and Clinical Key Features	Histopathology
Tricholemmal (sebaceous) cyst	• "Pilar cyst" or "isthmus-catagen cyst" • Female • Scalp (90%) • Nodule with no punctum, "shell out" at removal • Cells express keratin 10 and 17 • May be inherited as autosomal dominant trait	• Cyst lined by stratified squamous epithelium with no granular layer showing tricholemmal keratinization (i.e. pale cells increase in bulk and vertical diameter towards lumen); cholesterol clefts; calcifications; "scalloped-like" lining; eosinophilic-staining, compact keratin in lumen; perpendicularly oriented bundles of tonofibrils in the lining epithelial cells (feature of tricholemmal keratinization) • Pigmented variant of tricholemmal cyst (below)

Name	Predilection and Clinical Key Features	Histopathology
Proliferating and malignant tricholemmal cyst	• Possible variant of squamous cell carcinoma • Elderly females • Scalp (90%) • Large cysts (2–10 cm), usually solid or only partly cystic • Treatment is usually surgical excision	• Well-circumscribed cyst with lobular proliferation of squamous cells (often with palisading and some vitreous membrane formation) and focal cystic areas; some areas of tricholemmal keratinization (no granular layer)

Name	Predilection and Clinical Key Features	Histopathology
Onycholemmal cyst	• "Subungual epidermoid inclusions" • Dermis of nail bed • May be associated with onychodystrophy, clubbing, ridging, thickening, pigmentation, or no change in nail plate	• Free-lying cyst within the dermis of the nail bed; cyst contains onycholemmal keratin and calcification; no granular layer

Name	Predilection and Clinical Key Features	Histopathology
Hybrid cyst	• Cyst with both epidermal and tricholemmal cyst-like features, or a cyst with two different linings (epidermal, pilomatrixoma-like, tricholemmal) • Hybrid cysts with pilomatrical features associated with Gardner's syndrome 	• Often cystic structure with a sharp transition between an outer (upper) portion (i.e. epidermal) and an inner (lower) portion (i.e. tricholemmal keratinization) of the cystic lining • Hybrid cyst with pilomatrical features (pictures below)

Name	Predilection and Clinical Key Features	Histopathology
Hair matrix cyst	• Variant of epidermal cyst • Children and young adults	• Cyst wall with several layers of basaloid cells with a transition to squamous maturation near the lumen; small cystic spaces in wall
Pigmented follicular cyst	• Pigmented cyst clinically	• Cyst in the dermis with a narrow, pore-like opening to surface; epidermal-like lining (keratinization, rete ridges, and dermal papillae) and numerous luminal pigmented hair shafts
Cutaneous keratocyst	• Feature of basal cell nevus syndrome • Cysts with a thick brown fluid	• Cyst with a corrugated or festooned configuration with a lining of squamous epithelium; no granular layer; may contain vellus hairs
Vellus hair cyst	• Sporadic or autosomal dominant • Children to young adults • Chest and axillae • Multiple, small, asymptomatic papules • May spontaneously regress • Eruptive vellus hair cysts associated with steatocystoma multiplex and pachyonychia congenita, type II • Cells express keratin 17 • May coexist with trichostasis spinulosa (cluster of vellus hairs embedded in hair follicle)	• Small dermal cysts lined by stratified squamous epithelium; lumen with keratin and vellus hairs • Vellus hairs are doubly refractile with polarized light (picture above)

Name	Predilection and Clinical Key Features	Histopathology

Steatocystoma multiplex	• Sporadic > autosomal dominant
	• Young adults
	• Chest
	
	• Multiple (may be solitary) yellowish to skin-colored papules/cysts; oily discharge
	• Multiplex variant associated with Jackson–Lawler syndrome (pachyonychia congenita type 2):
	  • Autosomal dominant disorder with steatocystoma multiplex, ectodermal dysplasia, nail dystrophy, and keratoderma
	  • Keratin 17 mutation
		
		• Empty dermoid cyst (oily substance gone) with undulating stratified squamous epithelium; sebaceous glands in wall; corrugated, eosinophilic cuticle ("red roof"); may have vellus hairs
		
		• HP reminder: "stea- (stay) at the Red Roof Inn"

Name	Predilection and Clinical Key Features	Histopathology
Milium	• Milia develop congenitally, or associated with trauma, dermabrasion, topical steroids, bullous disorders, DLE, PXE, etc. • Any age • Cheek and forehead • Small (usually 1–2 mm), white papule, often multiple • Newborn milia variants: • Bohn's nodules (hard palate, buccal mucosa) = salivary gland remnants • Epstein's pearl (median palatal raphe) = trapped epithelium	• Small, superficial infundibular cyst with thinner wall (keratinizing stratified squamous epithelium); usually connected to eccrine sweat duct; may have vellus hairs or be connected to vellus hair follicle • Differs from comedones which are keratinous plugs in dilated pilosebaceous orifices
Comedo/ comedonal cyst	• Young adults • Face • Formed due to impaction of horny cells in the lumen of a sebaceous follicle • May be open ("blackhead") with a wide patulous orifice or closed ("white head") with a small orifice which is not always seen • May be familial	• Cystically dilated hair follicle containing abundant keratinous material. May have a patulous orifice or a narrow orifice (not always seen in H&E plane of section)

Name	Predilection and Clinical Key Features	Histopathology
Eccrine hidrocystoma	• Adult females • Periorbital area, face, trunk • Translucent, pale-blue, dome-shaped, cystic papules • Rarely develops to SCC	• Unilocular cyst wall with two layers of cuboidal epithelium with eosinophilic cytoplasm; often close to eccrine gland; no "decapitation" secretion
Apocrine hidrocystoma	• Middle-aged to older adults • Head and neck • Solitary, translucent or bluish hue lesion • May develop from Moll's gland of eyelid • Multiple cysts associated with Schöpf–Schulz–Passarge syndrome (autosomal recessive with PPK + eyelid apocrine hidrocystomas + hypodontia + hypotrichosis + hypoplastic nails)	• Multiloculated cyst with columnar cells with decapitation secretion (i.e. "pinch off" cytoplasm); flat basal layer of elongated myoepithelial cells

Name	Predilection and Clinical Key Features	Histopathology
Developmental cysts		
Bronchogenic cyst	• Present at or soon after birth as cyst or draining sinus • Males (4:1 ratio to females) • Midline near suprasternal notch • Appears as cyst or a draining sinus	• Respiratory, ciliated epithelial lining (pseudostratified columnar or cuboidal); keratin or mucin; sometimes surrounded by smooth muscle, mucous glands with interspersed goblet cells
Branchial cleft cyst	• Remnant of the branchial clefts • Children to young adults • Lateral neck • Cysts, sinus tracts, or skin tag appearance • Risk of SCC in long-standing lesions • Remnants of branchial cleft and typical location: • First pouch = angle of mandible • Second pouch = anterior border of sternomastoid muscle	• Stratified squamous and inner respiratory epithelial lining; heavy lymphoid tissue in wall • Differs from bronchogenic cyst by clinical location, common lymphoid follicles and stratified squamous epithelium and rarity of smooth muscle

Name	Predilection and Clinical Key Features	Histopathology
Thyroglossal cyst	• Midline of the neck • Deep lesions that move during swallowing	• Cyst with pseudostratified columnar to squamous epithelium; no adjacent smooth muscle mucous glands or cartilage • May contain thyroid follicles or lymphoid follicles
Thymic cyst	• Remnant of thymopharyngeal duct (third pouch) • Children to adolescents • Mediastinum, neck • Painless swelling in mediastinum or neck; often found posterior to thyroid's lateral lobe (left > right side)	• Various linings possible (respiratory and/or squamous lining); Hassall's corpuscles in wall; parathyroid tissue
Cutaneous ciliated cyst of the lower limbs	• Group of several variants of developmental cysts • Possible Müllerian origin • Lower limb of females (present shortly after menarche)	• Cyst with ciliated columnar or cuboidal lining; papillary projections into lumen; no glands or smooth muscle
Vulval mucinous and ciliated cysts	• Vestibule of the vulva (urogenital sinus origin)	• Pseudostratified ciliated columnar and/or mucinous epithelial lining
Median raphe cyst	• Midline developmental cyst from external urethral meatus to the anus (defective embryological closure of median raphe) • First three decades of life • Glans penis, ventral surface of penis • May be precipitated by trauma or infection	• Dermal cyst that does not connect with the surface or urethra; pseudostratified columnar to stratified squamous epithelium; possible mucous glands in wall

Name	Predilection and Clinical Key Features	Histopathology
Dermoid cyst	<ul><li>Subcutaneous cyst of sequestered ectodermal origin</li><li>Present at birth</li><li>Lateral angle of eye, forehead, neck</li></ul><ul><li>Asymptomatic, firm, non-compressible, non-pulsatile mass that does not transilluminate</li></ul>	<ul><li>Cyst with keratinizing squamous epithelium with attached pilosebaceous structures; sometimes smooth muscle in wall; lumen with hair shafts and keratinous debris</li></ul><ul><li>Hair shafts in lumen with keratinous debris</li></ul>

Name	Predilection and Clinical Key Features	Histopathology
Cystic teratoma	• Germ cell tumor made up of more than one cell type from more than one germ layer • Present at birth, often in glabella area or back • Varies from benign to malignant • Elevated AFP and HCG levels may indicate malignancy	• Various tissue types present from respiratory, thyroid, nerve, muscle, etc.
Omphalo-mesenteric duct cyst	• Periumbilical area remnant • Remnant may form subcutaneous cyst, umbilical polyp, umbilical sinus or enteric fistula • May be associated with Meckel's diverticulum	• Cyst connecting to skin with GI mucosa adjoining stratified squamous epithelium of adjacent skin; smooth muscle may be present in wall
Miscellaneous cysts		

Parasitic cysts	• Most important type is cysticercosis, the larval form of *Taenia solium*:
	  • Pork tapeworm
	  • Scolex has hooklets and two pairs of suckers
		• Cysticercosis: larva in cystic cavity; fibrosis in subcutaneous tissue; calcareous bodies (purple, oval calcified concretions)

Phaeomycotic cysts	• Subcutaneous cystic granuloma from infection by phaeohyphomycosis (pigmented hyphae) with brown walls • Often associated with foreign body (i.e. wood splinter) as source of infection	• Brown hyphae in dermis; suppurative granulomatous reaction; walled-off cystic space; foreign body (wood splinter)

Name	Predilection and Clinical Key Features	Histopathology
Digital mucous cyst	• Middle-aged to elderly females • Base of nail and dorsum of fingers • Solitary, dome-shaped, shiny, tense cystic nodule (resembles focal mucinosis) • A second type (myxoid cyst) overlies the DIP joint and resembles a ganglion cyst	• Mucinous pool with stellate fibroblasts (similar to focal mucinosis); may have cavity with myxoid connective tissue wall • Ganglionic variant comprises a cystic space with a fibrous wall; often small areas of myxoid change adjacent to wall; may be an attenuated synovial lining
Mucous cyst (mucocele) [Alcian blue (pH 2.5), colloidal iron]	• May result from rupture of a minor salivary duct • Lower lip, buccal mucosa • Translucent, white, or blue nodule with firm cystic consistency; may rupture	• "Mucosa + Cystic Space" • Possible sebaceous gland adjacent • Numerous neutrophils and eosinophils in cystic space or stroma (not true cyst since lacks lining) • Two types histologically: 1. Pseudocystic space with surrounding macrophages and vascular loose fibrous tissue 2. Granulation tissue with mucin, muciphages, and inflammatory cells

Name	Predilection and Clinical Key Features	Histopathology
Cutaneous metaplastic synovial cyst	• Solitary cyst that develops at sites of surgery or trauma (unrelated to joints or synovial structures) • Tender, subcutaneous nodule	• Intradermal cysts lined by a membrane resembling hyperplastic synovium; may only see slit-like space lined by synovium; may connect to surface
Pseudocyst of the auricle	• "Endochondral pseudocyst" • Middle-aged males • Upper-half or third of ear (usually unilateral) • No history of prior trauma, possibly due to ischemia	• "Hole in cartilage," intracartilaginous cavity without an epithelial lining; wall contains eosinophilic, amorphous material with small clefts; fibrosis in cavity • No inflammation (unlike relapsing polychondritis)

Name	Predilection and Clinical Key Features	Histopathology
Endometriosis	• Females • Umbilicus and sites of operation scars on lower abdomen • Bluish–black tumor that enlarges around menses; possible bloody discharge • Size affected by hormones at menses	• Endometrial glands (straight or tortuous, lined with pseudostatified columnar epithelium); fibrovascular stroma; basophilic rim with surrounding myxoid stroma around glands; extravasated RBC and hemosiderin

Name	Predilection and Clinical Key Features	Histopathology
Lymphatic cysts		
Cystic hygroma	• Variant of lymphangioma • Neonates to infants • Lower neck • Cystic swelling of the subcutaneous tissue • Associated with Down syndrome	• Lymphangioma with large cavernous spaces in subcutis lined by flattened endothelium; islands of connective tissue and smooth muscle around channels
Sinuses		
Congenital midline cervical cleft	• Birth • Located at ventral neck • Longitudinal opening along the midline neck, often weeping at birth, and then scar formation	• Cleft covered with stratified squamous epithelium overlying parakeratosis; dense fibrous tissue; sinus tract at caudal end lined with respiratory-type epithelium
Cutaneous dental sinus	• Result of chronic infection of dental origin • Face or neck • Intermittent, suppurative, chronic sinus tract • Rare association with SCC in epithelial lining.	• Sinus tract lined by heavily inflamed granulation and fibrous tissue; may have epithelial lining in part of tract • No grains seen as in actinomycosis

Name	Predilection and Clinical Key Features	Histopathology
Pilonidal sinus	• "Jeep disease" • Hirsute (hairy) males • Second decade (20s) • Sinus in sacrococcygeal region (most common location), umbilicus, axilla, scalp, eyelid, etc • Associated with SCC (rare) • *Note:* An interdigital Epilonidal sinus variant may occur in the finger webs of barbers' hands	• Sinus tract lined by granulation tissue; areas of stratified squamous epithelium in wall; chronic abscess cavity with hair shafts in the lumen • Hair shafts with granulation tissue (above)
Pits		
Congenital lower lip pits	• "Van der Woude syndrome" • Autosomal dominant (rare) • Vermilion zone of lower lip • Depressions and possible sinuses develop on lip (usually bilateral) • Associated with cleft lip and/or cleft palate	• Depression/invagination in epidermis with thinning in the base; parakeratosis on either side of pit; small fistula may lead from base of pit to underlying minor salivary gland; no significant inflammation
Preauricular sinus	• "Ear pits" • Common congenital abnormality (up to 1%) • Infants • Preauricular area • Small dell adjacent to external ear near ascending limb of helix • May be associated with hearing disorders and renal abnormalities • Branchio-oto-renal (BOR) syndrome is associated with preauricular sinuses; due to mutation in EYA 1 gene or SIX 5 gene	• Sinus lined by stratified squamous epithelium that may show some hyperkeratosis or parakeratosis; sebaceous gland may be present in wall; variable inflammatory infiltrate

Septal panniculitis differential:

"ASPEN Migration"
or
"Always Make Septal Panniculitis Easy Nowadays"

A = α1-antitrypsin deficiency

S = scleroderma/morphea*

P = polyarteritis nodosa (vasculitis)

E = erythema nodosum*

N = necrobiosis lipoidica*

Migration = migratory thrombophlebitis

* = septal panniculitis without septal necrosis

Erythema nodosum

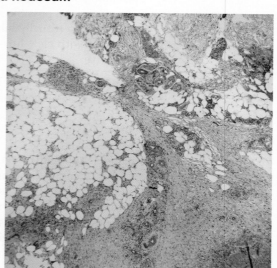

Name	Predilection and Clinical Key Features	Histopathology
Septal panniculitis without septal necrosis		
(Inflammatory reaction centered on the connective tissue septa of subcutaneous fat; inflammation of small venules)		

Erythema nodosum (EN)

- Young adults; women
- Anterior aspect of shin

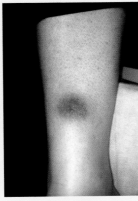 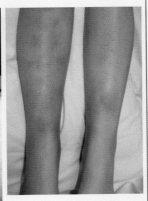

- Acute, painful red nodules on the shin; associated with fever, malaise, arthralgia (subsides 2–6 weeks)
- Associated with sarcoidosis, Sweet's syndrome, Behçet's disease, IBS, drugs (isotretinoin, OCPs, minocycline); infection (streptococcal #1 cause, coccidioidomycosis #1 cause of EN in south west USA)
- Löfgren's syndrome = acute sarcoidosis with EN + hilar lymphadenopathy + fever + arthritis + uveitis
  - *Note:* don't confuse with "Loeffler's syndrome" = eosinophilic pulmonary infiltrate associated with parasitic infections (i.e. hookworm)
- *"NoDOSUM" causes of EN:*
  - NO = no cause found
  - D = drugs (iodide, sulfonamide)
  - O = OCP
  - S = sarcoidosis, Löfgren's
  - U = ulcer (Behçet's, Crohn's > ulcerative colitis)
  - M = microbiology (infection)

- Septal panniculitis (widened septae) with paraseptal inflammatory wedges (neutrophils early, lymphocytes, histiocytes, possibly eosinophils); septal giant cells; Miescher's radial granulomas (small nodular aggregates of histiocytes around a central stellate cleft)

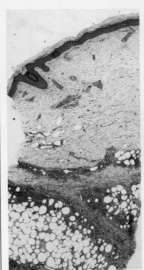 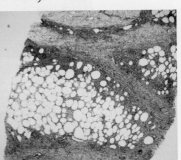

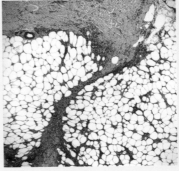 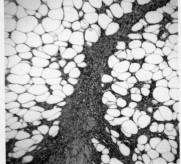

Name	Predilection and Clinical Key Features	Histopathology
Necrobiosis lipoidica [Sudan stain = lipids, VVG stain shows decreased collagen fibers, unlike scleroderma]	• Females in 30s and young insulin-diabetics • Legs (especially shins); 75% bilateral 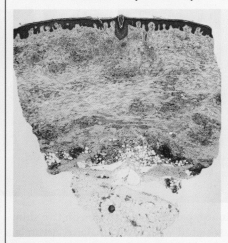 • Red papules with atrophic, shiny yellow–brown center and well-defined raised red-to-purple edge • May develop SCC in older lesions	• Fibrous septal widening; diffuse, palisading granuloma and necrobiosis (parallels epidermis, "cake-layer" like); perivascular infiltrate including plasma cells; necrotizing vasculitis; full dermis and diffuse/broad area; lipids in necrobiotic areas (no mucin) 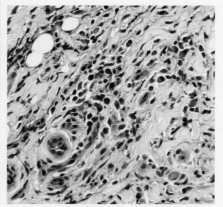 • Numerous plasma cells (above) 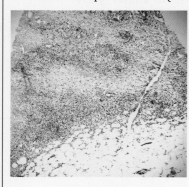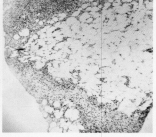

Name	Predilection and Clinical Key Features	Histopathology
Scleroderma/ subcutaneous morphea profunda [VVG stain shows normal collagen fibers, unlike necrobiosis lipoidica]	• If scleroderma involves only subcutaneous fat and/or fascia, then called morphea profunda or subcutaneous morphea • Autoimmune connective tissue disorder, causing excess collagen deposition • Women • Abdomen, sacral area, extremities • One or more ill-defined, deep sclerotic plaques • See p. 237 for more information on Scleroderma	• Thickening and hyalinization of collagen in the deep dermis and the septa/fascia; mixed inflammatory infiltrate with some multinucleate giant cells; possible lipomembranous changes. • Lymphoid collection (often with plasma cells) usually present at junction of thickened septa and fat lobules

Name	Predilection and Clinical Key Features	Histopathology
Lobular panniculitis (Inflammatory reaction present throughout the lobule, often some septal involvement also)		
Erythema induratum and nodular vasculitis	• Young, adult females • Calves (posterior lower leg) • Erythema induratum is possible infectious etiology, such as tuberculous origin or hepatitis C • Recurrent crops of tender, erythematous nodules on the calf	• Usually only deep inflammatory changes (mixed) and diffuse lobular panniculitis; granulomas (possibly tuberculoid with caseating necrosis of fat); vascular involvement of arteries and veins in fat

Name	Predilection and Clinical Key Features	Histopathology
Subcutaneous fat necrosis of the newborn	• Full-term infants (first 2–3 weeks) • Cheeks, shoulders, buttocks • Indurated, erythematous plaques and distinct nodule • Risk of hypercalcemia (1–4 months after resolution); possible thrombocytopenia • Associated with obstetrical trauma, hypothermia, asphyxia, anemia • Likely causes: • Trauma to fragile adipose tissue low in oleic acid and compromised circulation, then release of hydrolases leads to breakdown of unsaturated fatty acids • Associated with infant's high saturated-to-unsaturated fat ratio	• Needle-shaped clefts within fat cells and foamy histiocytes; calcification; fat necrosis; granulomatous infiltrate of mixed cells; normal epidermis
Sclerema neonatorum	• Premature infants (first week) • Often fatal disorder • Diffuse waxy, hard skin (sclerotic), which is dry and cold	• Similar to subcutaneous fat necrosis of newborn with: • Fine, needle-shaped crystal clefts in fat cells and foamy histiocytes (intracellular crystals of triglyceride) • Widened, edematous septae • But sclerema neonatorum shows little inflammation; while subcutaneous fat necrosis of newborn has granulomatous inflammation with mixed cells

Name	Predilection and Clinical Key Features	Histopathology
Cold panniculitis	• After exposure to severe cold • Infants, children (popsicles), and thighs of women riding horses in cold weather • Indurated, tender nodules or plaques	• Lobular panniculitis of mixed cells (neutrophils, lymphocytes and histiocytes); cystic spaces in fat due to fat cell rupture
Weber–Christian disease	• "Idiopathic lobular panniculitis" • Idiopathic panniculitis with systemic or visceral involvement (doubtful distinct entity) • Recurrent subcutaneous nodules/plaques, usually associated with fever	• Lobular panniculitis; numerous neutrophils early then foamy histiocytes and fat necrosis, then fibrosis

Name	Predilection and Clinical Key Features	Histopathology
α1-Antitrypsin deficiency	• Rare genetic disorder • Deficiency results in proteolytic activity causing emphysema, hepatitis, cirrhosis, angioedema due to deposition • Present in 30s and 40s • Trunk, proximal extremities • Tender, erythematous, indurated subcutaneous nodules that may become draining, ulcerated nodules • Possible Tx = IV α1-antitrypsin replacement	• Lobular (or septal) panniculitis with lots of neutrophils ("splaying of neutrophils" between collagen bundles in septae and dermis); fat necrosis with foamy macrophages; cystic spaces; necrosis and inflammation; fibrosis in later lesions; may have dissolution of dermal collagen with transepidermal elimination of "liquefied" dermis

Name	Predilection and Clinical Key Features	Histopathology

Cytophagic histiocytic panniculitis	• Chronic, recurring panniculitis with eventual multisystem involvement
	• Middle age to elderly
	• Usually fatal due to hemorrhagic diathesis from hemophagocytic syndrome
	• Legs
	• Ulcerated nodules or plaques, sometimes painful
	• Two variants:
	  1. Authentic panniculitis with cytophagic histiocytes
	    • May not progress to overt lymphoma
	  2. Subcutaneous panniculitis-like T-cell lymphoma (see pp. 357 and 759)
		• Lobular panniculitis with presence of sheets and clusters of histiocytes with prominent phagocytosis of red cells (hemophagocytic), white cells, and nuclear debris ("bean bag" cells)

Name	Predilection and Clinical Key Features	Histopathology
Panniculitis-like T-cell lymphoma	• Rare form of CTCL (CD8+ T cells) • Multiple subcutaneous tumors/plaques, often constitutional symptoms • α/β T-cell phenotype • See p. 759 for more information	• Variable admixture of pleomorphic small-to-large lymphoctyes and histiocytes infiltrating subcutis in a lobular panniculitis pattern; fat necrosis and karyorrhexis (fragmented nucleus) occur (see p. 759) • Lymphocytes surround fat cells (not specific, but good clue)

Name	Predilection and Clinical Key Features	Histopathology
Pancreatic panniculitis	• May precede underlying condition • Thighs, buttocks, lower extremities • Painful or asymptomatic subcutaneous nodule or indurated plaques • Labs = lipase, amylase • Associated with acute pancreatitis or pancreatic cancer (less common)	• Mixed lobular panniculitis; enzymatic fat necrosis with smudgy, "ghost-like" fat cells; basophilic deposits of calcium salts (fatty acids) at rim; neutrophilic infiltrate at margin • Saponification = basophilic granular calcium deposits due to lysed fat combining with calcium salts

Name	Predilection and Clinical Key Features	Histopathology
Lupus panniculitis	• "Lupus profundus" • Complication in cutaneous LE (1–3%) • Proximal extremities, lower back • Subcutaneus nodules or indurated plaques; may develop painful ulcers	• Lobular panniculitis with prominent lymphocytic infiltrate (possibly plasma cells and eosinophils); fibrous septae with lymphoid follicles (possibly germinal centers) • Possible LE changes in epidermis and dermis (50%); "mummified" or hyalinized around fat cells (looks like a pink, glassy rim) • Hyalinized fat cells (above) • Numerous lymphocytes (above)
Poststeroid panniculitis	• Children poststeroid use • Multiple subcutaneous nodules develop 1–35 days after high-dose steroid rapid withdrawal (uncommon with tapers)	• Sparing of septal vessels; needle-shape clefts in fat cells (similar to subcutaneous fat necrosis of newborn and sclerema neonatorum but differ clinically, especially with history and age)

Name	Predilection and Clinical Key Features	Histopathology
Lipodystrophy syndromes (Primary, idiopathic atrophy of subcutaneous tissue)		
Congenital generalized lipodystrophy	• Beradinelli–Seip syndrome • Seen at birth; autosomal recessive • Mutation = BSCL (AGPAT2 enzyme) and BSCL2	• Subcutaneous atrophy of fat cells; no inflammation
Acquired generalized lipodystrophy	• Lawrence–Seip syndrome • Develops in childhood • Associated autoimmune disease, infections	

Familial partial lipodystrophy	• Onset in puberty and facial sparing of lipoatrophy
	• Three types:
	  1. FPLD1 (Kobberling type) = LE only
	  2. FPLD2 (Dunnigan type): acromegalic facies, double chin
	  3. FPLD3 (mutation = PPARG)	

Acquired partial lipodystrophy (Barraquer–Simons disease)	• Female child (often after a fever or viral illness)
	• Typically, begins with symmetrical facial fat loss, progressing to upper trunk and arms fat loss
	
	• Often have low C3 level; risk of renal insufficiency
	• Associated with thyroid disease, dermatomyositis, acanthosis nigricans, myasthenia gravis, recurrent infections
	• Associated mutation = LMNB2
	• Variants:
	  • Weir-Mitchell type = face fat loss and atrophy on the arms, trunk
	  • Laignel–Lavastine = also fat loss of lower body
	  • Parry–Romberg syndrome = facial hemiatrophy
		• *Note:* lipodystrophy also seen at site of repeated insulin injections by diabetics

Localized lipodystrophy	• Annular or semicircular areas of atrophy; associated with post-injection, or pressure areas	

Name	Predilection and Clinical Key Features	Histopathology
HIV-associated lipodystrophy	• Usually due to protease inhibitors (especially indinavir), but also reverse transcriptase inhibitors • After 2–14 months on drugs, develop peripheral atrophy (face, extremity fat loss) and central obesity (abdominal fat) • Resolves usually after medication stopped	• Resembles non-inflammatory variant of lipodystrophy with atrophy of fat; except possible focal collections of lymphocytes and lipophages
Gynoid lipodystrophy	• "Cellulite" • Women (especially obese) • Buttocks, thighs, abdomen • Uneven distribution of subcutaneous adipose tissue	• Irregular, dimpled, "orange peel" skin surface; no specific or consistent histopathological features
Membranous lipodystrophy [PAS, Sudan black]	• Panniculitis that shows a characteristic lipomembranous (membranocystic) change • Associated with LE, erythema nodosum, Behçet's, etc.	• Lipomembranous changes; cysts lined by an amorphous, eosinophilic material with an arabesque (undulating) architecture

Name	Predilection and Clinical Key Features	Histopathology
Lipodermato-sclerosis	• "Hypodermatitis sclerodermaformis" or "scelerosing panniculitis" • Females • Medial ankle/lower leg • Circumscribed, indurated, inflammatory plaques; possible hyperpigmentation • Associated with venous insufficiency, arterial ischemia, chronic lymphedema, etc. • Possible Tx often includes compression stockings	• Similar to stasis dermatitis (superficially); fat necrosis, sclerosis, foamy macrophages, lymphocytes; widened septae; lipomembranous (membranocystic) changes with amorphous eosinophilic material lining cysts

Name	Predilection and Clinical Key Features	Histopathology
Factitial panniculitis	• Typically due to injection of substance (i.e. milk, urine) into subcutaneous fat	• Mixed septal and lobular panniculitis; sometimes suppurative; foreign body giant cells
Sclerosing lipogranuloma	• Form of factitial panniculitis • Due to tissue injection or implant leakage of oily (lipid) material, such as paraffin or liquid silicone • Augment areas, such as breasts, penis, calves • Painful, rubbery, indurated area; fistulas and ulcerations common • Photo of liquid silicone reaction after injection into calf areas	• "Swiss-cheese" appearance with fat cells disrupted and various sized cystic spaces surrounded by giant cells • Silicone (pictured above) • Lobular or mixed panniculitis; bands of hyaline fibrous tissue between fat cysts; septa contain scattering of lymphocytes, and lipid-containing macrophages and foreign body giant cells • Paraffinoma (pictured above)

Name	Predilection and Clinical Key Features	Histopathology
Traumatic fat necrosis	• Develop at site of trauma • Shins • Liquefaction of injured fat may occur and result in discharge through a surface wound	• Fat cysts with surrounding fibrosis; hemosiderin, collections of foam cells; mild patchy infiltrate; poorly circumscribed

Name	Predilection and Clinical Key Features	Histopathology
Encapsulated fat necrosis	• "Nodular-cystic fat necrosis" • Develops at site of trauma (infarcted area) • Solitary, whitish–yellow, 3–20 mm, mobile subcutis nodule	• Localized lobules of necrotic fat surrounded by thin fibrous capsule (usually hyaline); lipomembranous change common
Infective panniculitis	• Panniculitis due to infection (i.e. candidiasis, cryptococcosis, mycetoma, actinomycosis, chromomycosis, sporotrichosis, histoplasmosis); tick or brown recluse spider bites • Usually immunosuppressed patients (especially infection etiology) • Subcutaneous nodules	• Suppuration, granulomas or numerous eosinophils depending on etiology; heavy neutrophilic infiltrate

Name	Predilection and Clinical Key Features	Histopathology
Non-infective neutrophilic panniculitis	• Neutrophilic panniculitis occurs in early panniculitis without an infectious etiology (e.g. erythema nodosum, Behçet's, pancreatic panniculitis, factitial panniculitis)	• Neutrophilic lobular panniculitis; necrosis sometimes present; admixture of cells with chronicity
Eosinophilic panniculitis	• Non-specific entity with numerous eosinophils • Associated with erythema nodosum, vasculitis, parasite infection (e.g. *Gnathostoma spinigerum, Fasciola hepatica*), malignant lymphoma, narcotic dependency with injection granulomas	• Numerous eosinophils in a lobular panniculitis; sometimes flame figures or parasite present (*Gnathostoma* larva)
Calciphylaxis	• Chronic renal failure patient • Buttocks, abdomen, breasts, and extremities • Present as painful livedo reticularis and tender erythematous plaques (see Ch. 14, Cutaneous Deposits also) • Mortality rate = 60–80% • Possible Tx = sodium thioglycolate	• "Calcifying panniculitis" • Calcification in small blood vessels in dermis and subcutis with a lobular fat necrosis, intralobular calcification, and inflammatory infiltrate (neutrophils, lymphocytes, and foamy macrophages)
Miscellaneous lesions	• Panniculitis due to other conditions or situations: • Gout = urate crystals (see Ch. 14, Cutaneous Deposits) • Sarcoidosis and Crohn's disease = sarcoidal granulomas (see Ch. 7, Granulomatous Reaction Pattern) • Subcutaneous granuloma annulare or rheumatoid nodules = necrobiotic granulomas (See Ch. 7, Granulomatous Reaction Pattern) • Following jejunoileal bypass for obesity (5% patients)	

Name	Predilection and Clinical Key Features	Histopathology
Panniculitis secondary to large vessel vasculitis		
Cutaneous polyarteritis nodosa	• Benign form of polyarteritis nodosa (does not involve major arteries and organs like PAN) • Lower limbs • Painful, subcutaneous nodules in crops	• Vasculitis (fibrin in thick, vessel walls); inflammation (no necrosis in surrounding tissue)

Name	Predilection and Clinical Key Features	Histopathology

Superficial migratory thrombo-phlebitis	• Inflammation of veins, sometimes cord-like thickening
	• Lower limbs
	• Erythematous subcutaneous nodules or cord-like areas of induration
	• Associated with Behçet's disease, Buerger's disease, pancreatic carcinoma
	• *Note:*
	  • Trousseau's syndrome = acquired coagulopathy with migratory thrombophlebitis associated with internal malignancy
	  • Mondor's disease = sclerosing thrombophlebitis of the anterior chest wall or penis (associated with trauma, idiopathic, or rheumatologic disease)
		• Panniculitis limited to area immediately adjacent to the involved vessel in deep dermis or subcutaneous fat; thrombosis may be present
		
		• Assessment of the smooth muscle pattern is the most reliable method to differentiate an artery (continuous wreath of concentric smooth muscle) vs. a vein (bundled smooth muscle fibers with intermixed collagen)

Metabolic and Storage Diseases

Scurvy

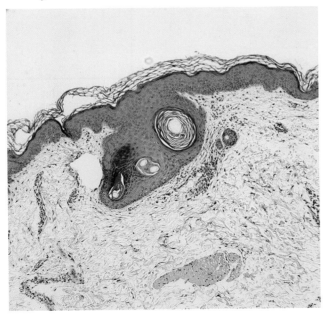

Name	Predilection and Clinical Key Features	Histopathology
Vitamin and dietary disturbances		
Scurvy [Perls' stains hemosiderin around follicles]	• Vitamin C (ascorbic acid) deficiency. This is a water-soluble vitamin for proline hydroxylation in collagen and normal hair growth • Dietary fad, alcoholics • Perifollicular hemorrhages, follicular hyperkeratosis, corkscrew hair, bleeding gums, poor wound healing, woody edema of the lower legs	• Extravasated RBCs around vessels in upper dermis; follicular hyperkeratosis; coiled, corkscrew hairs (photos below) • Perls' stain (above)
Vitamin A deficiency	• Fat-soluble vitamin • Malabsorption conditions • Dry and scaly skin with follicular keratotic papules (phrynoderma); night blindness	• Hyperkeratosis; keratotic follicular plugging; atrophic sweat glands

Name	Predilection and Clinical Key Features	Histopathology
Hypervitaminosis A	• Usually due to self-administration of excess amounts • Vomiting, diarrhea, desquamation of skin	• Non-specific histological findings
Vitamin K deficiency	• Fat-soluble vitamin necessary for hepatic synthesis and secretion of coagulation factors • Seen in liver disease, malabsorption • Bleeding to minor trauma (i.e. purpura, epistaxis, GI bleeding, hematoma)	
Vitamin B$_{12}$ deficiency	• Associated with poikilodermatous pigmentation	• Basal pigmentation and melanin incontinence
Pellagra (vitamin B$_3$ deficiency)	• Multisystem nutritional disorders due to niacin deficiency (nicotic acid, vitamin B$_3$) • Seen in dietary deficiency, malabsorption, chemotherapeutic agents (INH, 5-FU) and tryptophan metabolism abnormality (i.e. carcinoid syndrome, Hartnup disease (tryptophan absorption and transfer defect) • Initially, burning sensation in sun-exposed areas (dorsum of hand) which may form blisters; then intense hyperpigmentation with sharp margins and areas of desquamation; glossitis; angular cheilitis • Four Ds = dermatitis, diarrhea, dementia, death (if untreated)	• Non-diagnostic (hyperkeratosis, parakeratosis, epidermal atrophy with pallor of upper epidermis, basal hyperpigmentation)

Name	Predilection and Clinical Key Features	Histopathology
LYSOSOMAL STORAGE DISEASES		
Sphingolipidoses overall • Lysosomal storage diseases affecting complex lipid metabolism		
G_{M2}-gangliosidoses	• Hexosaminidase deficiency, build up fatty substance ganglioside G_{M2} • Two variants are: 1. Tay-Sachs = deposits limited to nervous system; psychomotor deterioration and blindness 2. Sandhoff's disease = gangliosides in almost all cells in body	
G_{M1}-gangliosidoses	• Autosomal recessive; lysosomal storage disorder with deficient β-galactosidase, build up of G_{M1}-ganglioside • Norman–Landing disease (pseudo-Hurler's syndrome) = infantile, severe form with gargoyle-like appearance, psychomotor regression, blindness, hirsutism, enlarged liver/spleen, hand/foot deformities	
Gaucher disease (glucosylceramide lipidosis)	• Deficient galactocerebroside (GBA gene); build up of glucocerebroside in mononuclear macrophage cells (Gaucher cell, "crumpled tissue paper" look); biopsies are negative for visible depositions • Type I (adult) = diffuse hyperpigmentation; bone pain; hepatomegaly; pingueculae ("eye bumps") • Type II (infantile) = hypertonicity, neck rigidity, HSM, fatal bronchopneumonia, collodion baby	
Fabry's disease (angiokeratoma corporis diffusum)	• X-linked recessive lysosomal storage disease • Deficient α-galactosidase A causing glycolipid to accumulate in blood vessels and organs • Multiple, deep red angiokeratomas in "bathing suit" distribution (spares face/scalp); whorled corneal opacities; cardio- and cerebrovascular disturbances; "Maltese cross" (birefringent lipid molecules) in polarized urine microscopy • Presents in late adolescence with recurrent fever and painful crisis in finger/toe (triggered by exercise, fever, stress, temperature changes); intermittent edema	• Angiokeratomas = large and small thin-walled vessels in upper dermis; small lipid deposits in endothelial cells • [PAS+, Sudan black; also material is birefringent under polarized light] • EM = intracytoplasmic inclusions with lamellar structure (endothelial cells, fibroblasts, but not Schwann cells)
Metachromatic leukodystrophy	• Deficiency in arylsulfatase A • Accumulation of metachromatic sulfatides in CNS and organs causing progressive psychomotor retardation • EM = "herring bone" inclusions in Schwann cells of myelinated nerves	
Krabbe's disease (galactosylceramide lipidosis)	• Autosomal recessive degenerative disorder with deficient galactocerebroside-β-galactosidase • Causes a build up of unmetabolized lipids in myelin sheath affecting nervous system (neurological symptoms in childhood)	
Disseminated lipogranulomatosis (Farber's disease)	• Autosomal recessive disorder with deficient ceramidase • Build up of lipid ceramide and products in joints, tissue, and CNS • By age 2–4 months = progressive arthropathy, subcutaneous nodules, hoarseness, lung disease	• EM = curvilinear bodies (Farber bodies) in fibroblasts and endothelial cells • "Banana-like" bodies in Schwann cells • "Zebra bodies" (vacuoles with transverse membrane) in endothelial cells, seen in storage diseases
Niemann–Pick disease	• Deficient sphingomyelinase causes sphingomyelin build up in organs; usually fatal in childhood • Type A and B mutation = SMPD-1: type A (most common) = xanthomas, HSM, psychomotor deterioration, cherry-red spot in eye, deafness • Type C mutation = cholesterol esterification	

Name	Predilection and Clinical Key Features	Histopathology
Oligosaccharidoses overall		
• Lysosomal enzyme deficiencies cause excess urinary excretion of oligosaccharides		
Sialidosis	• Deficiency of sialidase • Coarse facies, ataxia, myoclonus, and macular cherry-red spot	
Fucosidosis	• Autosomal recessive • Deficiency of lysosomal enzyme α-L-fucosidase: does not break down fucose glycolipids in cells • Early-onset psychomotor retardation; angiokeratomas present similar to Fabry's disease	
Mannosidosis	• α-Mannosidase deficiency • Results in mannose-rich oligosaccharide chains accumulating • Gargoyle-like facies; mental retardation; usually a benign course	
Mucolipidoses (ML) overall		
• Lysosomal storage diseases with features of mucopolysaccharidoses and sphingolipidoses		
I-cell disease (ML II)	• Autosomal recessive neurodegenerative disorder • Mutation = GNPTAB gene • Uridine-diphosphate-N-acetylglucosamine 1 phosphotransferase deficiency • Resembles Hurler syndrome • Short stature, facial dysmorphism, progressive mental/motor retardation, bony deformities	• Accumulate inclusion bodies with carbohydrates, lipids, and proteins dermis has increased oval or spindle-shaped cells, some with clear or foamy cytoplasm
Other lysosomal storage diseases		
Trimethylaminuria	• "Fish-odor syndrome" • Rare metabolic disorder characterized by a body malodor similar to decaying fish • Mutation = flarin-containing monoxygenase 3 (FMO3), resulting in trimethylamine accumulation	
Glycogenosis (type II)	• Disorder of glycogen storage with accumulation in tissues • Type II (Pompe's disease) has a deficiency of acid maltase	• Glycogen found in many cells
Neuronal ceroid-lipofuscinosis	• Progressive neurodegenerative disorder • Accumulation of ceroid or lipofuscin-like substance (CNS/organs)	• Affected cells contain yellow-brown pigment which is autofluorescent

Name	Predilection and Clinical Key Features	Histopathology
Miscellaneous metabolic and systemic diseases		
Acrodermatitis enteropathica	• Inherited disorder of zinc • Infancy (weaning-off-breast-milk age) • Transient zinc deficiency develops in cancers, premature infants on artificial feeding; breast-fed infants • Periorificial and acral crusted, eczematous eruption • Triad: 1. Alopecia 2. Diarrhea 3. Dermatitis • Clinical DDx = biotin deficiency (due to biotinidase deficiency or eating raw egg whites); early cystic fibrosis (perform sweat chloride test)	• Early lesions = increasing pallor of cells in upper epidermis; absent granular layer; confluent parakeratosis with overlying basket-weave stratum corneum; spongiosis and acanthosis; psoriasiform hyperplasia • Late lesions = confluent parakeratosis overlying psoriasiform hyperplasia; no significant epidermal pallor

Name	Predilection and Clinical Key Features	Histopathology
Necrolytic migratory erythema	• Cutaneous finding in glucagonoma syndrome (elevated glucagon levels, usually secondary to glucagon-secreting islet cell pancreatic tumor), zinc deficiency and hepatic disorders • Elderly (60s) • Trunk, groin, perineum, proximal legs • Skin finding = necrolytic migratory erythema, which is similar to TEN with waves of extending, intense annular erythema, flaccid bullae and superficial necrosis with skin shedding leading to flaccid bullae and erosions (resolves in 10–14 days) • Also see glossitis, stomatitis, anemia, weight loss	• "Red-white-blue" sign • Most common pattern = parakeratosis ("red"); pale ("white") vacuolated keratinocytes in upper epidermis; lower portion with normal epidermis ("blue"); necrosis; subcorneal or intraepidermal clefts; subcorneal pustules adjacent to necrotic areas

Name	Predilection and Clinical Key Features	Histopathology
Necrolytic acral erythema	• Acral location only, especially lower limbs • Strong association with hepatitis C • Eroded, erythematous to violaceous patches; later lesions become tender, flaccid blisters and erosions with hyperpigmentation • Possible Tx = may respond to oral zinc	• Similar to acrodermatitis enteropathica and necrolytic migratory erythema (pallor of upper epidermis, absent/decreased granular layer, parakeratosis)

Name	Predilection and Clinical Key Features	Histopathology
Hartnup disease	• Defective intestinal absorption of tryptophan and impaired renal tubular reabsorption of neutral amino acids • Pellagra-like skin rash (histopathology similar to pellagra), photosensitivity, cerebellar ataxia, mental disturbances	
Prolidase deficiency	• Autosomal recessive, inborn error of collagen metabolism • Recalcitrant leg ulcers, retardation, recurrent infections, premature graying of hair; risk of SCC in ulcers	
Tangier disease (familial HDL deficiency)	• Rare disorder of plasma lipid transport (deficiency of normal HDLs in plasma and accumulation of cholesterol esters in organs) • Pathognomonic = enlarged tonsils with orange–yellow striations and low plasma cholesterol level; almost absent HDL level	• Perivascular and interstitial foam cells (also lymphocytes and plasma cells); doubly refractile cholesterol esters in both intracellular and extracellular areas
Lafora disease (Unverricht's disease, myoclonic epilepsy)	• Fatal autosomal recessive degenerative disease with myoclonic epilepsy • Develop symptoms in adolescence • Triad = seizures, myoclonus, and dementia	• Lafora bodies seen in eccrine and apocrine excretory ducts (especially axillary skin) • Lafora bodies = PAS-positive, inclusion bodies within cells of skin (eccrine and apocrine ducts), neurons, heart, liver, muscle
Ulcerative colitis and Crohn's disease	• 10–20% develop skin manifestations • Most common cutaneous signs = erythema nodosum and pyoderma gangrenosum	• Crohn's = skin tags, fistulas, mucosal "cobble stoning," cheilitis granulomatosa • UC = vasculitis, thromboembolic phenomena
Whipple's disease	• Rare, multisystem, Gram+ bacterial infection (*Tropheryma whippelii*) • Hyperpigmentation of scars and sun-exposed skin; erythema nodosum; malabsorption; abdominal pain; arthritis and neurological manifestations	• Non-specific panniculitis with areas of foamy macrophages containing PAS-positive, diastase-resistant material (resembled small bowel biopsy)
Cystic fibrosis	• Defect in chloride ion channel gene • Cutaneous manifestations due to malnutrition (deficiency of protein, zinc, and fatty acids) • Erythematous, desquamating papules/plaques	• Non-specific; acanthosis, diminished granular layer with overlying parakeratosis; mild spongiosis; mild perivascular infiltrate

Diabetes mellitus manifestations

Name	Predilection and Clinical Key Features	Histopathology
Diabetes overall	• Vascular and neuropathic complications (atherosclerosis of large vessels, ischemia, reduced sweating, hair loss, sensory/motor/autonomic neuropathies) • Increased risk of infections (furuncles, *Pseudomonas* infection, *Candida albicans*, etc.) • Distinct cutaneous manifestations (necrobiosis lipoidica, scleredema, eruptive xanthomas, etc.) • Secondary diabetes (hemochromatosis, acanthosis nigricans, porphyria cutanea tarda, etc.)	
Diabetic microangiopathy	• Abnormal small vessels in organs/tissues (kidneys, eyes, skin)	• Thickening of small vessel walls with luminal narrowing (deposition of PAS-positive material in basement membrane)
Pigmented pretibial patches	• "Diabetic dermopathy" • Most common cutaneous finding (50%) in diabetes • Flat-topped, dull-red papules in pretibial area; become variably atrophic and hyperpigmented	• Early lesion = edema of papillary dermis; mild infiltrate; extravasated RBCs • Atrophic lesion = neovascularization of papillary dermis; sparse infiltrate; hemosiderin

Name	Predilection and Clinical Key Features	Histopathology
Bullous eruption of diabetes mellitus	• "Bullosis diabeticorum" • Rare condition associated with diabetes mellitus • Lower extremities • Asymptomatic blisters that often develop "overnight" • Associated with peripheral neuropathy • Heals usually within 2–6 weeks	• Intraepidermal or subepidermal blister; spongiosis; bullae contain fibrin and few inflammatory cells (no acantholysis and DIF negative)
Porphyrias with acute episodes and no cutaneous signs		
(Acute episodes = abdominal pain, neurological changes, and psychiatric disturbance)		
Acute intermittent porphyria (AIP)	• Autosomal dominant • Defect in uroporphyrinogen I synthase • No skin findings • Attacks often due to various factors, including drugs (barbiturates, sulfonamides, griseofulvin) • Labs = increased levels of porphobilinogen and ALA during and usually between attacks	
ALA-dehydratase deficiency porphyria	• Autosomal recessive • Deficiency of ALA-dehydratase • Resembles severe lead poisoning with overproduction of heme precursors	
Porphyrias with acute episodes and cutaneous signs		
(Cutaneous signs include painful, burning lesions to slowly developing fragility and blisters on sun-exposed areas)		
Hereditary coproporphyria	• Autosomal dominant • Deficiency of coproporphyrinogen oxidase • Labs = elevated urinary and fecal coproporphyrins; during attacks, porphobilinogen and ALA increased	
Variegate porphyria	• Autosomal dominant • Reduced activity of protoporphyrinogen oxidase (PPOX gene) by 50% or more • Develop clinical symptoms after puberty • Labs = elevated plasma porphyrin level and florescence at 626 nm • Other labs = elevated fecal protoporphyrin, coproporphyrin; during acute attacks, urinary ALA and porphobilinogen increased	

Name	Predilection and Clinical Key Features	Histopathology
Porphyrias with cutaneous signs only		
Congenital erythropoietic porphyria (Günther's disease)	• Autosomal recessive • Deficiency of uroporphyrinogen III cosynthase • Presents in infancy with red urine staining diapers pink in color; chronic photo-bullous dermatosis, erythrodontia (red discoloration of teeth); hypertrichosis, patchy scarring alopecia, deformities of hands • Severely mutilating, "werewolf-form" of porphyria • Labs = urine uroporphyrins and stool coproporphyrins	• More hyaline material in dermis than other variants

Name	Predilection and Clinical Key Features	Histopathology
Erythropoietic protoporphyria (EPP)	• Ferrochelatase deficiency (defect in terminal step of heme synthesis, occurs in mitochondria) • Autosomal dominant or autosomal recessive • Childhood • Acute photosensitivity with pain/burning; scarring of nose; radial scars around lips; risk of gallstones • Labs = protoporphyrin in blood/feces; normal urinary porphyrins • Reminder = "No PeePee (urine) in EPP"	• Hyaline material in and around blood vessels

Name	Predilection and Clinical Key Features	Histopathology

Porphyria cutanea tarda (PCT)	• "Tarda" = late adult onset
	• Deficiency = reduced activity of uroporphyrinogen decarboxylase
	• Dorsum of hands, light-exposed areas
	
	• Vesicles, milia malar hypertrichosis; vulnerable to mechanical trauma
	• Three major forms:
	  1. Familial (autosomal dominant)
	  2. Sporadic (hepatitis C, alcohol abuse, liver disease)
	  3. Toxic (hydrocarbons)
	• Labs = increased uroporphyrin in urine (8-carboxyl and 7-carboxyl porphyrins mainly) and plasma; increased isocoproporphyrin in feces
	• See p. 109 also
		• Subepidermal blister; festooning of dermal papillae; cell-poor inflammation; caterpillar bodies (eosinophilic, wavy, basement membrane material); hyaline material around blood vessel walls; dermal sclerosis in later lesions
		
		• DIF (image above) = linear IgG and C3 are "donut-like" around papillary dermal vessels (due to immunoglobulin deposits); granular and homogenous deposits of C5b-9 within blood vessels and possibly at the dermoepidermal junction are a characteristic PCT feature

Hepatoerythropoietic porphyria (HEP)	• Autosomal recessive • Severe variant similar to PCT • Deficiency of uroporphyrinogen decarboxylase (less activity of enzyme than PCT, so more severe) • Photosensitivity starts in childhood (not adulthood as in PCT) • Labs = similar to PCT, but elevated levels of RBC protoporphyrins also	

Pseudoporphyria	• Phototoxic bullous dermatosis similar to PCT (normal porphyrin in serum, urine, and feces)
	• Spontaneous skin fragility and blisters in sun-exposed areas (especially dorsum of hand)
	• In contrast to PCT, few patients develop hypertrichosis, hyperpigmentation or sclerodermoid features
	• Associated with NSAIDs/drugs (tetracycline, naproxen, furosemide, isotretinoin) and hemodialysis
	• "TIN LPN" acronym:
	  T = tetracycline
	  I = INH, isotretinoin
	  N = NSAIDs (naproxen)
	  L = Lasix (furosemide)
	  P = pyridoxine
	  N = nalidixic acid (fluoroquinolone)
		• Similar to PCT histologically
		• DIF = similar to PCT with depositions possible in or around dermal vessels, and at the dermoepidermal junction

19

Miscellaneous Conditions

Accessory tragus

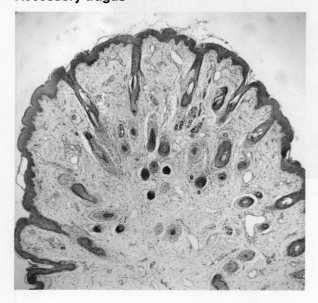

Name	Predilection and Clinical Key Features	Histopathology
Accessory tragus	• Present at birth • Preauricular region (possibly bilateral) and neck (anterior to sternomastoid muscle, called a "wattle") • Solitary, firm, rubbery, dome-shaped papule/nodule; appears "skin-tag-like" • Associated with Goldenhar syndrome (oculo-auriculo-vertebral spectrum) = first brachial arch abnormality with epibulbar dermoid cysts, auricular fistulas and accessory tragus; possible deafness	• Numerous, evenly-spaced vellus hair follicles in pedunculated papule/nodule; central core of fibroadipose tissue and central core of cartilage
Supernumerary nipple	• "Polythelia" • "Polymastia" = presence of nipple, areola and glandular tissue • 1% of population; slight female predilection • Anterior chest or abdomen usually along embryonic milk line (armpit-to-thigh) • Solitary, asymptomatic, slightly pigmented nodular lesion with small, central, nipple-like elevation • "Polythelia pilosa" = supernumerary nipple with only a small patch of hairs visible clinically • Possibly associated with congenital syndromes, such as Simpson–Golabi–Behmel syndrome (overgrowth, coarse facies, congenital cardiac/renal/skeletal anomalies, and embryonal tumors)	• Mild papillomatosis and hyperpigmentation; inverted pilosebaceous unit; increased smooth muscle laterally; often modified apocrine ducts (mammary glands and ducts) with decapitation secretion deep

Name	Predilection and Clinical Key Features	Histopathology
Accessory scrotum	• Scrotal skin outside normal location and without testicular tissue • Perineal region, inguinal region • Wrinkled epidermis with smooth muscle	
Cheilitis glandularis	• Chronic, recurrent, inflammation of minor salivary gland • Age 40s–70s (varies) • Lower lip • Enlarged lip (macrocheilia) with crusting and fissuring with a mucoid discharge, pin-point red macules	• Hyperkeratosis, focal parakeratosis, inflammatory crusting, edema • Often enlarged salivary gland with dilated excretory ducts
Omphalomesenteric duct remnant	• Umbilical lesion variant • Embryological remnant of the vitelline duct • Umbilical area • Red, pedunculated, papule; possible mucoid discharge • May form subcutaneous cyst, umbilical polyp, umbilical sinus, or enteric fistula • Omphalomesenteric duct cyst may be associated with Meckel's diverticulum	• Covered by epithelium which is usually small bowel or colonic type; usually abrupt transition from epidermis to intestinal or gastric epithelium

Name	Predilection and Clinical Key Features	Histopathology
Urachal remnant	• Umbilical lesion variant • Embryological remnant of the urachus • Present at birth • Umbilical area • May present as periumbilical dermatitis; possible passage of urine from umbilicus, if patent urachus	• Lined by transitional epithelium, sometimes smooth muscle bundles present
Fibrous umbilical polyp	• Umbilical lesion variant • Early childhood • Boys • Umbilical area • Nodule ranging from 0.4–1.2 cm	• Dome-shaped lesion with a stromal proliferation of moderately cellular fibrous tissue without significant inflammation; fibroblastic cells are plump to elongated with abundant pale pink cytoplasm; collagen is sparse to moderate; overlying epidermis has loss of rete ridges and basket-weave hyperkeratosis

Name	Predilection and Clinical Key Features	Histopathology
Relapsing polychondritis	• Autoimmune (often to type II collagen) rheumatologic disorder with recurrent inflammation of cartilaginous tissue • Middle-aged adult • Ears, nasal septum, tracheobronchial cartilage • Tenderness and reddening of both ears (spares earlobe), polyarthritis, ocular inflammation, vasculitis • Progressive destruction of cartilage with deformities (i.e. floppy ears, saddle nose) • 25% of deaths due to respiratory and cardiovascular complications • Associated with SLE, RA, psoriasis, Sweet's syndrome • MAGIC syndrome (mouth and genital ulcers with inflamed cartilage) = Behçet's disease + relapsing polychondritis	• Degeneration of cartilage/marginal chondrocytes with a decrease in basophilia of involved cartilage; perichondrial inflammation (especially neutrophils); older lesions show perichondrial fibrosis • DIF = Ig/C3 at chondrofibrous junction

Name	Predilection and Clinical Key Features	Histopathology

Acanthosis nigricans	• Axilla, neck, oral mucosa (25%)
	• Clinical associations:
	  • Endocrine (insulin-resistant diabetes, Prader–Willi syndrome, obesity)
	  • Paraneoplastic (carcinomas of GI, kidney, lymphoma)
	  • Familial (autosomal dominant)
	  • Idiopathic (obesity)
	  • Drugs (OCP, steroids, niacin)
	
	• Symmetrical, pigmented, velvety papillomatous plaques
	• May be associated with HAIR-AN syndrome, which is a multisystem disorder in women with hyperandrogenism (HA), insulin resistance (IR), and acanthosis nigricans (AN)
		• Marked hyperkeratosis, papillomatosis with "church spires;" valleys with hyperkeratosis and mild acanthosis; hyperpigmented basal layer; rete ridges do not appear elongated

Name	Predilection and Clinical Key Features	Histopathology
Confluent and reticulated papillomatosis (CRP)	• Puberty • Upper part of chest (sternum), intermammary region, and back • Asymptomatic, red-to-brown, verrucous papules with central confluence and reticulate pattern peripherally • More reticulated and stuck-on scale and less velvety than acanthosis nigricans • Possible Tx includes minocycline, isotretinoin	• Undulating hyperkeratosis, low papillomatosis; valleys with acanthotic down growths (similar to acanthosis nigricans, differs mainly clinically and CRP has dilated superficial dermal vessels)

Name	Predilection and Clinical Key Features	Histopathology
Acrokeratosis paraneoplastica	• "Paraneoplastic Bazex syndrome" • Violaceous erythema, keratoderma, and psoriasiform scaling on fingers and toes; later extension to ears and nose; skin changes often precede onset of cancer symptoms • Associated with cancers, especially esophageal cancer (usually supradiaphragmatic in origin) • *Note:* Not the same as Bazex syndrome (autosomal dominant disorder with follicular atrophoderma, hypohidrosis, facial BCCs, and pili torti)	• Histopathology is variable and often psoriasiform-like typically, also hyperkeratosis, focal parakeratosis, acanthosis, mild infiltrate

Erythroderma	• "Exfoliative dermatitis"
	• 60s (mean age); males
	
	• Cutaneous eruption causing pruritic erythema and exfoliation of almost all skin surfaces (>90%)
	• Possible common causes of erythroderma = "ID-SCALP":
	  • I = idiopathic
	  • D = drug allergy (i.e. phenytoin, INH, PCN, antimalarials, HCTZ)
	  • S = seborrheic dermatitis
	  • C = contact dermatitis
	  • A = atopic dermatitis
	  • L = lymphoma (i.e. mycoses fungoides) and leukemia
	  • P = psoriasis/PRP
		• HP = variable and often of little value

Papuloerythroderma of Ofuji	• Elderly males • Widespread erythematous, flat-topped papules with a sparing of body folds ("deck-chair" sign) • Often associated with underlying lymphoma or cancer	• Normal epidermis; slight acanthosis, spongiosis, and parakeratosis; perivascular infiltrate (lymphocytes, plasma cells, and eosinophils) • S100-positive dendritic cells abundant in dermis
Scalp dysesthesia	• Burning, stinging, or itching of scalp • Often associated with psychological stress • May be accompanied by telogen effluvium	

20 Cutaneous Drug Reactions

Terbinafine drug reaction

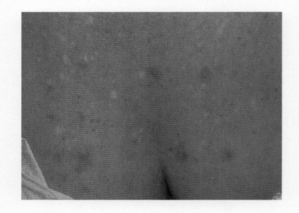

DRESS syndrome
(Drug rash with eosinophilia and systemic symptoms)

Name	Predilection and Clinical Key Features	Histopathology
Drug reactions overall		

• *Most common drug reactions:*
  1. Exanthematous reaction
  2. Urticaria
  3. Angioedema and fixed drug
• *Types of drug reactions:*
  • Type I (hypersensitivity) reaction (most significant type) = IgE mediated; causes anaphylaxis, urticaria, and angioedema
  • Type II (cytotoxic) reaction = not shown to clearly cause cutaneous reactions
  • Type III (immune complexes) = vasculitis, serum sickness, SLE-like drug reaction
  • Type IV (delayed hypersensitivity) reaction = rarely a cause of drug reactions
• *Clues to drug etiology:*
  • Eosinophils
  • Plasma cells
  • Activated lymphs
  • RBC extravasation
  • Apoptotic keratinocytes
  • Urticarial edema
  • Endothelial vessel swelling		

Clinicopathological reactions		
Exanthematous drug reaction (morbilliform)	• Most common drug reaction (40%) • Rash typically develops 1–3 weeks after drug given • Usually first appears on trunk, areas of pressure or trauma; then spreads to extremities symmetrically • Erythematous macules and papules/morbilliform (viral exanthem-like) • May include: penicillin, erythromycin, tetracyclines, gold, captopril, NSAIDs, ampicillin, thiazide, codeine, etc. • *Note:* exanthematous eruptions occur in 50–80% patients given ampicillin with mononucleosis, cytomegalovirus infection, or chronic lymphatic leukemia or who are also taking allopurinol	• Non-specific; spongiosis; vacuolar change; superficial perivascular inflammation with mixed infiltrate (lymphocytes, mast cells, occasional eosinophils, rarely plasma cells); apoptotic keratinocytes (Civatte bodies) in basal layer
Halogenodermas	• Includes iododerma, bromoderma, and fluoroderma due to ingestion of iodides, bromides, and fluorides • Face, neck, back, or upper extremities • Papulopustule which progresses to a vegetating, nodular lesion	• Pseudoepitheliomatous hyperplasia with intraepidermal and dermal abscesses with a few eosinophils
Drug hypersensitivity syndrome	• "DRESS syndrome" (Drug Rash with Eosinophils and Systemic Symptoms) • Often patient on anticonvulsants for 1–8 weeks • Generalized exanthem, fever, multi-organ toxicity, blood eosinophilia; often elevated liver enzymes • Common drugs implicated are phenytoin, carbamazepine, sulfonamides, allopurinol, dapsone, calcium channel blockers	• Non-specific histological findings

Name	Predilection and Clinical Key Features	Histopathology

Other clinicopathological reactions	• Numerous reactions possible, such as:
	  • Acanthosis nigricans = hormones and corticosteroids
	  • Acne = drugs, cosmetics, industrial chemicals
	  • Elastosis perforans serpiginosa = long-term penicillamine
	  • Erythema multiforme = sulfonamides, NSAIDs
	  • Fixed drug ("PABA"): pseudoephedrine and phenolphthalein, aspirin, barbiturates, antibiotics, and anti-inflammatory
	  • Hypersensitivity syndrome = phenytoin, dapsone, calcium channel blockers
	  • Hypertrichosis = minoxidil and oral contraceptives
	  • Infarction = first week of coumadin therapy
	  • Lipodystrophy = protease inhibitors
	  • Lichenoid drug = beta blocker, captopril, gold
	  • Neutrophilic eccrine hidradenitis = cytarabine
	  • Panniculitis/EN = OCPs, isotretinoin, minocycline, sulfa
	  • Pigmentation = antimalarials, tetracycline, amiodarone
	  • Pseudolymphoma = phenytoin, carbamazepine
	  • Psoriasiform drug reaction = beta blockers, lithium
	  • Pustular lesions = diltiazem, INH, cephalosporins
	  • Sclerodermoid lesions = polyvinyl chloride, bleomycin
	  • SLE-like reaction ("HIPP"): hydralazine, INH, procainamide, penicillamine
	  • SCLE-like reaction ("GATCH"): griseofulvin, ACE inhibitors, terbinafine, Ca channel blockers, HTCZ
	  • Toxic epidermal necrolysis (TEN) = sulfonamides, allopurinol, NSAIDs
	  • Ulceration = allopurinol, hydroxyurea	

Offending drugs

Name	Predilection and Clinical Key Features	Histopathology

Antibiotics	• Most common:
	  • Trimethoprim-sulfamethoxazole = urticarial reaction or exanthematous reaction
	  • Ampicillin = exanthematous reaction
	  • Amoxicillin = intertriginous eruption
	• *LOW* cutaneous side effects:
	  • Macrolides (erythromycin, azithromycin)
		• Other drugs:
		  • Fluoroquinolones = photosensitivity
		  • IV Vancomycin = "red man / red neck" syndrome
		  • Oral antifungals (terbinafine) = urticaria, erythema and pruritus

Non-steroidal anti-inflammatory drugs	• Reaction may vary from exanthematous to TEN
	  • Aspirin = acute urticaria, aggravates chronic urticaria
	  • Ibuprofen = vasculitis, urticaria, erythema multiforme, erythema nodosum
	  • Naproxen = fixed drug eruptions, vesiculobullous reaction	

Psychotropic drugs	• Reactions vary
	  • Lithium = acneiform eruption
	  • Chlorpromazine = blue–gray discoloration
	  • Chlordiazepoxide = exacerbation of porphyria	

Phenytoin sodium	• Broad spectrum of cutaneous reactions	
Gold	• Usually an eczematous or maculopapular reaction • May occur 2 years after initiation of therapy	
Retinoids	• Cutaneous side effects include: cheilitis, palmoplantar peeling, pyogenic granuloma-like lesions	
Cytotoxic drugs	• Various mucocutaneous complications possible: alopecia, stomatitis, ulceration, phlebitis, pigmentation, acral erythema, erythroderma, etc.	

Recombinant cytokines	• Granulocyte–macrophage colony-stimulating factor (GMCSF) > granulocyte colony-stimulating factor (GCSF)
	  • GMCSF = folliculitis, bullous pyoderma gangrenosum, erythroderma, etc.
	  • GCSF = Sweet's syndrome, bullous pyoderma gangrenosum, vasculitis, etc.
	• Erythropoietin = hirsutism, spongiotic reaction
	• Interferons (most common side effect of IFN-α = alopecia)
	• IL-2 = bullous disorders, erythema nodosum	

Intravenous immunoglobulin	• Eczema, alopecia, erythema multiforme, lichenoid dermatitis	
Protease inhibitors	• Lipodystrophy, maculopapular eruption, stria formation, excess granulation tissue of digits with paronychia	

Reactions to Physical Agents

Thermal burn

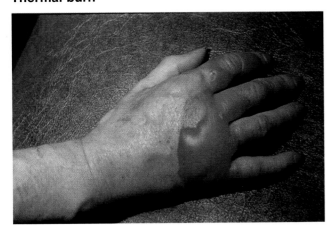

Name	Predilection and Clinical Key Features	Histopathology
Reactions to trauma and irritation		
Dermatitis artefacta	• Self-inflicted dermatosis, may not be consciously aware • Malingerers, mentally retarded, psychiatric issues • Clinical and histological appearance can vary tremendously; distribution and pattern often bizarre; lesions in different stages of healing 	
Dermatitis neglecta	• "Terra firma-forme" dermatosis, possibly due to inadequate frictional cleaning • Neck • Acquired, asymptomatic, pigmented plaque (acanthosis nigricans-look) that will not remove with gentle cleansing with soap and water, but removes when rubbed with alcohol	
Decubitus ulcer	• "Bedsore" in patients with extended time in bed • Pressure areas (sacrum, heels) • Classification and clinical stages: Stage I = non-blanchable erythema of intact skin Stage II = partial-thickness skin loss (blister, abrasion) Stage III = full-thickness skin loss; to the underlying fascia Stage IV = destruction to muscle, bone, etc.	• Early changes = dilated vessels and swollen endothelial cells; mast cells increased; necrotic epidermis and appendages; subepidermal bulla and necrosis; abundant fibrin • Re-epithelialization is slow and usually requires graft to area
Friction blister	• Heels and palms (areas with thick epidermis and firmly attached to dermis) • Recovery is rapid (days)	• Intraepidermal blister (below stratum granulosum); sparse or absent infiltrate • Differs from suction blister, which is subepidermal in location
Calcaneal petechiae	• "Black heel" or "talon noir" • Heels, palms (often bilateral and symmetric) • Painless, petechial eruption with a speckled, brown–black pigment • Often traumatic cause due to pinching force (i.e. sudden stopping in sports)	 • Lakes of hemorrhage in stratum corneum; hemoglobin (not hemosiderin) undergoing transepidermal elimination after extravasation from vessels in papillary dermis • Hemoglobin stain = benzidine stain or patent blue V stain

Name	Predilection and Clinical Key Features	Histopathology
Reactions to radiation		
• UVB = "sunburn cells" (apoptosis of keratinocytes), spongiosis, and later causes parakeratosis • UVA = no "sunburn cells," mild spongiosis		
Sunburn	• Due to ultraviolet exposure • Mainly due to UVB exposure • Red, tender patch; may blister	• UVB damage produces apoptosis of keratinocytes ("sunburn cells"), spongiosis, later causes parakeratosis; enlarged endothelial cells in superficial vessels; Langerhans cells in epidermis reduced in number • UVA does not result in "sunburn cells," and only mild spongiosis
Early radiation dermatitis	• Weeks after treatment • Red patches accompanied by edema with possible blistering or ulceration; later hyperpigmentation and epilation (hair loss)	• Vacuolated or necrotic keratinocytes; dermal edema; subepidermal blister; dilated vessels with swollen endothelial cells
Subacute radiation dermatitis	• Weeks to months after radiation	• Lichenoid tissue reaction with basal vacuolar change and apoptotic cells • Features similar to acute graft-versus-host disease • "Satellitosis" (satellite cell necrosis) = apoptotic ("dead") keratinocytes with lymphocytes in close apposition ("touching")

Name	Predilection and Clinical Key Features	Histopathology
Late radiation changes	• Years after treatment with >1000 rads • Poikiloderma (atrophy, telangiectasias, hypopigmentation, focal hyperpigmentation); loss of pilosebaceous appendages • Associated with increased risk of SCC (aggressive) and BCC, especially if >2000 rads	• "Morphea-like" + "radiation atypical fibroblasts" (large nucleus and cytoplasm) • Atrophy with loss of normal rete ridges; develops focal basal vacuolar change; dyskeratotic cells; swollen, hyalinized collagen with irregular eosinophilic staining in dermis; pilosebaceous structures absent but arrector pili muscle remains; dilation of vessels (telangiectasias)

Name	Predilection and Clinical Key Features	Histopathology
Reactions to heat and cold		
Thermal burns	• In children, mostly due to hot liquids • In adults, mostly due to flammable liquids • Usually classified as first, second, and third-degree burns according to extent of damage • Risk of secondary infection (especially Gram−), alopecia • Risk of SCC (20–40 years later) • Possible "delayed post-burn blister" (subepidermal blister occurring weeks to months after burn)	• First degree burn = necrosis of upper epidermis only (similar to a sunburn) • Second degree burn = vertical elongation of keratinocytes; necrosis of epidermis with crust of fibrin; possible pilosebaceous appendages destroyed (if deep type); eccrine glands undergo squamous metaplasia • Third degree burn = necrosis of entire skin and possibly underlying fat; inflammatory exudate at viable and non-viable border; arrector pili muscle lost; focal subepidermal clefts
Electrical burns	• May resemble third degree burn clinically • Severity varies depending on current, voltage, and extent of skin contact	• Cavity formation due to dermoepidermal separation; elongated, cytoplasmic processes extend from basal cells into cavity; vertical elongation of keratinocytes; homogenization of collagen in upper dermis; hemorrhage • Electrocautery effect (above)

Name	Predilection and Clinical Key Features	Histopathology
Frostbite	• Acral parts (fingers, toes), nose • White or blue–white skin color; blister forms 1–2 days after re-warming, followed days later by formation of hard eschar	• Necrotic tissue; inflammatory infiltrate at periphery
Cryotherapy effects	• Damage due to rapid cooling and formation of intracellular ice crystals; melanocytes sensitive to cold damage and result may be hypopigmentation • Liquid nitrogen = −196°C • Approximate temperature sensitivity ranges: • Melanocytes = −5°C • Hair follicles/glands = −20°C • Keratinocytes = −25°C • Fibroblasts = −30° to −35°C • Benign tumor = −25°C • Malignant tumor = −50°C	• Loss of cellular outline in epidermis and appears homogenized; subepidermal bulla formation
Polymorphous cold eruption	• Autosomal dominant disorder • Face and limbs • Non-pruritic, erythematous eruptions after exposure to cold air	• Superficial and deep mixed inflammatory infiltrate; predominantly neutrophils around eccrine sweat glands; no vasculitis

Name	Predilection and Clinical Key Features	Histopathology
Reactions to light		

Photosensitive genodermatoses	• Xeroderma pigmentosum: DNA repair defect
	• Cockayne's syndrome: ERCC8 or ERCC6 genes, excision-repair cross-complementing protein
	• Bloom's syndrome:
	  • "congenital telangiectatic erythema"
	  • RECQL3 gene
	• Hartnup disease: SLC6A19 mutation
	• Rothmund–Thomson syndrome:
	  • "poikiloderma congenitale"
	  • RECQ4 helicase gene
	• Smith–Lemli–Opitz syndrome:
	  • DHCR7 gene
	  • results in deficiency of 7-dehydrocholesterol reductase (final step in cholesterol biosynthesis)
	• Kindler's syndrome:
	  • KIND1 mutation
	  • Encodes kindlin-1 involved in the actin cytoskeleton	

Phototoxic dermatitis	• Damage from ultraviolet or visible radiation due to contact/ingestion of photosensitizing substance (energy released as returns to ground state) • Usually due to UVA range • Resembles sunburn with possible blister formation; followed by desquamation and hyperpigmentation • Possible phytophotodermatitis from plants with psoralen and other furocoumarins (especially celery, parsnip, carrots, limes/lemons) • Possible phototoxic reaction often due to topical and oral medications (furosemide, naproxen, doxycycline, thiazides, retinoids, etc.) • Photo-onycholysis is possible with tetracyclines, thiazides, captopril etc.	• "EM-like" + deep infiltrate • Topical agents cause = ballooning of keratinocytes in upper dermis; necrosis; apoptotic keratinocytes ("sunburn cells"); edema • If acute, then possibly only superficial inflammatory infiltrate • Bullous reaction (pseudoporphyria) appears as a subepidermal blister with rare inflammatory cells ("cell poor"), see p. 381

Name	Predilection and Clinical Key Features	Histopathology

Photoallergic dermatitis	• 24–48 hours after sun exposure and application of topical chemical, a pruritic, eczematous eruption develops
	
	• Requires:
	  1. Photosensitizing agent:
	    • fragrances: such as musk ambrette
	    • sunscreens with benzophenone
	    • benzocaine
	    • plants in *Compositae* family: such as daisy, dandelion, etc.
	    • drugs: itraconazole, B6, tetracycline, thiazides
	  2. Light
	    • especially UVA range
	  3. Delayed hypersensitivity response (type IV)
		• Similar to contact allergic dermatitis + deep infiltrate with spongiosis, spotty parakeratosis, some acanthosis; spongiotic vesicles; superficial and deep infiltrate

Hydroa vacciniforme	• Possible "scarring-variant" of PMLE • "Bazin's hydroa vacciniforme" • Sunlight (especially summer sunlight) provokes intermittent, bullous, scarring disorder with an unknown etiology • Childhood; male (resolves by adolescence) • Sun-exposed areas, especially face and dorsum of hands; varioliform scars and may lead to ear mutilation • Hours after sun exposure, symmetrical, clustered, pruritic/burning, red macules • Similar to eruption in EBV infection with increased lymphoma risk • Dietary fish oil may provide systemic photoprotection	• "PLEVA-like" • Necrosis; spongiosis that leads to intraepidermal vesicles with fibrin and inflammatory infiltrate serum in vesicles; superficial and deep infiltrate • DIF = scattered granular C3 at DE junction

Name	Predilection and Clinical Key Features	Histopathology
Polymorphic light eruption (PMLE)	• Sunlight-induced eruption after sun exposure • Due to UVA > UVB or visible light • 20s–30s (women) • Spring and early Summer; after puberty • Sun-exposed areas (dorsa of hands, forearms, face) • Patchy pattern of non-scarring, pruritic, erythematous papules, plaques on sun-exposed areas • Possible Tx = sun avoidance, UVB/PUVA, steroids, antimalarials • 50% cases with decreased sunlight sensitivity with time ("hardening")	• Papillary dermal edema with subsequent formation of vesicles (bullae); superficial and deep perivascular infiltrate (mainly lymphocytes) • No basal layer liquefaction degeneration; increased Langerhans cells (unlike typical sun exposure) • DIF = negative
Actinic prurigo	• Possible "persistent-variant" of PMLE • "Hutchinson's summer prurigo" or hereditary PMLE • Sunlight-induced eruption (especially UVA) • Childhood (female) • North American Indians and central America • Associated with HLA DR4 (80–90%); DRB1*0407 • Papular/nodular, pruritic, eczematous eruption on uncovered skin mainly (possibly some covered skin); cheilitis, conjunctivitis • Condition worse in summer	• Histology is not specific; irregular acanthosis, prominent telangiectasia, heavy infiltrate; lymphoid follicles • Cheilitis shows dense lymphocytic infiltrate with well-formed lymphoid follicles

Name	Predilection and Clinical Key Features	Histopathology
Chronic actinic dermatosis (Chronic photodermatoses)		
• Group of rare photodermatoses with persistent photosensitivity, marked predominance in older males • Presence of erythematous, edematous, and lichenified plaques in light-exposed areas		
Persistent light reaction	• Photosensitive reaction after withdrawal of photosensitizer (sensitive to agent and UVB) • Seen with halogenated salicylanilides, thiazide diuretics	• Epidermal spongiosis with focal parakeratosis and some acanthosis; moderately dense perivascular inflammatory cell infiltrate in the upper and mid-dermis
Photosensitive eczema	• Likely a photocontact allergic reaction (especially UVB) with unknown photoallergen	• Similar to photocontact allergic dermatitis with epidermal spongiosis and a superficial infiltrate
Actinic reticuloid	• Elderly • 10% have positive photo-patch test for *Compositae* family (daisy, dandelion, etc.) • Episodes of erythroderma-like picture involving non-exposed areas (sensitive to UVA/UVB and often visible light)	• Resembles cutaneous T-cell lymphoma, but mainly CD8+ in the epidermis, (unlike CTCL); superficial and deep lymphocytic infiltrate of CD4+ and CD8+ cells; large lymphoid T-cells; exocytosis of lymphocytes; "Pautrier-like" microabscesses
Brachioradial pruritus	• Rare, recurrent, localized, pruritic, solar dermatosis involving the brachioradial region • Possible association with cervical spine disease	• Normal appearing epidermis/dermis; marginal increase in mast cells

Cutaneous Infections and Infestations

22

Histological Pattern	Causes		
Histological patterns in infections and infestations			
Palisading granulomas	• Phaeohyphomycosis • Mycobacteriosis • Treponematosis • Sporotrichosis	• Cryptococcosis • Coccidioidomycosis • Cat-scratch disease	• Lymphogranuloma venereum • Schistosomiasis
Tuberculoid granulomas	• Tuberculosis • Tuberculids • Tuberculoid leprosy • Syphilis (late secondary or tertiary)	• Dermatophytosis (Majocchi's granuloma) • Cryptococcosis • Alternariosis • Histoplasmosis • Leishmaniasis	• Keloidal blastomycosis • Prototheriosis • Acanthamebiasis • Echinoderm injury • *Vibrio* and *Rhodococcus* infection
Suppurative granulomas	• Atypical mycobacterial infections • Lymphogranuloma venereum	• Blastomycosis-like pyoderma • Actinomycosis • Nocardiosis • Mycetoma	• Cryptococcosis • Aspergillosis • Deep fungal infections • Prototheriosis
Histiocyte granulomas	• Atypical mycobacteria • Lepromatous leprosy • Leishmaniasis	• Malakoplakia: Michaelis–Gutmann bodies in cytoplasm	
Histiocytes and plasma cells	• Rhinoscleroma • Syphilis • Yaws	• Granuloma inguinale (abscess also)	
Plasma cells predominate	• Syphilis • Yaws • Lymphogranuloma venereum	• Chancroid • Visceral leishmaniasis • Trypanosomiasis	• Arthropod bites (uncommon) • Vibrio infection
Eosinophils predominate	• Arthropod bites • Helminth infestation	• Cnidarian (coelenterate) contact	• Subcutaneous phycomycosis

Histological Pattern	Causes		
Neutrophils predominate	• Impetigo (subcorneal neutrophils) • Ecthyma • Cellulitis • Erysipelas (superficial edema) • Granuloma inguinale (microabscesses) • Chancroid (superficial neutrophils)	• Anthrax • Disseminated TB in AIDS patients • Erythema nodosum leprosum • Actinomycosis • Nocardiosis • Mycetoma • Flea bites • Lucio's phenomenon	• Yaws and pinta (intraepidermal abscess) • Blastomycosis-like pyoderma • Fungal kerion • Phaeohyphomycosis • Aspergillosis • Mucormycosis (infarction often)
Parasitized macrophages	• Rhinoscleroma • Granuloma inguinale • Lepromatous leprosy	• Histoplasmosis • Leishmaniasis	• Toxoplasmosis (pseudocysts) • *Penicillium* infection
Parasitized multinucleate giant cells and/or foreign body reaction	• Fungal infections • Prototheccosis	• Schistosomiasis • Demodex within tissues	• Mite infections
Superficial and deep dermal perivascular lymphocytic inflammation	• Leprosy (indeterminate) • Secondary syphilis (plasma cells)	• Arthropod bites • Coral reactions: often interstitial eosinophils	• Onchocerca dermatitis: microfilariae in lymphatics
Psoriasiform epidermal hyperplasia	• Chronic candidosis • Tinea imbricata	• Chronic dermatophytoses (rare)	
Pseudoepitheliomatous or irregular epidermal hyperplasia	• Amebiasis • Mucocutaneous leishmaniasis • Schistosomiasis • Yaws • Rhinoscleroma • Granuloma inguinale • Tuberculosis	• Vibrio infection • Deep fungal infections • Human papilloma virus infection • Milker's nodule and Orf • Blastomycosis-like pyoderma: oblique follicle, draining sinus	• Verrucous herpes/varicella in HIV • Toxoplasmosis (rare) • Chronic arthropod bite (rare)
Folliculitis and/or perifolliculitis	• Dermatophytoses • Pityrosporum folliculitis • Pyogenic bacterial infections	• Herpes simplex • Herpes zoster • Demodex infestation	• Larva migrans: eosinophilic folliculitis • Syphilis (rare)
Vasculitis	• Erythema nodosum leprosum • Lucio's phenomenon • Ecthyma gangrenosum • Necrotizing fasciitis	• Meningococcal/gonococcal septicemia • Cytomegalovirus infection: endothelial inclusion bodies • Spider bites	• Recurrent herpes: lichenoid lymphocytic vasculitis • Rickettsial infections: lymphocytic vasculitis • Papulonecrotic tuberculid
Tissue necrosis	• Ecthyma gangrenosum • Necrotizing fasciitis • Diphtheria • Anthrax • Tularemia • Cat-scratch disease • Rickettsial infection (eschar present)	• Severe Lepra reactional states • Scrofuloderma • *Mycobacterium ulcerans* infection • Papulonecrotic tuberculid • Chancroid (superficial necrosis only)	• Herpes folliculitis • Mucormycosis • Gnat, spider, and beetle bites • Acute tick bites • Stonefish/stingray contact • Orf • Amebiasis
Epidermal spongiosis	• Dermatophytoses • Candidosis • Cercarial dermatitis: eosinophils and neutrophils also • Larva migrans	• Chigger bites • Arthropod bites • Moth contact from genus *Hylesia* • Beetle contact	• Delayed reaction to cnidarians • Viral infections: herpesvirus-6, Coxsackievirus

Histological Pattern	Causes
Intraepidermal vesiculation	Ballooning degeneration and intranuclear inclusions: • Herpes simplex • Herpes zoster • Varicella • Orf and milker's nodule: pale superficial cytoplasm • Hand, foot, and mouth disease • Erysipeloid: superficial dermal edema • Beetle bites • Arthropod bites • Dermatophytoses • Candidosis
Parasite in tissue sections	• Helminth and arthropod infestations • Injuries from certain marine life
"Invisible dermatoses" (Section stained with H&E appears normal)	• Erythrasma • Pityriasis versicolor (spores and hyphae) • Dermatophytoses: compact orthokeratosis, neutrophils in stratum corneum, "sandwich sign" • Pitted keratolysis: crateriform defects, pits, pallor of stratum corneum, bacteria visible
Spindle cell pseudotumors	• Atypical mycobacteria • Histoid leprosy • Acrodermatitis chronica atrophicans

23 Bacterial and Rickettsial Infections

Bullous impetigo

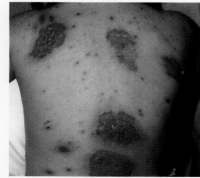
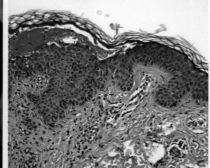

Name	Predilection and Clinical Key Features	Histopathology
Superficial pyogenic infections		
Common (non-bullous) impetigo [Gram stain]	• *Staphylococcus aureus* (#1 cause), also *Streptococcus pyogenes* • Red papules that develop a honey-crusted vesicle; nasal and perioral areas • Clinical test = anti-DNase B antibodies	• Subcorneal neutrophils with exocytosis through epidermis; Gram+ cocci; moderate inflammatory infiltrate in papillary dermis
Bullous impetigo [Gram stain]	• "Localized form of SSSS" resulting from the production in situ of staphylococcal epidermolytic toxin • Premature infants and chronic renal insufficiency adults (due to poor renal function which excretes toxin) • May be localized or generalized • Flaccid bullae forming "varnish-like" erosion • *S. aureus*, phage II (exfoliative toxin A targets desmoglein 1)	• Subcorneal blister with few neutrophils and acantholytic cells; Gram+ cocci; moderate infiltrate in papillary dermis • Due to local production of exfoliative toxin (as opposed to distant site in SSSS) • Gram stain showing bacteria (picture above right)

Name	Predilection and Clinical Key Features	Histopathology
Staphylococcal "scalded skin" syndrome (SSSS)	• "Ritter's disease" or "pemphigus neonatorum" in neonates • Usually infants and children <6 • Face, neck (not mucosa typically, like SJS/TEN) • Preceding URI, conjunctivitis, or carrier state • Sudden onset of skin tenderness and scarlatiniform eruption then large, flaccid bullae; positive Nikolsky sign; desquamation of large areas • *S. aureus*, phage II; exfoliative toxins A and B (more often type B) (toxin targets desmoglein 1)	• No bacteria visible; subcorneal splitting (granular layer) of epidermis with sparse neutrophils and few acantholytic cells; sparse mixed infiltrate in dermis • Due to distant site production of exfoliative toxin
Staphylococcal toxic shock syndrome	• 15–35 years old • Seen with tampon usage in menstruating women; wound infections • Erythrodermic, macular rash, sudden fever, Systemic systems (F/C/N/V), shock; mucosal inflammation • Negative blood culture since due to toxin • Strain of *S. aureus* releases TSST-1 (acts as "superantigen" seen in menstrual causes) and enterotoxins B and C (seen in 50% of non-menstrual causes)	• Foci of spongiosis with few neutrophils; degenerate keratinocytes; superficial perivascular/interstitial mixed infiltrate; vasculitis but lacks fibrin
Streptococcal toxic shock syndrome	• Adults • Occurs in setting of a deep soft tissue infection (50% of cases have unknown source) • Severe pain in extremity (different to *Staph.* TST); fever; shock, organ failure • Positive streptococcal bacteremia (60%) • Group A streptococci (*S. pyogenes*) exotoxin and M protein act as "superantigens" to immune system • Tx = supportive; often includes clindamycin (may inhibit bacterial toxin production)	• Similar to ecthyma gangrenosum with necrosis of epidermis/dermis; hemorrhage in dermis; mixed inflammatory infiltrate; vasculitis
Perianal streptococcal dermatitis	• "Perianal cellulitis" • Child (7 months to 8 years); possibly after URI • Perianal area • Well-demarcated, erythema perianally with desquamating scale; may precipitate guttate psoriasis • Group A β-hemolytic streptococci	

Name	Predilection and Clinical Key Features	Histopathology
Ecthyma	• Means "pustule" • Infection that extends partially into dermis (deeper than impetigo) • Children • Extremities • Often due to Group A streptococci (*S. pyogenes*) • Vesicopustule that develops "punched-out" necrotic base • No systemic symptoms	• Gram+ cocci; ulceration of skin with inflammatory crust; heavy infiltrate of neutrophils in reticular dermis (base of ulcer)
Ecthyma gangrenosum	• Severe variant of ecthyma • Often seen in immunosuppressed patients with septicemia • Due to *Pseudomonas aeruginosa* • Purpuric macule that becomes hemorrhagic bulla then an ulcer with central gray–black eschar; septicemia causes fever, hypotension, tachycardia also	• Numerous Gram− bacteria; necrosis of epidermis/ dermis; hemorrhage in dermis; mixed inflammatory infiltrate; vasculitis

Name	Predilection and Clinical Key Features	Histopathology
Deep pyogenic infections (cellulitis)		
Erysipelas	• Type of superficial cellulitis involving the deep dermis and lymphatics • Lower extremities, face • Well-defined, tender erythema with an elevated border and spreads rapidly; possibly vesicles at edge of lesion; + lymphadenopathy • Often due to Group A streptococci (*S. pyogenes*) • Possible Tx = PCN or erythromycin (PCN-allergy)	• Subepidermal edema with possible vesiculobullous lesion formation; heavy infiltrate of neutrophils (but no abscesses)
Erysipeloid	• "Diamond skin disease" • Meat and fish handlers • Web area of fingers; hands, but spares terminal phalanges • Red area involving finger web areas; possible systemic variant • Due to *Erysipelothrix rhusiopathiae* (Gram+), contaminates dead organic matter (meat, fish) • Possible Tx = PCN or erythromycin	• Massive edema of papillary dermis overlying a diffuse, mixed infiltrate
Blistering distal dactylitis	• Uncommon infection localized to the volar fat pad of distal phalanx of fingers/toes • Due to massive subepidermal edema • Most commonly due to Group A streptococci	

Cellulitis	• Poorly demarcated dermal and subcutaneous infection
	
	• Tender, erythematous, ill-defined area (rubor, dolor, calor, tumor), may be due to:
	  • *Staph. aureus* (children)
	  • *Haemophilus influenzae* B (child's facial area)
	  • group A streptococci (adults)
	  • *Vibrio vulnificus* (extremity)
	  • *Pasteurella multocida* (cat bites)
	  • *Eikenella corrodens* (fist fight, human bite)
		• Similar erysipelas with edema and heavy infiltrate; infiltrate involves subcutis and may lead to a septal panniculitis

Name	Predilection and Clinical Key Features	Histopathology
Necrotizing fasciitis	• Rare form of cellulitis ("flesh-eating bacteria") involving deeper tissue and possibly the muscle • Legs • Poorly defined erythema; serosanguineous blisters; necrosis; Possible systemic symptoms • Mixed infection (#1 cause), group A streptococci (10%), *Pseudomonas*, *Staphylococcus*, etc. • Fournier's gangrene = necrotizing fasciitis involving perineum/scrotum, usually in elderly men	• Vasculitis with inflammation of vessel walls; thrombi; mixed inflammatory cells; necrosis of epidermis, dermis, and upper subcutis
Clostridial myonecrosis ("gas gangrene")	• Deep anaerobic cellulitis (muscle and soft tissue necrosis) • Elderly (diabetes or vascular disease); postoperative GI surgery • Foul smelling, painful necrotic nodule, toxic, brown-fluid bullae; sometimes crepitus • *Clostridium perfringens*, toxins (α-toxin and perfringolysin) damage deeper tissue	
Progressive bacterial synergistic gangrene	• "Meleney's ulcer" • Usually in operative wounds • Indurated, ulcerated areas with a gangrenous margin • Mixed growth of peptostreptococcus and *Staph. aureus* or Enterobacteriaceae	
Erosive pustular dermatosis	• Elderly • Sun-damaged scalp • Widespread erosions and crusted papules that result in scarring alopecia	
Blastomycosis-like pyoderma	• Large verrucous plaque studded with multiple pustules and draining sinuses • *Staphylococcus aureus* and *Pseudomonas* are often isolated from tissue	• Heavy infiltrate with small abscesses; few granulomas; pseudoepitheliomatous hyperplasia; intraepidermal microabscesses; in some variants solar elastosis

Name	Predilection and Clinical Key Features	Histopathology
Corynebacterial infections (Gram+ bacilli)		
Diphtheria	• Rare cutaneous infection in tropics • "Punched-out" ulcer with well-defined, irregular margins; gray slough covering base; possibly severe lymphadenitis • *Corynebacterium diphtheriae* (Gram+), more commonly causes pharyngitis with a pseudomembrane	• Necrosis of epidermis and dermis; bacilli visible; necrotic base
Erythrasma [PAS, methenamine silver, Giemsa]	• Superficial, localized bacterial infection in moist areas and skin folds • Elderly, diabetics, and obese individuals • Axilla, groin, and often in toe webs of diabetics • Irregular, well-defined, red patch with a fine scale that develops a brown patch, often asymptomatic • Due to *Corynebacterium minutissimum* (Gram+ diphtheroid) • Wood's lamp shows coral–red fluorescence (due to bacteria creating water-soluble coproporphyrin III) • Possible Tx = topical erythromycin or 1% clindamycin (may treat orally for multiple plaques)	• Often normal appearance (one of "invisible dermatosis") • Gram and PAS stain reveal rod-like bacteria in the superficial stratum corneum
Trichomycosis	• Axillary and pubic hair bacterial infection • Hair shafts with yellow–brown concretions; red staining sweat, odor • Usually due to *Corynebacteria tenuis* (normal flora), and possibly other species • Possible Tx = shave hair, antibacterial soap/peroxide	

Name	Predilection and Clinical Key Features	Histopathology
Pitted keratolysis [Methenamine silver stain]	• Superficial bacterial infection of stratum corneum that causes pitting on feet (rarely hands/palms) • Hot climate; moist feet (i.e. hyperhidrosis) • Plantar surface of feet, especially pressure points • Multiple, painless, "punched-out" depressions on feet; possibly brownish discoloration causing dirt-impregnated appearance; odor • Often due to *Kytococcus sedentarius* (old name, *Micrococcus sedentarius*) and *Corynebacterium* species which produce proteases that degrade keratin	• Multiple crateriform defects in stratum corneum with areas of pallor; base and margins of pits have fine filamentous and coccoid organisms

Name	Predilection and Clinical Key Features	Histopathology
Neisserial infections		
Meningococcal infections	• Infants (6–12 months) and young adults • Increased risk if asplenia or C5, 6, 7, 8 deficiency • Erythematous macules, nodules, petechiae; hemorrhagic lesions if purpura fulminans • *Neisseria meningitidis* • Possible Tx = IV PCN or chloramphenicol (PCN-allergy); consider treating contacts with prophylactic rifampin	• Acute vasculitis with fibrin thrombi and extravasation of fibrin; neutrophils in and around vessels

Gonococcal infections (GC)	• *Neisseria gonorrhea* (Gram negative diplococci with fibrillar pili)
	• Variants:
	  • Acute, classic GC (urethritis)
	  • Disseminated GC (acral necrotic, hemorrhagic pustule, fever, oligoarthritis
	  • Ophthalmia neonatorum
	  • Extragenital GC
	• Fitz–Hugh–Curtis syndrome: PID (pelvic inflammatory disease) + perihepatitis (RUQ pain)
		• Pustules and epidermal necrosis; extravasated RBCs and thrombi; possibly Gram negative intracellular diplococci found

Mycobacterial infections		
Tuberculosis overall	• *Mycobacterium tuberculosis* (acid-fast bacilli or AFB) • May have cutaneous involvement by either exogenous exposure or internal contiguous involvement	
Primary tuberculosis	• "Tuberculosis chancre" • Primary exogenous infection in a non-sensitized host, i.e. no previous exposure • Weak immunity • Painless, red–brown papule that ulcerates ("tuberculoid chancre"); regional lymphadenopathy (LAD)	• Mixed infiltrate (neutrophils, lymphocytes, and plasma cells); superfical necrosis and ulceration; later tuberculoid granulomas with possible caseation necrosis • AFB easily found; but few if granuloma develops

Name	Predilection and Clinical Key Features	Histopathology
Lupus vulgaris	• Hematogenous spread from distant TB site (#1 type of reinfection TB) • Strong immunity • Young adults • Head and neck, penis • Multiple, brown–red papules forming a plaque with "apple-jelly" appearance with diascopy • May develop contractures, lymphedema, SCC	• Dermal tuberculoid granulomas with little/no caseation; prominent Langhans cells; AFB not usually found
Tuberculosis verrucosa cutis	• "Warty tuberculosis" • Exogenous reinfection in a sensitized host (most common skin TB) • Strong immunity • Back of hand/finger, legs • Solitary, purulent verrucous plaque; occupational contact typically (e.g. autopsy)	• Hyperkeratosis and hyperplasia of epidermis; intraepithelial neutrophilic microabscesses; caseating granulomas; AFB may be found

Name	Predilection and Clinical Key Features	Histopathology
Scrofuloderma	• Contiguous, direct extension to skin from underlying focus (i.e. node or bone) • Low immunity • Neck, submandibular area • Undermined ulcer or discharging sinus; bluish borders; surrounding induration; dusky, red color • Atypical mycobacteria are often the cause	• Epidermis atrophic or ulcerated; underlying abscess surrounded by mainly histiocytic infiltrate; granulomas at periphery of necrotic tissue; AFB found in smear but not always in tissue Fite stain (above)

Name	Predilection and Clinical Key Features	Histopathology
Orificial tuberculosis	• Spread by autoinoculation from advanced internal TB (usually lung) • Low immunity • Shallow ulcers in mouth	• Ulceration with underlying caseating granuloma • Numerous AFB found
Disseminated miliary cutaneous tuberculosis	• Hematogenous spread from lungs, meninges, etc. • Low immunity • Children and immunosuppressed • Disseminated, small, red macules/papules that become necrotic and form small ulcers	• Numerous AFB in a neutrophil abscess surrounded by histiocytes

Tuberculids (Id reaction)	• Hypersensitivity reaction to TB antigens due to distant active infection elsewhere; as a result, not able to isolate bacteria in lesions. High immunity, but also allergic sensitivity to bacteria
	• Variants:
	  1. Papulonecrotic eruption (most common):
	    • children
	    • extremities, buttocks
	    • recurrrent, dusky-red papules with necrosis; heal with varioliform scars
	    • HP = ulceration and "V-shaped" area of necrosis; surrounding palisade of histiocytes and inflammatory cells; well-formed granulomas; vasculitis
	  2. Erythema induratum of Bazin:
	    • women (90%)
	    • lower legs, especially calves
	    • bluish–red plaques and nodules
	    • HP = lobular panniculitis (difficult to distinguish from nodular vasculitis)
	  3. Lichen scrofulosorum
	    • children to young adults
	    • trunk area
	    • asymptomatic, perifollicular and lichenoid-like papule
	    • HP = perifollicular and eccrine inflammation; granulomas (not lichenoid in appearance)	

Name	Predilection and Clinical Key Features	Histopathology
Atypical (non-tuberculous) mycobacteria		
Mycobacterium ulcerans infection [Ziehl–Neelsen]	• "Buruli ulcer" • Children to young adults • Central Africa (wetlands) • Lower part of legs • Papule/pustule that forms a painless ulcer with an undermined edge • *M. ulcerans* produces an exotoxin that results in an ulcer • Possible Tx = often excision	• Extensive "coagulative" necrosis in dermis and fat with little inflammation; extracellular AFB present
Mycobacterium marinum infection	• "Swimming pool granuloma" • Hands, elbows, knees • Solitary, verrucoid nodules/plaques; 1–2 weeks after trauma in water environment • May form "sporotrichoid" appearance with lesions along lymphatics • Organism in pools, aquariums, and brackish water • Organism unable to multiply at higher internal temperature, so stays in the skin	• Epidermis varies (ulceration, acanthosis, pseudoepitheliomatous hyperplasia); abscesses and poorly formed granulomas with no caseation; chronic inflammatory infiltrate

Name	Predilection and Clinical Key Features	Histopathology
Mycobacterium fortuitum and chelonae/ abscessus	• Group of rapid growers including *Mycobacterium fortuitum, M. chelonae*, and *M. abscessus* • Found in soil, dust, and water • Most common form = post-injection abscess • Multiple erythematous nodules in distal extremity or "sporotrichoid-like" pattern	• Ill-defined granulomas with necrotic foci; bacilli easily seen in clusters

Name	Predilection and Clinical Key Features	Histopathology
Mycobacterium avium intracellulare	• Slow grower; found in water, soil, and dairy products • Found in water, soil and dairy products • Immunocompromised hosts • Causes chronic pulmonary infection; multiple purulent leg ulcers	 • Fite stain (photo above)

Name	Predilection and Clinical Key Features	Histopathology
Leprosy or "Hansen's disease"		
Mycobacterium leprae, Gram+ obligate intercellular bacteria, which are acid-fast and stain with Fite stain and Ziehl–Neelsen stain • Spreads to close contacts by aerosol spread from nasal or oral mucosa; incubation average = 5 years • Infects mainly skin, nasal mucosa, and peripheral nerves (parasites live in macrophages and Schwann cells); found in cool skin areas (grows at 35°C): if affecting nerves, then first sensation lost = temperature sensation • May grow *M. leprae* in mice footpads and nine-banded armadillo • Prevalent in tropical countries; India has two-thirds of the cases		
Indeterminate leprosy	• Initial infection with type of response not declared • Limbs • Solitary, hypopigmented or faintly red lesion; sensation normal • Heals spontaneously but in 25% progresses to develop one of determinate types described below	• Superficial and deep lymphocytic infiltrate around vessels, nerves, and dermal appendages; prominent mast cells (high suspicion needed for diagnosis) 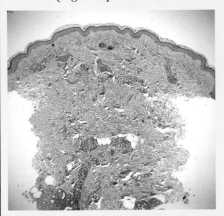 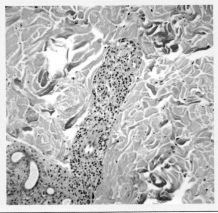

Name	Predilection and Clinical Key Features	Histopathology
Borderline leprosy (BB)	• Immune response beginning, but not definitive • Unstable form • Numerous lesions; asymmetric lesions with ill-defined margins on erythematous or copper-colored patches often annular; moderate decreased sensation	• Poorly defined epithelioid granulomas lacking Langhans giant cells; uninvolved subepidermal zone (grenz zone); AFB present
Borderline-lepromatous leprosy	• More lesions, shiny and less well-defined • Collections of macrophages rather than epithelioid cells; grenz zone present; variable lymphocytes	

Name	Predilection and Clinical Key Features	Histopathology
Lepromatous leprosy (LL)	• "Low cell-immunity + numerous bacilli" • TH2 (antibody-mediated) response, especially IL-4, IL-5, IL-10, IL-13 • Incubation = 10 years • Generalized, symmetric, macular lesions; no loss of sensation; normal sweating in area; lateral eyebrow alopecia; saddle-nose deformity	• Diffuse infiltrate of foamy macrophages in dermis with a grenz zone; numerous AFB in macrophages or large clumps (globi) • Virchow cells are macrophages with bacilli • Numerous organisms in dermis and nasal secretions Virchow cells (above)
Borderline-tuberculoid leprosy	• More numerous and smaller lesions than tuberculoid leprosy • Hypoesthesia and hair growth impairment in lesion common	• Grenz zone (unlike tuberculoid leprosy); tubercle formation less evident and less nerve destruction than tuberculoid leprosy

Name	Predilection and Clinical Key Features	Histopathology
Tuberculoid leprosy (TT)	• "Strong cell-immunity + no bacilli seen" • TH1 (cell-mediated) response, especially IFN-γ, IL-2, IL-12 • #1 type in India and Africa • Neural involvement common (especially greater auricular, common peroneal, ulnar, radial, and posterior tibial) • Incubation = 4 years • Few, well-demarcated asymmetric lesions (<3); usually single, red plaque with atrophic center; lesions may be hypohidrotic and hairless • Decreased sensation and enlarged nerve may be seen	• Non-caseating epithelioid granulomas in papillary dermis and around neurovascular structures; Langhans giant cells; no grenz zone; do not see organisms (>50% cases)
Tuberculoid leprosy (TT)	• "Strong cell-immunity + no bacilli seen" • TH1 (cell-mediated) response, especially IFN-γ, IL-2, IL-12	

Name	Predilection and Clinical Key Features	Histopathology
Histoid leprosy	• Nodular variant of lepromatous leprosy • Numerous brown papules and nodules on apparently normal skin	• Mimics a fibrohistiocytic tumor with spindle-shaped cells in a storiform pattern; circumscribed nodular lesion; numerous AFB in cells
Lepra reaction or type I reaction	• Cause = type IV hypersensitivity reaction • Occurs in borderline leprosy when a shift ("upgrade" or "downgrade") occurs toward another type • Seen in patients during first 6 months of treatment, pregnancy, stress, etc. • Increased erythema, edema, inflamed lesions, tenderness • Possible Tx = prednisone	• Edema, increased lymphocytes
Erythema nodosum leprosum or type II reaction	• Cause = immune complex-mediated vasculitis • Seen in 25–70% of lepromatous leprosy patients • Extremities, face • Bright red, painful nodules on extremities and face • Possible Tx = thalidomide	• "Erythema nodosum + vasculitis" • Edema of papillary dermis; mixed infiltrate; vasculitis • DIF = C3 and IgG in dermal vessels' walls

Name	Predilection and Clinical Key Features	Histopathology
Lucio's phenomenon	• "Small vessel vasculitis + thrombotic phenomenon" • Diffuse non-nodular form of lepromatous leprosy • Mexican ethnicity • Hemorrhagic ulcers form as a result of necrotizing vasculitis or vascular occlusion due to endothelial swelling/thrombosis	• Necrotizing vasculitis of vessels in upper and mid-dermis; or possible endothelial swelling and thrombosis of vessels without a vasculitis
Miscellaneous bacterial infections		
Anthrax ("Woolsorter's disease")	• Animal handlers, terrorists • Purpuric macule/papule on exposed area • Forms vesicle which ulcerates and forms painless central black eschar (differs from Brown recluse bite that is painful) • *Bacillus anthracis* (95% cutaneous, 5% inhaled/GI) • Edema toxin (increased cAMP, causes edema and impairs neutrophil function); lethal toxin (increases TNF-α, IL-1) • Tx = antibiotics; do not treat by surgical excision due to risk of spreading	• Necrosis of epidermis/upper dermis; hemorrhage; dilated vessels; sparse infiltrate; spongiosis; large, square-cut bacteria in chains

Name	Predilection and Clinical Key Features	Histopathology
Brucellosis	<ul><li>"Malta fever"</li><li>Farmers; ingesting non-pasteurized goat milk/cheese</li><li>5–10% brucellosis patients have cutaneous involvement</li><li>Varies clinically = disseminated papulonodular eruption, maculopapular rash, or erythema nodosum-like lesions; fever, headache, arthralgia, hepatosplenomegaly; malodorous perspiration (pathognomonic)</li></ul>	<ul><li>Variants:<ul><li>Papulonodular = lymphocytes, histiocytes; focal granulomas</li><li>Maculopapular = non-specific with mild infiltrate in upper dermis</li><li>Erythema nodosum-like = septal panniculitis with infiltrate into fat lobules; plasma cells</li></ul></li></ul>
Yersiniosis	<ul><li>*Yersinia pseudotuberculosis*, *Y. enterocolitica*</li><li>Erythema nodosum-like lesions, erythema multiforme-like</li></ul>	<ul><li>Erythema nodosum-like = septal panniculitis with extension into fat lobules; necrotizing vasculitis</li></ul>
Granuloma inguinale [Warthin–Starry, Wright, and Giemsa stains]	<ul><li>"Donovanosis"</li><li>*Klebsiella granulomatis* (old name = *Calymmatobacterium granulomatis*)</li><li>Papule that becomes a painless, beefy, red ulcer (very vascular) without lymphadenopathy (LAD)</li><li>Possible Tx = doxycycline × 3 weeks</li></ul>	<ul><li>Ulcerated; plasma cells and macrophages in base of ulcer; prominent vessels; margins with pseudoepitheliomatous hyperplasia; Donovan bodies (mononuclear cells with intracytoplasmic vacuoles packed with bacteria); Giemsa or Leishman stains</li></ul>
Chancroid [Giemsa or Warthin–Starry stains]	<ul><li>*Haemophilus ducreyi* ("railroad track" or "school of fish" appearance)</li><li>Painful, irregular-edged ulcer with tender, suppurative LAD</li><li>Possible Tx = azithromycin or ceftriaxone</li><li>Watch for co-infection with HSV and syphilis</li></ul>	<ul><li>Broad ulceration, base of ulcer with three zones:<ol><li>Tissue necrosis, fibrin, RBC and neutrophils</li><li>Vascular proliferation, prominent endothelial and mixed infiltrate cells</li><li>Deepest zone with plasma cells, lymphocytes</li></ol></li></ul>

Name	Predilection and Clinical Key Features	Histopathology
Rhinoscleroma [Warthin–Starry, PAS, Gram stains]	• Opportunistic infection of nasal airways • Endemic in parts of Africa, Asia, and Latin America • Non-specific rhinitis with purulent discharge; then hypertrophy of membranes with a nodular stage, scarring and then deformities ("Hebra-nose" deformity) • Due to *Klebsiella rhinoscleromatis*	• Granulomatous reaction pattern • Mikulicz cells (pictured above) = macrophages with vacuolated cytoplasm • Plasma cells with Russell bodies (pictured above), which are eosinophilic, inclusions containing immunoglobulins

Name	Predilection and Clinical Key Features	Histopathology
Tularemia	• "Rabbit fever" • Laboratory workers with animals • Ulceroglandular variant is most common (papule formation at rabbit or tick bite location with ascending lymphangitis and nodule formation along lymphatics, fever) • Possible Tx = streptomycin (possibly Jarisch–Herxheimer reaction) • *Francisella tularensis* (Gram− bacterium) • Transmitted by: • bite (deer fly or tick) or • contact with infected rodent/rabbit	• Ulcer with necrosis; adjacent epidermis is acanthotic with spongiosis; do not see causative organism
Listeriosis	• Rare infection of neonates, elderly, immunocompromised • Papular/pustular or purpuric lesions; bacteremia with/without meningitis • *Listeria monocytogenes* (Gram+ bacterium)	• Mild spongiosis with lymphocyte exocytosis; pustular lesions with neutrophils; mixed infiltrate; Gram+ coccobacilli in macrophages
Cat-scratch disease [Silver stains, such as Warthin–Starry]	• Site of cat scratch • Papule or crusted nodule followed 2 weeks later with regional LAD; possible systemic symptoms • *Bartonella henselae* (binds to feline RBCs, invades endothelium, produces an endothelium cell-stimulating factor)	• Zone of necrosis in upper dermis; surrounded by mantle of macrophages and lymphocytes; granulomas; necrobiosis

Name	Predilection and Clinical Key Features	Histopathology
Bartonellosis (Carrion's disease)	• *Bartonella bacilliformis*, invades RBCs and forms Rocha–Lima inclusions • Peru, Columbia • Transmission: *Lutzomyia sand fly* (old name *Phlebotomus*) • Variants: • Oroya fever = fever, hemolytic anemia • Verruga peruana = If survive Oroya fever, develop benign, disfiguring verruga lesions	
Trench fever	• "Five day fever" or "Quintan fever" • *Bartonella quintana* • Transmission: human body louse • Relapsing at 5-day intervals, headache, malaise, pain in long bones, macular rash • Seen mainly during WWI, but now urban areas, especially in poor living conditions	
Bacillary angiomatosis	• "Disseminated cat-scatch fever" • Immunocompromised patients • Caused by infection with *Bartonella henselae* or *B. quintana*, which produce an endothelial cell-stimulating factor • Red vascular papule • Possible Tx = erythromycin (macrolide)	• Clumps of bacilli; subcutaneous vascular proliferations with plump endothelial cells

Name	Predilection and Clinical Key Features	Histopathology

Malakoplakia
 	
[von Kossa stain, Perls' stain, PAS]
	• Acquired inflammatory, granulomatous condition usually involving a urogenital tract (bladder) infection, but may also involve skin in perianal, inguinal, and abdominal area
	• Cutaneous malakoplakia seen in patients who are immunocompromised and/or defect in macrophage function
	• Rarely cutaneous = perianal, inguinal areas
	• Yellow to pink papule/plaque; may have drainage of abscess/sinus
	• Possibly due to acquired defect in destruction of phagocytosed bacteria (especially *Escherichia coli, Staph. aureus*) and inadequate bacterial death by macrophages/monocytes exhibiting defective phagolysosome activity (partially digested bacteria)
		• Chronic inflammatory process with closely packed macrophages with von Hansemann cells and Michaelis–Gutmann bodies:
		  • von Hansemann cells:
		    • foamy histiocytes with fine eosinophilic cytoplasmic granules and the cells stain with CD68, lysozyme, and α1-antitrypsin
		    • PAS-positive diastase-resistant inclusions
		  • Michaelis–Gutmann bodies:
		    • "targetoid," pale-blue, laminated, intracytoplasmic, phagolysosome concretions within histiocytes
		    • result from partially digested bacteria accumulated in macrophages and lead to deposition of calcium and iron on residual bacterial glycolipids
		    • von Kossa and Perls' stain show Michaelis–Gutmann bodies

"Sago palm" disease	• "Sepik granuloma" (from Sepik district of New Guinea) • Extremities, face • Multiple cutaneous nodules on extremities, face • Follows injury by sago palm (*Metroxylon*)	• Diffuse dermal mixed infiltrate with large foamy histiocytes; amorphous pink material with gray, round dots (Gram+ organism, unable to culture or identify)
Chlamydial infections		
Psittacosis	• Pneumonia illness from infected birds; may develop various cutaneous symptoms (morbilliform rash, erythema nodosum, etc.) • *Chlamydia psittaci*	

Lymphogranuloma venereum	• *Chlamydia trachomatis* serovars L1-3
	• More common in Asia, Africa, South America
	
	• Painless lesion + inguinal lymphadenopathy (LAD)
	• "Groove sign" = LAD above/below Poupart ligament (forms groove appearance)
	• Possible Tx = doxycycline × 3 weeks
		• Three clinical stages:
		  1. Primary = papule, vesicle (not usually biopsied)
		  2. Secondary = regional LAD, buboes with draining sinus
		  3. Tertiary = rectal strictures, fistula, genital elephantiasis
		
		• Second stage has characteristic lesion in lymph nodes: stellate abscess with poorly formed palisade of epithelioid cells and histiocytes; sinus formation; fibrosis in later lesions

Name	Predilection and Clinical Key Features	Histopathology
Rickettsial infections		
• *Rickettsia* = Gram negative bacilli (intracellular only) • Targets endothelial cells causing a vasculitis • Possible Tx for infections = tetracycline/doxycycline		
Rocky Mountain spotted fever [Giemsa stain, *Rickettsia* DIF best]	• Vasculitis caused by infection of endothelial cells • *Rickettsia rickettsii* • Transmission by ticks: *Dermacentor andersoni* or *variabilis* tick • Acute fever and morbilliform rash with central petechiae (starts acral and then spreads centripetally) • Possible Tx = doxycycline (consider even in children <8) or chloramphenicol (especially in pregnancy)	• Vasculitis (due to vascular endothelium invasion by bacteria) with extravasated RBC and thrombi; dermal edema; epidermal necrosis and spongiosis at initial bite location

Name	Disease	Organism	Mode of Transmission
Rickettsia, spotted fever group	Rocky Mountain spotted fever	*R. rickettsii*	*Dermacentor* tick bite
	Boutonneuse fever or Mediterranean spotted fever	*R. conorii*	Tick bite
	Rickettsialpox	*R. akari*	Mite bite (house mouse); spotted fever that is not due to a tick bite
	Siberian tick typhus	*R. sibirica*	Tick bite
	Queensland tick typhus	*R. australis*	Tick bite
Rickettsia, typhus group	Epidemic typhus	*R. prowazakii*	*Pediculus humanus corporis* (body louse) feces
	Murine typhus	*R. mooseri* (*typhi*)	Flea feces
	Scrub typhus	*Orientia tsutsugamushi* (formerly *Rickettsia*)	Mite (chigger)
	Endemic typhus	*R. typhi*	Rat flea (*Xenopsylla cheopis*)
Q fever	• Cause = *Coxiella burnetii* (no longer classified as *Rickettsia*) • Transmission = aerosol • Do not usually result in cutaneous lesions		

Name	Predilection and Clinical Key Features	Histopathology
Miscellaneous infections		
Glanders	• Horse handlers, veterinarians • *Burkholderia mallei* (Gram− bacterium) (old name *Pseudomonas mallei*) • Bacterium produces an exotoxin • Multiple, purulent nodules along the lymphatic vessels ("farcy buds"); lymphadenopathy and fever; may cause pulmonary infection with cough and discharge • Can be fatal, if untreated • Possible Tx: • Antibiotics (such as streptomycin, tetracycline) • Excision	Diagnosed by clinical laboratory tests and clinical suspicion
Melioidosis	• "Whitmore's disease" • Similar to glanders • *Burkholderia pseudomallei* (Gram− bacterium), (old name *Pseudomonas pseudomallei*) • Bacterium found in soil and water	

24 Spirochetal Infections

Secondary syphilis

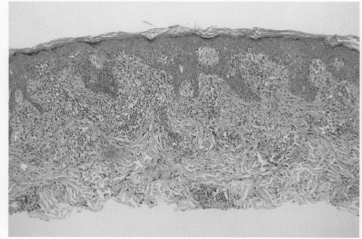
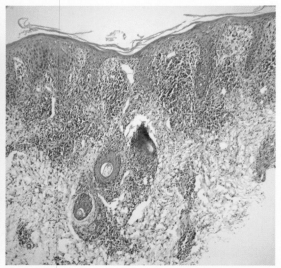

Name	Predilection and Clinical Features	Histopathology
Treponematoses (Syphilis = *Treponema pallidum*)		

Congenital syphilis	• Usually a result of transplacental infection of the fetus from an infected mother
	• Early congenital syphilis:
	  • Prematurity, low birth weight, rhinorrhea, and mucocutaneous lesions
	  • Macular rash, vesiculobullous or scaling lesions
	  • Predominantly on the palms and soles
	• Late congenital syphilis:
	  • Interstitial keratitis, neurosyphilis, bone and cardiovascular disease
	  • Hutchinson's notched incisors, Mulberry molars	

Primary syphilis	• 2–6 weeks after infection with *Treponema pallidum* • Genital area • Painless papule with clean base; fever; non-tender lymphadenopathy (not suppurative) • Heals with stellate or nondescript scar • Possible Tx = PCN intramuscularly (IM)	• Chancre: ulceration of epidermis; plasma cells; diffuse infiltrate; endothelial swelling of vessels; acanthosis at periphery; numerous spirochetes (especially near vessels) • Warthin–Starry stain, or darkfield microscopy aid diagnosis

Name	Predilection and Clinical Features	Histopathology
Secondary syphilis	• Occurs up to 6 months after chancre heals • Occurs anywhere on body, including palms and soles • "Great imitator" clinically • May present as: generalized, non-pruritic papulosquamous rash (80%); lichenoid rash; condylomata lata; "moth-eaten" alopecia; hypomelanosis ("necklace of Venus") • Possible Tx = PCN IM	• Varies tremendously histologically: • Plasma cells/endothelial swelling may be sparse/absent • May be lichenoid, psoriasiform, granulomatous, etc. • *T. pallidum* may be identified with silver stains such as Warthin–Starry stain or by immunoperoxidase techniques
		• Organism highlighted by staining (photo above)

Name	Predilection and Clinical Features	Histopathology
Latent syphilis	• 70% latent for life • Non-infectious stage with bacteria inactive in nodes, spleen • Early (<1 year of infection) and late (>1 year of infection) stages • Late latent stage may have negative RPR	

Tertiary syphilis	• 33% develop tertiary syphilis
	• Features:
	  • Gummas (50%),
	  • Cardiovascular (25%): especially endarteritis
	  • Neurosyphilis (25%): tabes dorsalis, Argyll Robertson pupils
	• Possible Tx = PCN IM + probenecid; or aqueous PCN then benzathine PCN
		• Tuberculoid granuloma with or without caseation; plasma cells; fibrosis; do not usually see spirochetes

Endemic syphilis (bejel)	• Contagious disease in Middle East (especially Euphrates Valley) • Virtually eradicated with public health measures • Clinically similar to yaws (see below); "mucous patches" in mouth/pharynx; skin and bone lesions	• Histopathology similar to yaws (see p. 438)

Name	Predilection and Clinical Features	Histopathology

Yaws
[Warthin–Starry stain]
	• "Frambesia"
	• Contagious, tropical, non-venereal infection
	• Teenager
	• Tropical areas
	• Lower extremities
	• Red, painless papule that ulcerates; may form tracts to bone lesions
	• Bone lesions
	• No other systemic symptoms
	• *Treponema pallidum pertenue*
	• (Same serology tests as syphilis)
	• Stages:
	  1. Primary stage = papule forms chronic ulcerating papillomatous mass
	  2. Secondary stage = widespread lesions with a discharge
	  3. Tertiary stage (years) = chonic gummatous ulcers usually on face or over long bones (with involvement common);
		• Primary and secondary lesions = prominent hyperplasia with scale crust (pink–red color on H & E); intraepidermal abscess; heavy mixed infiltrate (including plasma cells)
		• [Warthin–Starry stain finds organism in epidermis, unlike *T. pallidum* in upper dermis]

Pinta	• "Carate"
	• Contagious non-venereal infection (cutaneously)
	• Caribbean, central/South America
	• *Treponema pallidum carateum*
	• Skin-to-skin transmission
	• Overlap of clinical stages common:
	  • Cutaneous lesions only (no systemic involvement)
	  • Small macule/papule surrounded by red halo that forms plaques with variety of colors
	  • Later stage forms symmetric, depigmented, vitiligo-like lesions
	
	• Secondary stage (pictured above)
		• Primary and secondary lesions = hyperkeratosis, parakeratosis and acanthosis; exocytosis of inflammatory cells; mixed superficial and perivascular infiltrate (including plasma cells); treponemes found in upper epidermis (rarely in dermis)
		• [Warthin–Starry stain finds organism in epidermis, unlike *T. pallidum* in upper dermis]

Name	Predilection and Clinical Features	Histopathology
Borrelioses		
Erythema chronicum migrans	<ul><li>"Lyme disease"</li><li>*Borrelia burgdorferi*</li><li>Transmission: Ticks (*Ixodes scapularis* or *dammini*)</li><li>May develop to multisystem disease (Lyme) and involve joints, CNS, cardiac</li><li>Centrifugally spreading erythematous lesion at tick bite site (within 3 months)</li><li>Possible TX = Doxycycline (children, Amoxicillin)</li></ul>	<ul><li>Suuperficial and deep perivascular and interstitial infiltrate (mainly lymphocytes); some plasma cells; eosinophils prominent adjacent to bite location [Warthin-Starry stain (find along DEJ)]</li></ul>
Acrodermatitis chronica atrophicans	<ul><li>Third or late stage manifestation of European lyme disease</li><li>Europe (rarely seen in US)</li><li>Elderly and females</li><li>*Borrelia afzelii* (most common cause)</li><li>Initially, soft, painless, bluish–red discoloration with swelling on distal extremities and around joints</li><li>Months to years later form red–brown discoloration and thin, "cigarette paper-like," translucent skin (atrophic phase); may form juxta-articular fibrotic nodules or bands on extensor surfaces (elbows, knees)</li><li>Associated with lymphoma</li></ul>	<ul><li>Early stages = superficial and deep lymphocytic infiltrate (some histiocytes, plasma cells); accentuation around vessels and adnexa; vacuoles that resemble fat cells in upper dermis</li></ul> <ul><li>Later stages = atrophy of dermis and epidermis (loss of rete ridges); loss of elastic fibers and pilosebaceous follicles; nodules show homogeneous collagen enclosing islands of fatty tissue</li></ul>
Borrelia-associated B-cell lymphoma	<ul><li>Lymphoma may occur in skin affected by acrodermatitis chronica atrophicans</li><li>20% of cutaneous B-cell lymphomas can identify *Borrelia burgdorferi* present</li></ul>	

25 Mycoses and Algal Infections

Chromoblastomycosis

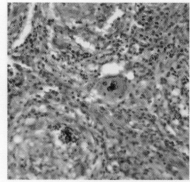
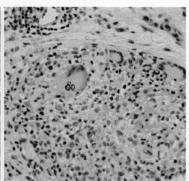

Common fungus stains

- PAS = stains cell wall purple
- Gomori–Grocott methenamine silver (GMS) stain = stains fungi black against a green background
- Mucicarmine or alcian blue stain capsules (i.e. *Cryptococcus neoformans*)
- Calcofluor white = imparts bright fluorescence to fungi under fluorescence microscopy

Name	Predilection and Clinical Key Features	Histopathology
Superficial filamentous infections		
Dermatophytoses overall	• Tinea has hyphae without budding yeast • Ability to invade	• Three genera: • *Epidermophyton* • *Microsporum* • *Trichophyton* • Ecological groups: • Anthropophilic • Zoophilic • Geographic
Tinea capitis	• Most common cause = *T. tonsurans*, *T. violaceum* • Children • Varies clinically; mild erythema with scaling to pustules and folliculitis on scalp; alopecia • Endothrix infection ("black dot" hair stubs), such as *T. tonsurans* and *T. violaceum*; does not fluoresce with Wood's lamp • Ectothrix fungi may fluoresce green, such as *M. canis* or *M. audouinii*	• Perifollicular neutrophils; spongiotic epidermis; may develop suppurative folliculitis or a granulomatous process • Endothrix with fungus seen in the hair shaft (above)

Name	Predilection and Clinical Key Features	Histopathology
Kerion	• Most common cause = *T. verrucosum*, *T. tonsurans* • Scalp • Boggy, violaceous, pustular plaque due to strong inflammatory response by host to fungi • Result of hypersensitivity reaction to the dermatophyte infection	• Heavy infiltrate present with perifollicular neutrophils or mixed infiltrate
Favus	• Most common cause = *T. schoenleinii* • Child in developing countries • Yellow crusts (scutula) overlying erythematous base; may result in localized alopecia • Infection may persist for life	• Heavy infiltrate with fungal elements
Tinea incognito	• Atypical tinea clinical presentation due to use of topical steroids 	• Similar to other tinea infections with visible fungal elements
"Id reaction"	• Secondary allergic eruption on the body (e.g. palms) palms due to a distant dermatophyte infection (especially tinea pedis)	

Name	Predilection and Clinical Key Features	Histopathology
Tinea faciei	• May be due to *T. rubrum*, *T. mentagrophytes*, *M. gypseum*, *T. tonsurans* • Facial erythema with scaling	• *T. rubrum* (most common cause) • Three changes in stratum corneum: 1. Neutrophils in epidermis 2. Compact orthokeratosis 3. "Sandwich sign" • Also see spongiosis, perifollicular neutrophils, variable inflammatory infiltrate • Commonly use GMS or PAS stains to highlight fungi
Tinea barbae, tinea corporis, and tinea cruris	• Most common cause = *T. rubrum* > *T. mentagrophytes* • Often common in groin area = *E. floccosum* • Scaly, erythematous plaques with central clearing	
Tinea pedis (athlete's foot)	• Swimmers, military personnel, marathon runners • Most commonly due to *T. rubrum* and *T. mentagrophytes* var. *interdigitale* • Scaling border, possible maceration/fissures	
Tinea manuum	• Tinea of the palms • Most common cause = *T. rubrum* • Diffuse palmar scaling with accentuation in the creases; usually accompanied by tinea pedis and onychomycosis ("two feet and one hand syndrome")	 • GMS Stain (photo above)
Tinea imbricata	• South America, South Pacific • Unique type of tinea corporis with concentric, scaly, polcyclic rings • Due to *Tinea concentricum*	• Numerous hyphae and spores in the thickened stratum corneum; underlying epidermis may show psoriasiform hyperplasia

Name	Predilection and Clinical Key Features	Histopathology
Majocchi's granuloma	• "Tinea folliculitis" • More common on the lower legs of females who are immunocompromised • Nodular, plaque-like lesion around ruptured follicles • Most common cause = T. *rubrum*, M. *canis*	• Perifollicular and dermal granulomas; chronic inflammation; reactive lymphoid follicles; fungal elements may take several forms, including yeasts, bizarre hyphae, mucinous coatings, or sometimes sparse • PAS stain (above)

Name	Predilection and Clinical Key Features	Histopathology

Onychomycosis
[GMS or PAS stain]
	Variants:
	1. Distal lateral superficial onychomycosis (DLSO)
	  • Most common cause = T. *rubrum*
	
	2. Proximal superficial onychomycosis (PSO)
	  • Most common cause = T. *rubrum*
	
	3. White superficial onychomycosis (WSO)
	  • Most common cause = T. *mentagrophytes*
	
	4. *Fusarium* onychomycosis
	  • Risk in immunocompromised patients
		• Fungal infection of the nail (40% due to dermatophytes)
		• Fungal elements seen mostly in the deeper portion of the nail plate; GMS or PAS stain will highlight the organism
		
		• GMS stain (above)

Dermatomycosis	• Fungal infections of hair, nails, or skin by non-dermatophytes with filamentous forms	

Name	Predilection and Clinical Key Features	Histopathology
Yeast infections		
Candidiasis (or candidosis) overall	• Candida has pseudohyphae (yeast in a row) and budding yeasts • Stain with PAS, GMS	
Acute superficial candidosis	• Affects moist areas, skin folds • Vesicles, pustules, and crusted erosions with beefy-red appearance; "satellite lesions"	• Neutrophils in stratum corneum; spongiform pustules or subcorneal pustules; pseudohyphae and budding yeasts in corneum
Chronic mucocutaneous candidosis	• Most common cause = C. *albicans* • Persistent mouth, vaginitis, skin, and nail infections (paronychia) • Associated with immunodeficiency and endocrinopathy syndromes (one with hypoparathyroidism and/or hyperadrenalism, and another with hypothyroidism)	• Similar to acute superficial candidosis, but more epidermal acanthosis; scale crust; spores and hyphae easily found
Disseminated systemic candidosis	• Immunosuppressed and debilitated patients, also patients with hematological disorders and neutropenia • Trunk area • Erythematous, papulonodular rash on trunk • Often due to C. *tropicalis*	• Microabscesses in upper dermis, sometimes centered on vessels; few budding yeasts may be found

Name	Predilection and Clinical Key Features	Histopathology
Candidosis of the newborn	• Congenital cutaneous candidosis: • birth or first few days • generalized erythematous macules and papulopustules (intrauterine infection) • Neonatal candidosis: • first 2 weeks of life • oral and perioral lesions (acquired during delivery) • Infantile gluteal granuloma: • specific role of candida is uncertain: diaper dermatitis is part of the spectrum • discrete granulomatous lesions in diaper area (picture below) 	
Oral candidosis	• "Thrush" • Infants, debilitated adults • May be initial manifestation of AIDS • Irregular white patches and plaques in the mouth	• Epithelial hyperplasia (characteristic feature)
Genital candidosis	• Vaginal candidosis common • Thick, creamy vaginal discharge	
Periungual candidosis	• Women who immerse hands often or are immunocompromised • Fingers (especially middle finger of dominant hand) and nails • Initially, develop paronychia with secondary penetration of keratin by fungi	
APECED	• "Autoimmune Poly-Endocrinopathy-Candidiasis-Ectodermal Dystrophy" or "Whitaker syndrome" • Type I polyglandular autoimmune syndrome • Associated with Candidiasis, hypoparathyroidism, and adrenal failure (Addison's) • Mutation = AIRE gene (autoimmune regulator)	

Name	Predilection and Clinical Key Features	Histopathology

Cryptococcosis
 	
[PAS (yeast) and alcian blue (capsule)]
	• Immunosuppressed
	• Face, neck, forearms
	• Found in dried bird (especially pigeon) and bat excreta
	• Enters body usually by respiratory tract
	
	• Purulent or necrotic nodule or plaque
	• Also may cause pulmonary granulomas and meningoencephalitis
		• Variable histology
		• Dense infiltrate with mulitnucleate giant cells containing organisms with prominent capsule; "shotgun" appearance to dermis due to mucin
		• *Cryptococcus neoformans* (doubly refractile under polarized light)
		
		• Histological stains:
		  • Central yeast = stains with PAS, silver methenamine, Fontana–Masson
		  • Capsule = stains with alcian blue, mucicarmine, and Indian ink

Name	Predilection and Clinical Key Features	Histopathology
Pityriasis versicolor [PAS, GMS]	• Upper trunk, upper arms • Red–brown (light skin) to hypopigmented (darker skin) to hyperpigmented and slightly scaly macules • Yellow fluorescence with Wood's lamp • Often due to *Malassezia globosa* (old name *M. furfur*) • Hypopigmentation due to production of dicarboxylic acid (i.e. azelaic acid) which is a competitive inhibitor of tyrosinase, causing loss of pigment • Hyperpigmentation may be due to large melanosome production, orthokeratosis, and the presence of organisms	• Hyphae and budding yeasts in stratum corneum; normal epidermis; see "spaghetti and meatballs" appearance of spores and hyphae • *Malassezia* has two forms in the yeast phase: ovoid (*Pityrosporum ovale*) and spherical (*P. orbiculare*)

Name	Predilection and Clinical Key Features	Histopathology
Pityrosporum folliculitis [PAS, GMS]	• Females (>30 years old) • Upper trunk, upper arms • Often due to *Malassezia globosa*, *M. furfur* • Associated with seborrheic dermatitis, pityriasis versicolor, Down syndrome, and pregnancy • Erythematous follicular papules and pustules; possibly pruritic	• Dilated follicle; often plugged with keratin and debris • Budding yeast in follicle (no hyphae)
Trichosporonosis	• Rare generalized blood-borne infection in immunocompromised patient, especially in leukemia/lymphoma • Purpuric papules with central necrosis; usually fatal • Due to *Trichosporon asahii* (formerly *T. beigelii*)	• Numerous slender hyphae and budding yeasts in dermis/vessel walls

White piedra	• Yeast-like fungus
	• Scalp, face, public area
	• South America
	• White to tan-colored gritty nodules along the hair shaft (less adherent than black piedra)
	• Common causes:
	  • *Trichosporon ovoides* (formerly *T. beigelii*)
	  • *Trichosporon inkin*
	  • See also p. 319
		• Nodule consists of numerous spores around

Name	Predilection and Clinical Key Features	Histopathology
Systemic mycoses		
North American blastomycosis [PAS, GMS]	• "Gilchrist's disease" • *Blastomyces dermatitidis* (dimorphic fungus) • Adults • In United States, most cases along Mississippi, Missouri, and Ohio river basins and the Great Lakes • Face • Crusted verrucous plaques with an annular pustular border, possible central healing • Causes lung infections (#1), spreads to GI, brain, and skin • Primary skin inoculation rare • Clinical variants: • Pulmonary • Disseminated • Primary cutaneous	• Mixed pyogenic and granulomatous inflammation; pseudoepitheliomatous hyperplasia; microabscesses; diffuse mixed infiltrate; spores have broad-based bud (seen in giant cell or tissue)
North American blastomycosis	• "Gilchrist's disease" • *Blastomyces dermatitidis* (dimorphic	• Culture morphology: • 30°C = "lollipop" conidia (pear-shaped, pyriform) • 37°C = thick, double-contoured cell wall with broad-based buds

Name	Predilection and Clinical Key Features	Histopathology
Coccidioido-mycosis [PAS, GMS; not mucicarmine]	• "Valley fever" • *Coccidioides immitis* (dust-borne, "barrel-shaped" arthrospores) • Most virulent of fungi (extremely infectious arthroconidium) • South-east USA, Mexico • Face • Self-limiting, flu-like lung infection (#1); possible febrile illness; hypercalcemia • Red, verrucous nodules (especially on face); erythema nodosum occurs in 20% with pulmonary infections	• Pseudoepitheliomatous hyperplasia; diffuse suppurative granulomatous reaction (non-caseating granulomas); large, thick-walled spherules (average 50 μm) with granular cytoplasm or endospores • Culture morphology: • 30°C = barrel-shaped arthroconidium • 37°C = tissue-dimorphic (require special broth to convert) • DDx: rhinosporidiosis, which has larger (average 200 μm) spherules and the cell wall stains with mucicarmine, unlike coccidioidomycosis

Name	Predilection and Clinical Key Features	Histopathology
Paracoccidioido-mycosis	• "South American blastomycosis" • *Paracoccidioides brasiliensis* (dimorphic fungus in soil) • Latin America • Mucocutaneous areas • Causes lung infection, regional lymphadenopathy, mucocutaneous ulcerations, and verrucous plaques • Clinical variants: • Primary pulmonary disease with subsequent mucocutaneous ulcerations (if disseminated) • Primary mucocutaneous (especially if chew on stick/leaves) • Primary cutaneous (verrucous plaques)	• Pseudoepitheliomatous hyperplasia; dermal infiltrate; granulomas; spores have multiple buds ("mariner's wheel") • H & E stain (above) and GMS stain (below) at same location • Difficult to see fungi as "mariner's wheel" without staining • Culture morphology: • 30°C = "lollipop" (pyriform) conidia, similar to blastomycosis • 37°C = cerebriform ("coral-like") with large "mother" yeast and budding "daughter" yeast with narrow neck ("mariner's wheel")

Name	Predilection and Clinical Key Features	Histopathology
Histoplasmosis [PAS, GMS]	• "Darling's disease" • Mainly a pulmonary infection (rarely primary skin inoculation) • South-eastern USA • *Histoplasma capsulatum* (dimorphic soil fungus) • Self-limiting, flu-like lung infection (#1), cutaneous spread uncommon unless immunocompromised • Reservoir is bird and bat guano • Disseminated histoplasmosis in a transplant patient (above) • Diffuse, crusted, ulcerated nodules, papules; may appear "molluscum-like" • Possible Tx = amphotericin B, itraconazole, voriconazole	• Epithelioid granulomas with numerous parasitized macrophages by small ovoid yeast-like organisms with surrounding clear halo ("pseudocapsule") • GMS stain (pictured below) • Culture morphology: • 30°C = spiny macroconidia ("tuberculated") • 37°C = cerebriform ("coral-like") with round budding yeasts with narrow necks

Name	Predilection and Clinical Key Features	Histopathology
Infections by dematiaceous (pigmented) fungi		
Chromomycosis	• "Chromoblastomycosis" • Caused by *Fonsecaea* (#1 cause), *Phialophora*, *Cladosporium* species • Often follows superficial trauma • Extremities • Scaly papule slowly expands to annular, verrucous plaques • Systemic infections rare	• Pseudoepitheliomatous hyperplasia; hyperkeratosis; mixed dermal infiltrate; no caseation (tuberculoid granulomas); microabscesses; golden-brown sclerotic bodies/Medlar bodies ("copper pennies", clusters of brown spores) in the dermis

Name	Predilection and Clinical Key Features	Histopathology
Phaeohypho-mycosis	• "Dark-filamentous-fungi" (i.e. *Alternaria, Curvularia, Pseudallescheria boydii*) • Distal extremities • Often follows superficial trauma (especially wood splinter or vegetable matter) • Solitary subcutaneous cyst or nodular, cystic, or verrucous lesion	• Brown, filamentous hyphae (not copper penny spores) • Walled-off cystic space (central necrotic debris); suppurative granulomatous reaction; may see foreign body (wood splinter)

Name	Predilection and Clinical Key Features	Histopathology
Sporotrichosis	• "Rose gardener's disease" • *Sporothrix schenckii* (yeast form causes lesions) • Hands, forearms • Nodules and pustules after inoculation (rose thorns, sphagnum moss, splinters) • *Note:* epithelioid sarcoma may appear clinically similar • Possible Tx = itraconazole or potassium iodide (iodide has risk of GI upset and thyroid suppression)	• Pseudoepitheliomatous hyperplasia; diffuse mixed dermal infiltrate; granulomas (tuberculoid, histiocytic, and suppurative); extracellular • "Sporothrix asteroid" (hyaline material is immune complexes on fungal surface); round/oval/cigar-shaped spores (difficult to see even with PAS or GMS stain)

Name	Predilection and Clinical Key Features	Histopathology
Tinea nigra palmaris	• Tropics • Palm of fingers, especially if hyperhidrosis • Slowly enlarging, brown to black macule or patch (may resemble a melanocytic macule) • Typically caused by *Hortaea werneckii*, a superficial pigmented mycosis of the stratum corneum	• Numerous brown hyphae present in superficial layers • No inflammatory reaction • Clue: "holes" in stratum corneum (contain fungi)
Alternariosis	• *Alternaria alternata* (plant pathogen) • Face, forearm, hands, knees (exposed areas) • Chronic crusted nodules, pustules, or ulcers • Accidental human infection	• Non-caseating granulomas; microabscesses; intraepidermal abscesses; thick scale crust with neutrophils; septate hyphae and spores (epidermis/dermis)

Name	Predilection and Clinical Key Features	Histopathology
Mycetoma and morphologically similar conditions		
Mycetoma	• Chronic granulomatous infection • Tropics (west Africa, India, South America) • Feet ("Madura foot") • Initially, a subcutaneous nodule that forms a draining, painless nodule (6–12 months), ulceration, fibrosis; may cause bone deformity • Clinical triad ("TED"): 1. Tumefaction (swelling) 2. Exudate of grains 3. Draining sinuses • Possible Tx = surgical excision, systemic antifungal, or antibiotics • Two main etiology groups: 1. Actinomycetic mycetoma: • Aerobic filamentous bacteria, such as: • *Nocardia brasiliensis* (#1) = pale grains • *Actinomadura pelletieri* = red grains 2. Eumycotic mycetoma/true fungi, such as: • *Madurella mycetomatis* = black grains	• Suppurative granulomas with "sulfur granules" (large colonies of bacteria/fungi); mixed infiltrate; fibrosis; grains vary in color depending on etiology • Eumycotic mycetoma (fungal elements visible)

Name	Predilection and Clinical Key Features	Histopathology
Nocardiosis [H & E, Gram stains]	• Immunocompromised patients • Aerobic Gram+ bacteria (not a fungus) • Primary skin infection may cause mycetoma, "sporotrichoid-like" or abscess/ulcer lesions • Possible Tx = sulfonamides • May cause septicemic infections (especially of pulmonary origin) or one of three types of primary cutaneous infection (mycetoma, lymphocutaneous, or superficial cutaneous infection)	• Dense neutrophil infiltrate in deep dermis/subcutis; abscesses; necrosis; hemorrhage; "sulfur granules"

Name	Predilection and Clinical Key Features	Histopathology
Actinomycosis [Giemsa, PAS, Gram stain]	• Chronic (possibly fatal) bacterial infection similar to fungal lesions • May occur anywhere on body, including cervicofacial, thoracic, or abdominal regions • Fluctuant swellings, draining sinuses, subcutaneous abscesses • Variants may cause actinomycetoma, "lumpy jaw," GI actinomycosis possible • *Actinomyces israelii* (Gram+ bacterium), which is an endogenous source (i.e. mouth flora) • Similar to mycetoma, so discussed in this location although due to a bacterium	• Abscess of neutrophils, mixed infiltrate, granules (sclerotic), bacteria granules (sulfur granules are clumps of basophilic organisms) • PAS stain (above) • Gram stain (above) • Splendore–Hoeppli phenomenon = eosinophilic border due to immunoglobulins (Ab); also seen with *Staph. aureus*, *Proteus*, *Pseudomonas*, and *E. coli* (due to Ab and debris; is not specific)

Name	Predilection and Clinical Key Features	Histopathology
Botryomycosis [Gram stain]	• "Bacterial pseudomycosis" • Chronic bacterial infection with discharge of granules • *Staphylococcus* (#1 cause), *Pseudomonas*, *Proteus* • Hands, feet, head, inguinal and gluteal areas • Large swollen plaque with ulcers, nodules; discharging sinuses of small whitish granules • Appears "Mycetoma-like" so discussed in this location although due to a bacterium	• Small, basophilic, "sulfur granules" due to bacteria present in center of suppurative zone with surrounding eosinophilic zone; *(no filaments present as with mycetoma)*

Name	Predilection and Clinical Key Features	Histopathology
Zygomycoses		
Mucormycosis [H & E, PAS, GMS]	• Opportunistic fungi which "love" sugar (soil and decaying vegetables) • Diabetics who are immunocompromised • *Rhizopus*, *Mucor* and *Absidia* (Non-septate hyphae branching at 90° angles) • Tender, indurated, large plaque with a dusky center; often necrotic	• Variation in appearance (possibly sparse infiltrate, granulomatous pyoderma, ulceration) • Broad, ribbon-like, non-septate hyphae with 90° branching ("Moose antlers"); may invade vessel walls
Subcutaneous phycomycosis	• Deep fungal infection by various non-septate fungi (often *Basidiobolus* and *Conidiobolus*)	• Smudgy eosinophilic material around hyphae (Splendore–Hoeppli like); granulomas with possible abscesses and necrosis

Name	Predilection and Clinical Key Features	Histopathology
Hyalohyphomycoses (unpigmented, septate)		
Hyalohyphomycoses Overall	• Group of opportunistic infections with the fungi growing in tissue in hyphal elements that are unpigmented, septate, and branched or unbranched • Includes *Schizophyllum commune*, *Acremonium*, *Fusarium*, *Penicillium*, and *Scedosporium*	• Oval yeast with cross walls; parasitized macrophages

Name	Predilection and Clinical Key Features	Histopathology
Fusariosis	• Neutropenic patients (i.e. transplant and burn patients) • Often due to *Fusarium solani* • Superficial and systemic infection possible • Numerous skin lesions possible, including red or gray macules, pustules, nodules, vasculitic lesions, etc. • May cause onychomycosis also	• Septate hyphae at 45° branching (similar to Aspergillosis) • Heavy acute and chronic infiltrate in dermis and/or subcutis. Dermal necrosis may be associated with mycelia invasing blood vessels) • Culture = looks like "clumps of bananas"
Penicilliosis	• AIDS patients (inhaled from bamboo rats) • South-east Asia (Thailand, Hong Kong) • Thermal dimorphic fungi (*Penicillium marneffei*) • "Molluscum-like" lesions, fever, lymphadenopathy, pulmonary disease • Possible reservoir: bamboo rat	• Oval yeast with cross walls; parasitized macrophages
Aspergillosis [Silver methenamine stains best]	• Opportunistic infection (immunocompromised, especially cancer patients) • Lung infection (#1), rarely involves skin (hematogenous spread) • Violaceous plaques or nodules that rapidly progress to necrotic ulcer with a black eschar	• Septate, 45° branching hyphae (often in vessels); variation in appearance due to host response (granulomas, abscesses, fungal masses)

Name	Predilection and Clinical Key Features	Histopathology
Miscellaneous mycoses		
Lobomycosis [H & E, PAS]	• "Lobo's disease" or "keloidal blastomycosis" • Rare, chronic fungal disease (also infects Atlantic bottlenose dolphins) • Central and South America • Ears, exposed areas • *Lacazia loboi* (old name *Loboa loboi*) • Slow-growing keloid-like nodule or ulcerated verrucous plaque • 10% with lymph node involvement; association with SCC (chronic lesions)	• Extensive granulomatous infiltrate; "sieve-like" appearance due to numerous unstained fungal cells free and in macrophages; thick cell wall, "lemon-shaped" fungi, often in chains of globose cells

Name	Predilection and Clinical Key Features	Histopathology
Rhinosporidiosis [Mucicarmine stains cell walls]	• India, South America • Nasal and pharyngeal mucosa • Red, friable, pedunculated, or polypoid nodule • Organism = *Rhinosporidium seeberi*	• Large "raspberry-like" sporangia (average 200 μm) with numerous endospores; spores mature from the periphery to the center of the sporangia; mixed infiltrate; granuloma formation • DDx: coccidioidomycosis, which has smaller (average 50 μm) spherules and does not stain with mucicarmine, like rhinosporidiosis cell wall
Pneumocystosis [Methenamine silver, Giemsa, Wright stains]	• Immunosuppressed host (AIDS) • External auditory canal, other skin areas • More commonly causes lung infections (pneumonia) • Skin infection rare: pedunculated polypoid lesion (especially ear) or friable, necrotic papules/nodules; may have "molluscum contagiosum-like" lesions • Parasite: *Pneumocystis jiroveci* (formerly *P. carinii*) • No longer considered a protozoan, now a fungus • Possible Tx = TMP-SMX, pentamidine (antifungals do not resolve)	• Perivascular mantle of amphophilic, foamy to finely stippled material (similar to pulmonary pneumocystosis)

Name	Predilection and Clinical Key Features	Histopathology
Algal infections		
Prothecosis [H & E, but best seen with PAS, GMS]	• Immunocompromised • Often due to traumatic inoculation • Infection due to achloric algae (*Prototheca wickerhamii* is most common) • Eczematous, herpetiform, or papulonodular lesions forming plaques • Possible visceral dissemination	• "Soccer ball-like" morula (sphere with endospores) due to multiple septations in organism (sporangia); chronic granulomatous reaction with mixed infiltrate; necrosis

26

Viral Diseases

DNA viruses ("HAPPy")

H = herpes virus (HSV, VZV, CMV, EBV); see figure
H = hepadnavirus (hepatitis B)
A = adenovirus
P = papovavirus (HPV)
P = poxvirus (molluscum, smallpox, Orf, milker's nodule)
P = parvovirus B19 (only single-stranded DNA virus): think "slap cheeks with one DNA" (single-stranded)

RNA viruses

Paramyxovirus (measles, mumps), picornavirus (Coxsackie), rhabdovirus (rabies), retrovirus (HIV), togavirus (rubella)

Herpes simplex virus (HSV)

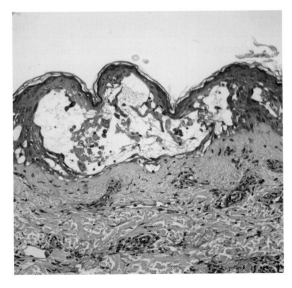

Name	Predilection and Clinical Key Features	Histopathology
Poxviridae		

• Double-stranded DNA virus, causing intracytoplasmic inclusions:
   • Oval or cylindrical-shaped virus = molluscum contagiosum and Orf
   • Brick-shaped viruses = other poxviridae viruses		

Cowpox	• Viral disease of cattle (reservoir may be cat, rodent) • Milkers • Hands, forearm, face • Pustular eruption with slight fever and lymphadenitis • Disseminated cowpox (above)	• Similar to variola (see below) with cytoplasmic eosinophilic inclusion bodies and a dermal lymphocytic infiltrate
Kaposi's varicelliform eruption	• Generalized eruption variant in atopic dermatitis individuals, Darier's disease, burns, etc. • Resembles eczema herpeticum (see p. 475); currently, eczema herpeticum and eczema vaccinatum are grouped together as Kaposi's varicelliform eruption	
Vaccinia	• Smallpox vaccine virus (laboratory-developed member of poxvirus group) • Vesicular papule which gradually dries up producing a crust and leaves a scar • "Eczema vaccinatum" = patients often with a history of eczema who form disseminated skin infection after vaccination	• Similar to variola with intracytoplasmic inclusion bodies (not intranuclear inclusion bodies, otherwise similar to herpes simplex, zoster, and varicella)

Variola (smallpox)	• Centripetal eruption (extremities-to-trunk) of umbilicated papules; vesicles, pustules (lesions at same stage); heals with scarring
	• Two types:
	  1. Variola major (severe form with significant fatality rate)
	  2. Variola minor (mild form with fatality <1%)
		• Intraepidermal vesicles with eosinophilic, intracytoplasmic inclusion bodies (Guarneri bodies); diffuse dermal lymphocytic infiltrate; rare multinucleate cells

Name	Predilection and Clinical Key Features	Histopathology
Molluscum contagiosum	• DNA poxvirus ("brick-shaped") • Children, adolescents • Head, neck, flexural areas, genitalia • Dome-shaped, umbilicated, waxy papule • Often spontaneous regression in approximately 1 year	• Crater filled with hyperplastic squamous epithelium; Henderson–Patterson bodies or "molluscum bodies" (intracytoplasmic inclusions that push nucleus/granules aside in cells above the basal layer) • Henderson–Patterson bodies (picture above) have the nucleus pushed aside by the intracytoplasmic inclusions

Name	Predilection and Clinical Key Features	Histopathology
Milker's nodule	• Paravaccinia poxvirus • Transmitted from udders of infected cows • Hand • Red–violaceous, eroded/crusted nodule (various stages also) • Regresses with a scar in 6–8 weeks	• Similar to Orf (see below), except not usually full-thickness necrosis as in Orf; pink-colored inclusions

Name	Predilection and Clinical Key Features	Histopathology
Orf	• "Ecthyma contagiosum" • Paravaccinia poxvirus • Hands, forearms • Mature lesion is a nodular lesion with central umbilication and erythematous halo (goes through various stages) • Regresses in 7 weeks • Primarily a disease of young sheep and goats, often involving lips and perioral area	• Histology depends on the stage • Vacuolated superficial epidermis with pink intracytoplasmic inclusion bodies; full-thickness necrosis; "finger-like," downward projections into dermis; numerous vessels; dense lymphocytic infiltrate (neutrophils); papillary dermal edema; inclusion bodies in keratinocyte's cytoplasm • Electron micrograph of virus: demonstrates a cylindrical-shaped viral capsule with a "cross-hatched" appearance

Name	Predilection and Clinical Key Features	Histopathology
Herpesviridae (Double-stranded DNA virus, causing intranuclear inclusions)		
Herpes simplex virus (HSV)	HSV-1: • Children • Lips, perioral area HSV-2: • After puberty • Genital area • Painful, grouped, clear vesicles; heal without scarring • Virus latent in sensory ganglia during remission	• Intraepidermal vesicles; necrosis; ballooning degeneration; steel-gray nuclei with peripheral margination of chromatin, intranuclear inclusions (Cowdry type A or Lipshutz bodies); acantholysis; multinucleated keratinocytes • *Note:* Intraepidermal vesicles form due to ballooning degeneration ("swelling" of infected cells causes secondary acantholysis) and reticular degeneration (hydropic swelling with eventual rupture of cell) • Late changes include hair follicle involvement (picture below) • Three Ms of HSV cellular effects: • Margination of chromatin (specific finding) • Multinucleate giant cells • Molding of nucleus

Name	Predilection and Clinical Key Features	Histopathology
Eczema herpeticum	• Generalized infection of skin with HSV • Most commonly in association with atopic dermatitis • Condition is currently grouped into Kaposi's varicelliform eruption (see p. 470) • Extensive vesicles and crusted papules on the body 	• Same as HSV histologically
Varicella (HHV-3)	• "Chickenpox" • Childhood • Successive crops at different stages of development (papule, vesicle, crust, healing) (unlike smallpox which has lesions at the same stage of development) • Congenital varicella infection = greatest risk if maternal infection occurs during first trimester	• Indistinguishable from HSV histologically

Name	Predilection and Clinical Key Features	Histopathology
Herpes zoster (HHV-3)	• "Shingles" • Adults • Reactivation of latent varicella virus • Most common sensory ganglia involved are the lumbar and thoracic nerves • Fever and pain, then papules and vesicles develop which crust • *Ramsey–Hunt syndrome* = tinnitus, facial paralysis, vesicles of tympanic membrane/external ear (geniculate ganglion of the facial nerve, CN VII)	• Same as HSV histologically

Name	Predilection and Clinical Key Features	Histopathology
Cytomegalovirus (CMV)	• HHV-5 • Immunocompromised or neonates • Various skin manifestations including maculopapular eruption, urticaria, etc. • "Blueberry muffin" baby (dermal erythropoiesis, also in congenital rubella) • One of TORCH syndromes • Congenital CMV = #1 cause in US of congenital deafness and mental retardation • Leading cause of blindness (retinitis) in AIDS patients • Possible Tx or prophylaxis = ganciclovir	• Enlarged endothelial cells in dermal vessels due to virus, appear like "owl's eye" cells (halo around pink, eosinophilic intranuclear inclusions); may have intranuclear and intracytoplasmic inclusions

Name	Predilection and Clinical Key Features	Histopathology
Epstein–Barr virus (HHV-4)	• 10% of EBV patients get an erythematous, macular, or maculopapular rash (especially with ampicillin or amoxicillin) • *Clinical triad* = fever, pharyngitis, and lymphadenopathy • Associated with Gianotti–Crosti syndrome (#1 cause in US), oral hairy leukoplakia, mononucleosis, Kikuchi's disease (histiocytic necrotizing lymphadenitis)	• Non-specific changes; mild perivascular infiltrate of inflammatory cells
Human herpesvirus-6 (HHV-6)	• "Roseola infantum" or "exanthem subitum" • Infants • Cutaneous eruptions resembling measles or rubella; high fever then morbilliform rash (after fever); common cause of fever-induced seizures • Possibly associated with DRESS syndrome (drug reaction with eosinophilia and systemic symptoms) • Reactivation of virus in immunocompromised patient may lead to fevers, pneumonitis, encephalitis, bone marrow suppression	• Spongiosis, spongiotic vesicles, lymphocyte exocytosis, edema
Human herpesvirus-7 (HHV-7)	• Infant • Possibly associated with pityriasis rosea and roseola	

Human herpesvirus-8 (HHV-8)	HHV-8 is associated with:
	1. Kaposi's sarcoma variants:
	  • Classic KS:
	    • elderly Mediterranean or Ashkenazi Jews
	    • purple–red plaque on lower extremity
	  • Immunosuppressed KS = transplant or ciclosporin patients:
	    • similar to AIDS-related Kaposi's
	  • African endemic KS in children and young adults:
	    • mainly infects lymph nodes (lymphadenopathy) > skin
	    • fatal in 2 years
	  • African endemic KS in adults:
	    • nodular (usually benign course), florid and infiltrative variants
	  • AIDS-related KS:
	    • strong association with HHV-8
	    • often gastrointestinal involvement also
	2. Multicentric variant of Castleman's disease:
	  • Non-clonal disease of the lymph nodes (widespread involvement) with angiofollicular hyperplasia
	  • See Chapter 40, Cutaneous Non-lymphoid Infiltrates
		
		• Kaposi's sarcoma (see also p. 712)

Name	Predilection and Clinical Key Features	Histopathology
Papovaviridae (Papillomaviridae)		

- Double-stranded DNA virus which infects the basal layer keratinocytes and replicates in the nucleus
- Contains capsid which protects from degradation (does not contain a viral capsule) Early (E) genes:
  - HPV E6 can degrade p53 and cause the p53 to not inhibit the G1 cell cycle (causing the suprabasal keratinocytes to continue cell cycle)
  - HPV E7 can bind under phosphorylated pRB (retinoblastoma) causing the E2F protein to induce synthesis of DNA genes
- Late (L) genes 1 and 2 encode for the capsid (L1 capsid protein is the major capsid protein and used in the HPV vaccine for HPV-6, -11, -16, -18)

Name	Predilection and Clinical Key Features	Histopathology
Verruca vulgaris	<ul><li>"Common warts"</li><li>HPV-1, HPV-2, and HPV-4</li><li>Child to adult</li><li>Fingers, exposed areas</li></ul> 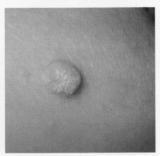 <ul><li>Hard, rough-surfaced papule; may contain "black dots" which are thrombosed vessels</li></ul>	<ul><li>"Sharp" papillomatosis, hyperkeratosis, columns of parakeratosis overlying papillomatous projections, often with small hemorrhages in columns; hyper-granulosis (keratohyaline granules) in "valleys", acanthosis; inward turning of elongated rete ridges (arborization); koilocytes (vacuolated, superficial keratinocytes with "raisin-like" pyknotic nuclei)</li></ul> 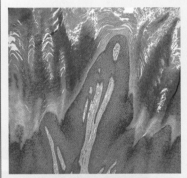 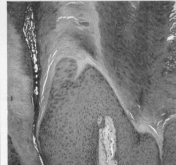 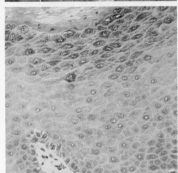 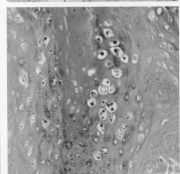 <ul><li>Hypergranulosis in "valleys" with visible koilocytes</li></ul>

Name	Predilection and Clinical Key Features	Histopathology

Palmoplantar warts	• HPV-1, HPV-2, and HPV-4
	• Palm, sole
	
	• Painful lesion, usually either:
	  • Mosaic warts:
	    • superficial variant
	    • form large plaque lesions
	  • Myrmecia:
	    • deep variant
	    • resemble "anthill" due to sloping sides and central depression
	
		• Similar verruca vulgaris, except more of lesion is deeper to plane of skin surface and invades into dermis
		
		• Plantar wart
		
		• Myrmecia wart

Ridged wart	• Nodular variant of palmoplantar warts • Associated with HPV-60 • Hands and feet • Nodular lesions that do not disrupt the dermatoglyphics (retention of the surface ridge pattern) as do other wart lesions	• Verruca in appearance histologically, but often shows more acanthosis, but only mild papillomatosis

Name	Predilection and Clinical Key Features	Histopathology
Verruca plana	• "Flat warts" • HPV-3 and HPV-10 • Children to young adults • Dorsum of hands, face • Flesh-colored or brownish, flat-topped papules	• Similar to verruca vulgaris, except minimal or no parakeratosis
Butcher's warts	• HPV-7 (remember, Butcher has 7 letters) • People who handle raw meat	• Similar to common verruca vulgaris histologically

Epidermodysplasia verruciformis (EDV)	• "Lewandowsky–Lutz dysplasia"
	• Inherited disorder with widespread HPV and possible SCC risk
	• Usually autosomal dominant
	• Infancy to childhood
	• Two forms:
	  1. HPV-3 (HPV-10):
	    • multiple flat, wart-like lesions
	    • possible disturbed cell-mediated immunity
	    • no tendency to malignancy
	    • histology resembles flat warts
	  2. HPV-5 (HPV-8):
	    • family history
	    • usually develop actinic keratosis in 30s
	    • malignant potential (SCC)
	    • appear as plane warts and red–brown patches
	• Mutations = EVER1 (TMC6) and EVER2 (TMC8) genes (possibly involve PSORS2 region of EVER2/TMC8 genes)
		• HPV-3-induced lesions: appear similar to plantar warts histologically
		• HPV-5-induced lesions: large cells with blue–gray cytoplasm ("bubbly blue") and perinuclear halo in the upper epidermis

Name	Predilection and Clinical Key Features	Histopathology
Condyloma acuminatum	• "Genital warts" • HPV-6 and HPV-11 • Anogenital region • Fleshy, exophytic papule or plaque	• Marked acanthosis, vacuolated koilocytes; may be "SCC-like" • If podophyllin treated within 48 hours of biopsy, appears histologically as: • epidermal pallor • degenerate keratinocytes • increased mitotic figures
Buschke–Löwenstein tumor	• Giant condylomata acuminata, variant of condylomatous carcinoma • Anogenital area • Large exophytic lesion	• Marked acanthosis, vacuolated koilocytes

Name	Predilection and Clinical Key Features	Histopathology
Focal epithelial hyperplasia	• "Heck's disease" • HPV 13, HPV-32 • Eskimos, Native Americans • Mucosa of lips and cheeks • Multiple soft, pink, or white papules on oral mucosa • Reminder: 12 letters + ' in Heck's disease = 13 (HPV-13)	 • Mucosal hyperplasia with acanthosis and clubbing of broad rete pegs; pallor of epidermal cells (especially upper layers); koilocytes

Name	Predilection and Clinical Key Features	Histopathology
Bowenoid papulosis	• HPV-16, HPV-18 • Sexually active young adults • Glans penis, vulva • Solitary or multiple verruca-like, red–brown or whitish papules in genital area • Low risk of invasive SCC • Often resistant to treatment and may have protracted course, especially if poor immunity	• Close histological resemblance to squamous cell-in-situ • Full-thickness epidermal atypia and loss of architecture; mitoses frequent (often in metaphase); dyskeratotic cells; small, dark basophilic, inclusion-like bodies in upper epidermis
Parvoviridae		
Parvovirus B19 virus overall	• Single-stranded DNA virus (other DNA viruses are double-stranded) • Infects erythroid progenitor cells • May cause erythema infectiosum or papular-purpuric gloves and socks syndrome (see below)	
Erythema infectiosum	• "Slapped cheek" disease or fifth disease • Caused by parvovirus B19 • Children (age 4–10) • Spread by respiratory droplets • Clinical: • After the onset of viral prodrome: malar erythema develops and then maculopapular rash followed by a reticulated-like, lacy rash on extremities: • may return with physical exercise for a period • Typically benign: • but associated with miscarriages, hemolytic anemia, etc. • associated with fetal hydrops in pregnant women, especially if mother infected in first 20 weeks	
Papular-purpuric gloves and socks syndrome	• Caused by parvovirus B19 • Also seen with Coxsackie virus and HHV-6 • Young adults • Pruritic erythema of the palms/soles with petechia and purpura; edema	

Name	Predilection and Clinical Key Features	Histopathology
Picornaviridae		
Hand, foot, and mouth disease	• Coxsackie A16, enterovirus 71 • Hand, foot, and mouth • Febrile illness with circular vesiculopustules in the anterior parts of the mouth and creases in hands and feet • Associated with Gianotti–Crosti syndrome	 • Intraepidermal vesicles with reticular degeneration (hydropic swelling and rupture); few balloon cells; necrosis; mild perivascular infiltrate; no multinucleate cells or inclusion bodies
Herpangina	• Coxsackie virus A and B • Children aged 3–10 • Soft palate, uvula, and pharynx • Fever with painful erosions on soft palate, uvula, and pharynx • Think of "only mouth disease, not hand and foot"	
Togaviridae		

Rubella	• "German measles" or third disease:
	  • Mild fever
	  • Posterior auricular and occipital lymphadenopathy
	  • Erythematous rash starts on face: cephalocaudad spread
	  • Forchheimer's spots = petechiae on soft palate
	  • Peripheral blood contains Turk cells (atypical lymphocytes in rubella)
	  • Congenital rubella:
	    • non-immune pregnant woman spread to fetus
	    • risk of miscarriage, cataracts, deafness, patent ductus arteriosus	

Ross River and Barmah Forest viruses	• Australia and Oceana area • Transmitted by mosquitoes • Diffuse maculopapular erythematous eruption: predominantly on limbs and trunk • Fever and joint pain	

Name	Predilection and Clinical Key Features	Histopathology
Flaviviridae		
West Nile fever/ encephalitis	• East Africa; appearing in North America • Main reservoir = birds (crow family): transmitted by culicine mosquito • 80% of patients have no signs or symptoms • Small number (1 in 150) develop severe neurological disease (especially in individuals over 50) • Specific marker = multifocal chorioretinitis • Fever, malaise, eye pain, and headache • Predominantly on extremities, palms, and soles • Non-blanching, punctate, erythematous macules and papules that spread centripetally	
Dengue fever	• Tropical and subtropical regions of Asia and Africa • Acute febrile illness, myalgia, retro-orbital pain, headaches, diffuse, erythematous rash with areas of normal skin within diffuse erythema ("islands of white in sea of red") • Transmission = *Aedes aegypti* mosquito • Four serotypes of dengue virus; although lifelong immunity from serotype, if infected with different serotype may develop more severe variant dengue hemorrhagic fever (DHF) or dengue shock syndrome (DSS)	• Mild perivascular infiltrate of lymphocytes in the superficial dermis; variable red cell extravasation • Diagnosis is made by serological tests, viral isolation, or PCR-based detection of viral antigen
Hepatitis C virus	• Possible skin manifestations (15% of patients): • Vasculitis • Pigmented purpuric dermatosis • Lichen planus • Erythema nodosum • Erythema multiforme • Necrolytic acral erythema • Pruritus • Symmetric polyarthritis with livedo reticularis • Sporadic porphyria cutanea tarda	
Paramyxoviridae		
Measles	• "Rubeola": • RNA paramyxovirus • Exanthem spread in cephalocaudad manner • Triad of three Cs and K: • Cough • Coryza • Conjunctivitis • Koplik's spots (Gray–white papules on buccal mucosa, appear before rash during prodrome)	
Retroviridae		
Human immunodeficiency virus (HIV)	• Retrovirus that infects and destroys CD4+ T lymphocytes by apoptosis • Cutaneous manifestations: • Most common = pruritic papular eruption • Viral (molluscum contagiosum, HSV, verruca vulgaris, oral hairy leukoplakia) • Bacterial (mycobacteria, bacillary angiomatosis) • Fungal (candidosis, dermatophytosis, histoplasmosis, cryptococcosis, mucormycosis, *Penicillium marneffei*) • Neoplasms (Kaposi's, cutaneous lymphomas, skin cancers) • Dermatoses (psoriasis, seborrheic dermatitis, vasculitis, idiopathic pruritus, PCT)	

Name	Predilection and Clinical Key Features	Histopathology
Infective dermatitis of children due to human T-lymphotrophic virus type 1 (HTLV-1)	• Japan, Caribbean, and sub-Saharan Africa • Scalp, axillae, groin, external ear, retroauricular region • Eczema-like appearance, dermatopathic lymphadenopathy likely due to breastfeeding as the virus origin • HTLV-1 can cause adult T-cell leukemia/lymphoma	• Similar to atopic dermatitis histologically
Other viral diseases		
Hepatitis A virus	• Rarely skin manifestations • May cause a photo-accentuated eruption, accompanied by deposition of IgA in endothelial cells of upper dermis • May develop Gianotti–Crosti syndrome and a vasculitis	

Hepatitis B virus	• Skin manifestations:
	  • Serum sickness-like prodrome with urticarial or vasculitic lesions
	  • Polyarteritis nodosa
	  • Essential mixed cryoglobulinemia
	  • May cause papular acrodermatitis of childhood (Gianotti–Crosti syndrome)
	  • Photo-localized pustular eruption (rare)	

Name	Predilection and Clinical Key Features	Histopathology
Gianotti–Crosti syndrome	• "Papular acrodermatitis of childhood" • Children • Localized to face and extremities (spares trunk) • Non-relapsing, erythematous, papular rash, lasting 3 weeks; lymphadenopathy, acute hepatitis • Associated with EBV (#1 cause in US), hepatitis B, hepatitis A, Coxsackie, cytomegalovirus	• May show three tissue reactions (spongiotic, lichenoid, and lymphocytic vasculitis)
Kikuchi's disease	• "Histiocytic necrotizing lymphadenitis" • Young adult Japanese females • Rash (morbilliform, urticarial, maculopapular, etc.), fever, lymphadenopathy • Possible viral etiology (HHV-6, HHV-8, EBV, etc.)	• Appears "SLE-like" with a lichenoid interface reaction
Unilateral laterothoracic exanthem	• "Asymmetric periflexural exanthem of childhood" • Childhood • Axillae and lateral trunk • Unilateral eruption close to axilla with a centrifugal spread; spontaneous resolution; "Statue of Liberty" sign (raise arm and see rash on lateral thoracic area) • Likely viral etiology (possibly associated with parvovirus B19)	• Superficial perivascular lymphocytic infiltrate (often "tight cuffs" around vessels)
Kawasaki disease	• "Mucocutaneous lymph node syndrome" • Children under 5 years of age (usually under 2) • May have viral etiology • High fever + bilateral conjunctivitis, oropharyngeal changes, cervical lymphadenopathy • Peripheral changes (rash, peeling on hands/feet), exanthem • Risk of coronary aneurysms • Possible treatments = IVIG and aspirin	

Name	Predilection and Clinical Key Features	Histopathology
Rhabdovirus ("Bullet-shaped" virion)		
Rabies	• Deadly viral infection (*Lyssavirus*) spread by infected animals • Anxiety, drooling, convulsions, muscle spasms, death • No cutaneous manifestations • No cure at this time	• Best cutaneous location for skin biopsy to diagnose is the nuchal skin (look at cutaneous nerves for virus)

27 Protozoal Infections

Leishmaniasis

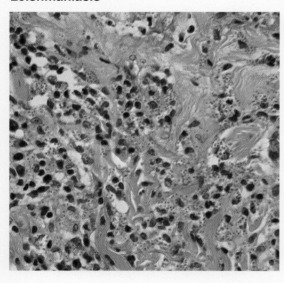

Name	Predilection and Clinical Key Features	Histopathology
Amebae		
• Single-celled organism with trophozoite and cyst stages • Motility by pseudopods		
Amebiasis	• GI infection with cutaneous involvement rare (0.3%); usually a complication of amebic colitis • Tropics • Perianal area, thighs, genital area • Parasite: *Entamoeba histolytica* • Reservoir: humans • Painful ulcers, fistulas, or nodules; irregular ulcer covered with a gray slough; unpleasant odor (may resemble SCC clinically) • Possible Tx = metronidazole	• Ulceration with necrosis in base; pseudoepitheliomatous hyperplasia; granulation tissue; organisms have eccentric nucleus, prominent nucleoli and granular, eosinophilic cytoplasm with phagocytosed RBCs
Acanthamebiasis	• Free-living amebae of soil and water • Immunocompromised and AIDS patients • Parasites: *Acanthamoeba* and *Naegleria* • Pustular, chronic ulcerating or nodular lesions; meningoencephalitis (major clinical feature)	• Tuberculoid granulomatous lesion in deep dermis; vasculitis; organisms present in tissue are large and have a thick cell wall in either trophozoite or cyst form
Flagellates		
(Group of protozoa that move with a flagella)		
African trypanosomiasis	• "African sleeping sickness" • Africa • Parasite: *Trypanosoma brucei* • Transmission: tsetse fly (especially *Glossina* spp) • "Trypanosome chancre" forms after bite (painful, boil-like lesion), fever • Winterbottom's sign = posterior cervical lymphadenopathy • Later, edema of hands, feet and face; fleeting erythematous maculopapular rash develops (often circinate), called trypanid • Possible Tx = suramin, pentamidine	• Superficial and deep infiltrate with lymphocytes and prominent plasma cells; organisms seen in exudate
American trypanosomiasis	• "Chagas disease" • South America, Texas • Parasite: *T. cruzi* (bug's fecal contamination at bite site) • Transmission: reduvid or kissing bug (*Triatoma*, "tiger-stripes") • Typically, visceral smooth muscle involvement (cardiac failure, GI megacolon); no significant skin lesions, but possibly macular and ulcerative eruption due to parasitosis of skin • Romana sign (unilateral, periorbital edema due to conjunctival entry) • Possible Tx = nifurtimox	• Similar to HP as African trypanosomiasis
Leishmaniasis		
• Host: rodents, dogs • Transmission: sandfly (especially *Phlebotomus*) • Diagnostic modalities: skin biopsy, Novy–McNeal–Nicolle (NNN) medium; Montenegro test (leishmanin intradermal skin test), PCR • Possible Tx = pentavalent antimalarial drugs, such as meglumine antimonate and sodium stibogluconate (cardiotoxic, QT prolongation)		

Name	Predilection and Clinical Key Features	Histopathology
Cutaneous leishmaniasis	• Chronic, self-limited granulomatous disease; may resolve spontaneously with scarring • Papule forms into ulcerated lesion with rolled borders ("volcano sign") • *Leishmaniasis recidivans:* • Dry, erythematous plaques (especially on face) that recur at the periphery of the original ulcer; appear psoriasiform • Old world leishmaniasis: • *L. tropica* (Asia and Africa) • Sandfly (*Phlebotomus*) • New world leishmaniasis: • *L. mexicana* (central and South America) • Sandfly (*Lutzomyia*)	• Massive dermal infiltrate of lymphocytes, giant cells, plasma cells, etc.; pseudoepitheliomatous hyperplasia; small tuberculoid granulomas; "marquee sign" (organisms localize at periphery of macrophages); amastigote with kinetoplast seen in dermal macrophages as intracytoplasmic bodies next to a purple dot • Kinetoplast appears as an oval body near the nucleus and functions as a mitochondrial structure with its own DNA

Name	Predilection and Clinical Key Features	Histopathology
Mucocutaneous leishmaniasis	• Central and South America • Tongue, nasopharynx • Vegetating, verrucous, sporotrichoid lesions (may develop months to 25 years later) • Main cause: *Leishmania braziliensis*	• Similar to acute cutaneous form; tuberculoid granulomas; pseudoepitheliomatous hyperplasia; presence of necrosis with a reactive response (favorable prognosis) • Espundia (*L. braziliensis*) = destructive cutaneous changes that may develop 25 years after apparent clinical cure
Visceral leishmaniasis	• "Kala-azar" or 'black fever" • Tropical countries, Indian subcontinent • Fever, anemia, hepatosplenomegaly; erythema (face); hyper-or hypopigmented macules (trunk); nodules (face, limbs) • Main cause: *L. donovani*	• Dense inflammatory infiltrate beneath an atrophic epidermis (lymphocytes, plasma cells, eosinophils, etc.); follicular plugging • Leishman–Donovan bodies [Giemsa stain or Weigert iron hematoxylin stain]
Disseminated leishmaniasis	• "Primary diffuse cutaneous leishmaniasis" • Anergic individuals • Widespread nodules and macules, without ulceration or visceral involvement	• Infiltrate is almost entirely composed of parasitized macrophages, with scant lymphocytes
Other flagellates		
Trichomoniasis	• Usually caused by *Trichomonas vaginalis* • Cutaneous infection rare (usually genital infection, especially median raphe of penis) • Underlying cyst or tract usually present	• Trichomonad demonstrated on pus drained from abscess
Giardiasis	• Associated with GI infection by *Giardia lamblia* • Urticaria and angioedema (often associated with infection), atopic dermatitis, papulovesicular eruption	• No specific findings; condition clears with treatment of the infection
Coccidia (Contaminated food and water; important in immunosuppressed patients)		

Toxoplasmosis	• Two variants:
	  1. Acquired (immunosuppressed)
	  2. Congenital (one of TORCH infections)
	• One of TORCH infections = toxoplasmosis, "other," rubella, cytomegalovirus, herpes virus
	• Parasite: *Toxoplasma gondii*
	• Host: cats
	• Fever, lymphadenopathy, ocular disease, encephalitis, skin manifestations, include morbilliform, purpuric, urticarial, nodular lesions
	• Possible Tx = sulfadiazine + pyrimethamine
		• Superficial and mid-dermal perivascular lymphohistiocytic infiltrate; parasites in macrophage cytoplasm; pseudoepitheliomatous hyperplasia

Sporozoa		
Babesiosis	• Immunocompromised or splenectomy patients • Transmission: tick bites transmit the hema-protozoan of genus *Babesia* • Flu-like symptoms, cutaneous lesions rare (possibly annular erythema similar to necrolytic migratory erythema)	• May be similar to necrolytic migratory erythema; subcorneal pustulation with adjacent parakeratosis
Miscellaneous		
Pneumocystosis	• No longer considered a protozoan, now a fungus (See Ch. 25, p. 467) • *Pneumocystis jiroveci* (formerly *P. carinii*)	• Perivascular mantle of amphophilic, foamy to finely stippled material (similar to pulmonary pneumocystosis)

28 Marine Injuries

Jellyfish stings

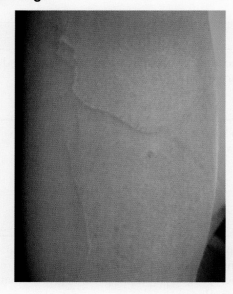

Seabather's eruption

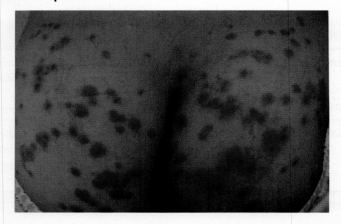

Name	Key Features	Photos and Additional Information
Cnidarians	• Portuguese man-of-war, box jellyfish, corals • Have nematocysts that contain toxins	 Portuguese man-of-war
Molluscs	• Scallops, oysters, slugs, squid, cone shells, some octopus	

Echinoderms	• Sea urchins, starfish, sea cucumbers
	• Sea urchin:
	  • spines break off and release neurotoxin, causing immediate burning pain, then edema and erythema
	  • may form granulomas later	

Sponges	• Especially "fire sponge" (*Tedania ignis*):
	  • contact causes severe vesicular dermatitis
	  • Bermuda fire sponge may cause contact erythema multiforme	

Seaweed	• *Lyngbya* species (Cyanobacteria):
	  • release toxin in water causing dermatitis, intraepidermal vesiculation
	• *Alcyonidium hirsutum* (moss animal):
	  • produce colony known as sea chervil or Dogger bank moss
	  • pruritic vesiculobullous dermatitis ("Dogger bank itch" seen in fishermen)	

Venomous fish	• Venomous spines can produce severe systemic reactions that are potentially fatal • Stonefish (most dangerous in group) has a potent neurotoxin • Stonefish and stingray can produce tissue necrosis	
Swimmer's itch	• Freshwater swimming (exposed area) • Parasite: freshwater cercarial larvae (schistosome) • Host: waterfowl (humans are accidental infection)	• Clinical: red, pruritic papules in uncovered areas due to skin penetration by cercaria; self-limiting (week) • HP: dermal edema, sparse perivascular eosinophils and neutrophils
Seabather's eruption	• Saltwater swimming (covered area) Parasite: • Larval form of thimble jellyfish *Linchi unguiculata*: Florida coastal waters • Sea anemone *Edwardsiella lineata*: Long Island coastal waters	• Clinical: red, pruritic papules in clothed areas (under swimsuit) due to trapped larvae that have nematocysts (stinging cells) triggered by mechanical pressure or osmotic change; self-limiting (week) • HP = superficial and deep perivascular and interstitial infiltrate of lymphocytes, neutrophils, and eosinophils

29 Helminth Infestations

Onchocerciasis

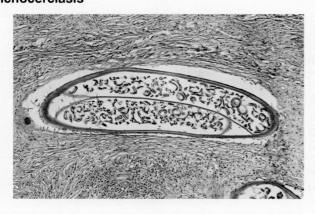

Cutaneous larva migrans

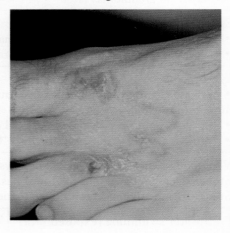

Name	Predilection and Clinical Key Features	Histopathology
Trematode (fluke) infestations		
Schistosomiasis	• Parasite: cercarial larvae of flukes (trematodes) • Larvae in aquatic snails • Red, pruritic papules from cercaria burrowing; later migrate to veins and site of predilection; may produce verrucous nodules or ulcers in the genital or perianal areas Three major species: 1. *Schistosoma mansoni* (egg with lateral spine in stool): • rarely extragenital cutaneous manifestations • prefer portal and mesenteric veins • Africa, Caribbean, South America 2. *S. haematobium* (egg with apical spine in urine): • perineal lesions • predilection for pelvic/bladder veins • Africa and Near East 3. *S. japonicum* (egg with *NO* spine found in stool): • urticarial lesions • predilection for veins in small intestines • Far East • Possible Tx = praziquantel	• Intraepidermal spongiosis with exocytosis of eosinophils and neutrophils; genital/perianal lesions show prominent pseudoepitheliomatous hyperplasia; dermis with numerous ova (not see adult worms) and granuloma formation
Cestode (tapeworm) infestations		
Cysticercosis	• Pork tapeworm • Accidental infestation • Chest wall, upper arm, thighs • Parasite: *Taenia solium* (pork tapeworm), scolex with hooklets and two pairs of suckers • Transmission: uncooked pork • Asymptomatic, subcutaneous nodules composed of white cystic structure with an outer membrane containing a clear fluid and a cysticercus larva attached to one end	• Larva found; fibrous tissue reaction in the subcutaneous tissue with a moderate chronic inflammatory cell infiltrate (variable eosinophils); may contain a few scattered giant cells • Diagnosis made by appearance of scolex on larva (hooklets and two pairs of suckers)
Sparganosis	• Rare tapeworm larvae infestation • Tropics • Parasite: *Spirometra* species (no scolex) • Subcutaneous nodule that slowly migrates	• Subcutaneous fibrosis and inflammatory mixed infiltrate (including eosinophils); worm or larvae in cystic cavity with a flattened structure with longitudinal and horizontal muscle bundles ("checkboard" appearance), basophilic calcareous corpuscles (characteristic feature of cestodes)

Name	Predilection and Clinical Key Features	Histopathology
Nematode infestations		

Onchocerciasis	• Tissue-dwelling nematode
	• Tropical Africa, Yemen
	• Larvae mature to worms and form non-tender, subcutaneous nodules containing worms; microfilariae in lymphatics and migrate to dermis
	• May affect and cause:
	  • Eyes:
	    • "river blindness", #2 cause of blindness
	  • Pruritic, papular rash with hypopigmentation ("leopard skin")
	  • Hyperpigmentation and lichenification:
	    • "lizard" or "elephant" skin
	• Parasite: *Onchocerca volvulus*
	• Transmission: *Simulium* black fly
	• Possible Tx = ivermectin
		• Subcutaneous nodule with dense fibrous tissue; eosinophils; worms with paired uteri; microfilariae in female worm or free in dermis

Dirofilariasis	• Dog heartworm • Mediterranean region • Parasite: *Dirofilaria* worm • Transmission: mosquito • Solitary, erythematous, and tender nodule at site of the worm	• Center of nodule contains degenerating, tightly-coiled worm with a thick, laminated cuticle; intense mixed inflammatory infiltrate (including eosinophils)

Name	Predilection and Clinical Key Features	Histopathology
Cutaneous larva migrans	• "Creeping eruption" • Feet, buttocks, hands • Parasite: hookworms of *Ancylostoma braziliense* (dogs and cats), *Necator* (humans), etc. • Serpiginous, urticarial plaques moving • 1–2 cm/day movement, but only in epidermis (since hookworm lacks collagenase to travel deeper)	• Small cavities in epidermis corresponding to larva track with superficial mixed infiltrate (including eosinophils); spongiosis; intraepidermal vesicle with eosinophils; edema; usually do not see larva
Larva currens	• "Racing larva" • Cutaneous strongyloides (*Strongyloides stercoralis*): • Serpiginous urticarial plaque moving 10 cm/hour (quick) on groin/buttocks, trunk • May cause widespread petechiae and purpura • Usually cause little cutaneous reaction as they migrate through skin to the vessels in order to reach the lungs	
Dracunculiasis	• Dracunculiasis means "affliction with little dragons" • "Guinea worm disease" • Nematode: *Dracunculiasis medinensis* • Reservoir: drinking water with copepods ("water fleas") • Blistering lesion due to migration of worm, which will eventually be extruded through rupture of the bleb	• Anterior end of migration surrounded by granulation tissue containing mixed inflammatory infiltrate; fibrosis and inflammation deeper

30 Arthropod-induced Diseases

Tick

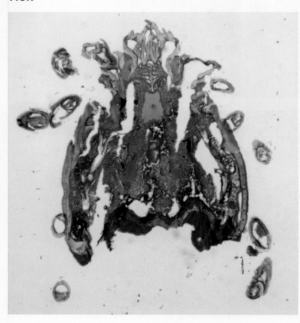

Name	Predilection and Clinical Key Features	Histopathology
Arachnids		
Scorpion bites	• Acral areas usually • Throbbing indurated lesions that may form purpura, bullae, necrosis, etc. • Possible lymphadenitis, systemic symptoms	• Neutrophilic vasculitis with hemorrhage to an arterial wall necrosis to an eschar-covered ulceration and necrosis
Jumping spider	• Pain, no systemic symptoms • Main venom: hyaluronidase • "Jumping spider jumps HIGH" (hyaluronidase)	• Neutrophilic vasculitis with possible hemorrhage; may ulcerate with subcutaneous necrosis; usually eosinophils present
Wolf spider	• Pain, lymphangitis, eschar; bite often secondarily infected • Main venom: histamine • "Wolf spider is furry and HISSES a lot" (histamine)	
Black widow (*Latrodectus mactans*)	• Pain (no necrosis of lesion), cramps, paralysis; due to uncontrolled neurotoxin release • Main venom: lactotoxin neurotoxin • "Black widow is CRAZY lady" (neurotoxin)	
Brown recluse (*Loxosceles reclusa*)	• "Violin spider" (fiddle shape on back) • "Red-white-blue" sign (erythema, ischemia, and necrosis) • Main venom: sphingomyelinase-D • "Brown recluse SPHINGS in the dark" (sphingomyelinase causes hemolysis and necrosis)	• Necrotic lesion with epidermal and superficial dermal necrosis

Name	Predilection and Clinical Key Features	Histopathology
Tick bites	• May cause local erythema due to embedded mouthparts and may transmit diseases	• Mouthparts below an intradermal cavity; moderate mixed infiltrate • If chonic, may form granuloma with superficial and deep infiltrate • Neutrophils often prominent in recent bites
	• Soft ticks (*Argasidae* family)	• *Ornithodoros* species = relapsing fever, Q fever
	• Hard ticks (*Ixodidae* family)	• *Ixodes scapularis* = black-legged teardrop shape: • lyme disease, granulocytic ehrlichiosis, babesiosis (malaria-like) • *Dermacentor* species (wood tick) = possible "tick paralysis" (rapidly resolves with tick removal): • Rocky Mountain spotted fever • attach typically to head and neck • *Amblyomma americanum* ("lone star tick" due to white dorsal spot on female): • ehrlichiosis, Rocky Mountain spotted fever, lyme • attach typically to legs

Name	Predilection and Clinical Key Features	Histopathology
Demodicidosis	• Common human follicle mite • Face • Implicated in rosacea, blepharitis, and folliculitis • *Parasite = Demodex mite:* • *Demodex folliculorum* = found in hair follicle • *Demodex brevis* = found in sebaceous glands	• Follicular dilation; dense homogeneous eosinophilic material around mites; folliculitis; perifollicular inflammation 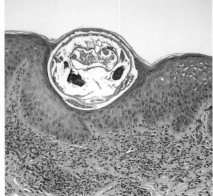

Scabies	• Axilla, groin, finger webs, nipples, trunk
	
	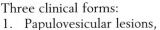
	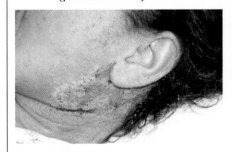
	
	• Extremely pruritic papules, vesicles, or burrows (female creating to deposit eggs)
	• Parasite = *Sarcoptes scabiei* mite (life cycle of 30 days, lays 60–90 eggs)
	• Three clinical forms:
	  1. Papulovesicular lesions,
	  2. Persistent nodules
	  3. Crusted or "Norwegian" scabies (picture below)
		• Eggs, mites, or scybala (brown feces) in stratum corneum; spongiosis; spongiotic vesicles; subepidermal bullae; superficial and deep mixed infiltrate with eosinophils; exocytosis of eosinophils and some neutrophils
		
		• Crusted or "Norwegian" scabies (pictured below)
		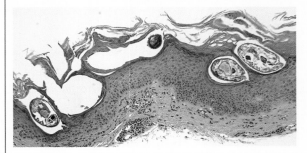

Name	Predilection and Clinical Key Features	Histopathology
Cheyletiella dermatitis	• Non-burrowing mite on dogs, rabbits, cats (called "walking dandruff" on animals) • Chest, proximal extremities (sites of close proximity to pet) • Pruritic dermatitis with grouped, erythematous papules or papulovesicles	• Focal epidermal spongiosis at bite; superficial and mid-dermal mixed infiltrate (including eosinophils); may form vesiculobullous lesions
Other mite lesions (small arachnids)	• Food mites and grain itch mites • Grocery and cheese mite • Paper mites (stored papers and old books) • *Trombicula* (chiggers) • House mouse mite (rickettsial pox) • Various mites may produce urticarial, red papules	• May produce similar appearance to mild arthropod reactions
Insects		
Human lice (pediculosis)	• Lice are blood-suckers and inject saliva that produces an allergic reaction and pruritus • May transmit: • epidemic typhus (*Rickettsia prowazekii*) • relapsing fever (*Borrelia recurrentis*) • trench fever (*Bartonella quintana*)	
	• Head lice (*Pediculus humanus capitis*)	• Infect scalp hair • Empty nit (above)
	• Body lice (*Pediculus humanus corporis*)	• Reside on host and clothing
	• Pubic lice (*Phthirus pubis*)	• "Crab lice" • Infect pubic, axillary hair, or eyebrows

Name	Predilection and Clinical Key Features	Histopathology
Bedbugs	• (Red–brown-colored bug with a flat oval body) • *Cimex lectularius* • Associated with unwashed linen and dirty, dilapidated housing • Urticarial, vesicular lesions with a "breakfast–lunch–dinner" linear bite pattern • Feed at night • May transmit hepatitis B, Chagas' disease	• Variable edema of upper dermis with mixed perivascular infiltrate; interstitial eosinophils
Myiasis	• Fly larvae infestation • Feet and forearms • Furuncle-like appearance with an ulcer formation as larvae work out and fall to ground • Parasite: larvae (maggots) of flies (*Diptera* order) 	• Small cavity possibly containing developing larvae (encased in thick cuticle with widely spaced spines on surface); heavy mixed infiltrate (including eosinophils)

Name	Predilection and Clinical Key Features	Histopathology
Tungiasis	• Central and South America • Feet (since poor-jumping flea) • Nodule or papule • Parasite: pregnant female, sand flea *Tunga penetrans*	• Flea with exoskeleton and ova below stratum corneum in epidermis/dermis; mixed inflammatory infiltrate; hyperkeratosis; acanthosis; ulceration; mass of eggs may be seen in the stratum corneum

Other insect bites	• Numerous insects can cause skin reactions:
	  • *Lytta vesicatoria* ("Spanish fly") = blister beetle in southern Europe that produces cantharidin
	  • Mosquitoes
	  • Biting gnats
	  • Fleas
	  • Moths and butterflies
	
	• Deer fly bites (above)
	
	• Ant bites (above)
		• "Wedge-shaped" infiltrate (below)
		
		• May have prominent papillary dermal oedema with superficial and deep infiltrate (often some eosinophils)

Exaggerated bite reactions	• Leukemia patient (especially chronic lymphocytic leukemia) • Exuberant papules, vesiculobullous lesions develop • Possible Tx = dapsone	• Eosinophilic spongiosis; vesiculation; full-thickness necrosis; intraepidermal and subepidermal vesicles; superficial and deep infiltrate

Tumors of the Epidermis

Warty dyskeratoma

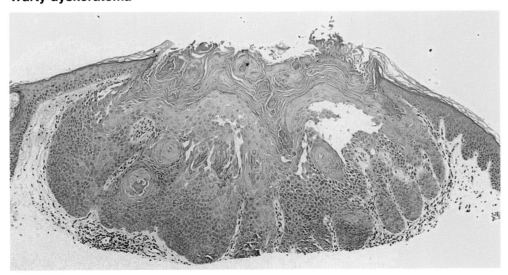

Name	Predilection and Clinical Key Features	Histopathology
Epidermal and other nevi		
Epidermal nevus	• Developmental malformation (congenital hamartoma) • Birth to early childhood • Neck, trunk, extremities • Linear, warty, brown or pale plaque • BCC or SCC may arise in epidermal nevi • Associated with Proteus syndrome, nevus comedonicus • Variants: • "Ichthyosis hystrix" = large, disfiguring nevi with bilateral distribution on trunk and whorl-like pattern • Epidermal nevus syndrome = epidermal nevi (especially ILVEN variant) with neurological, ocular, and skeletal abnormalities	 • Hyperkeratosis; flat, broad papillomatosis; thickened granular layer; acanthosis; slight increase in basal melanin pigment; multiple variable patterns seen; often look "hyperkeratotic SK-like"

Name	Predilection and Clinical Key Features	Histopathology
Inflammatory linear verrucous epidermal nevus (ILVEN)	• Clinicopathological subgroup of epidermal nevi • Early age of onset • Lower extremities • Presents as pruritic, linear eruption along lines of Blaschko • Lesion resembles linear psoriasis clinically and histologically • Associated with epidermal nevus syndrome and burn scars	• Psoriasiform hyperplasia; alternating parakeratosis (overlying agranulosis) and orthokeratosis (overlying hypergranulosis with depressed "cup-like" appearance); mild perivascular infiltrate in upper dermis; variable spongiosis
Nevus comedonicus	• Rare abnormality of infundibulum of hair follicle • Birth to middle age • Face, trunk, neck (usually unilateral) • Unilateral, grouped, or linear open comedones (central keratotic plug) • Alagille syndrome = autosomal dominant disorder with arteriohepatic dysplasia; may be associated with nevus comedonicus	• Dilated keratin-filled invaginations of the epidermis; possible atrophic sebaceous and pilar structure or small lanugo hair present
Familial dyskeratotic comedones	• Autosomal dominant • Childhood to adolescence • Trunk, extremities • Multiple comedones develop	• Follicle-like invagination in the epidermis; filled with laminated keratinous material; dyskeratotic cells in walls of invagination (especially at base)

Name	Predilection and Clinical Key Features	Histopathology

Pseudoepitheliomatous hyperplasia

- Irregular hyperplasia of epidermis, follicular infundibula, and acrosyringium with prominent acanthotic down growths; pale cells with abundant cytoplasm but no significant atypia or mitoses

Granuloma fissuratum	<ul><li>"Spectacle-frame acanthoma"</li><li>Lateral aspect of nose bridge, retroauricular region</li><li>May appear BCC-like, but groove corresponding to point of contact with spectacles aids diagnosis</li></ul> 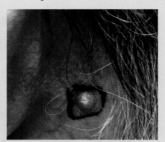 <ul><li>Painful or tender firm, flesh-colored or pink nodule with a grooved central depression at point of pressure/friction</li></ul>	<ul><li>Focal "LSC-like" in appearance (not "granuloma-like"); marked acanthosis with broad, elongated rete pegs; mild hyperkeratosis; central depression with attenuated or ulcerated epidermis; prominent granular layer; telangiectasias with inflammatory infiltrate</li></ul> 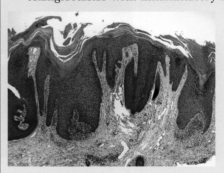 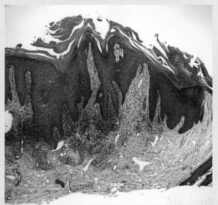
Prurigo nodularis	<ul><li>"Picker's nodule"</li><li>Extensor aspects of arms, trunk, face (areas within reach to "pick")</li></ul> 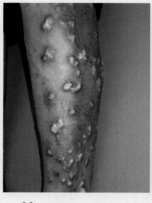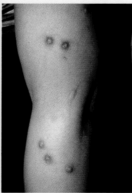 <ul><li>Numerous, persistent, intensely pruritic, firm, pink, localized nodules</li><li>May have underlying cause</li></ul>	<ul><li>"Localized LSC-like"</li></ul> 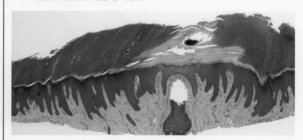 <ul><li>Prominent hyperkeratosis with focal parakeratosis; marked irregular acanthosis (often pseudoepitheliomatous); hypergranulosis; vertical orientation of collagen in dermal papillae; perivascular lymphocytic infiltrate</li></ul> 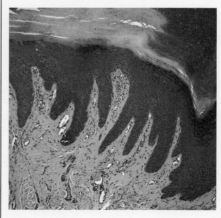

Name	Predilection and Clinical Key Features	Histopathology
Acanthomas		
• Benign tumors of epidermal keratinocytes ("tumor of acanthosis")		
Epidermolytic acanthoma	• All ages • Solitary, verrucous-like papule • Decreased keratin 1 and 10	• Epidermolytic hyperkeratosis (i.e. hyperkeratosis, vacuolar degeneration); bluish, "moth-eaten" keratinocytes with hazy borders, vacuoles, and cytoplasmic eosinophilic inclusions

Name	Predilection and Clinical Key Features	Histopathology
Warty dyskeratoma	• Middle age to elderly • Head and neck • Solitary papule with an umbilicated/pore-like center on sun-damaged skin	• "Isolated cup" of Darier's disease • Cup-shaped or comedo-like invagination of epidermis with down growths; hyperkeratosis, parakeratosis, dyskeratotic keratinocytes (including corps ronds and grains) and acantholysis
Acantholytic acanthoma	• Elderly men • Trunk area • Solitary, asymptomatic keratotic papule/nodule • Multiple lesions in renal transplant patients	• "Focal acantholysis without dyskeratosis" (similar to localized Hailey–Hailey) • Exophytic, hyperkeratosis, papillomatosis, and acantholysis

Name	Predilection and Clinical Key Features	Histopathology
Seborrheic keratosis (SK)	• "Senile warts" • First appear in middle age • Chest and almost any body part, except palms/soles • Sharply, demarcated, gray–brown to black, "stuck-on," greasy, verrucous-like" papule • Irritated seborrheic keratosis (above) • *Note:* Endothelin-1 (keratinocyte-derived cytokine) stimulates melanocytes and thought to cause melanization of seborrheic keratoses	• Epidermal proliferation (hyperkeratosis, papillomatosis, acanthosis); horn pseudocysts; abundant melanin; possible "squamous eddies" (nests of squamous cells); "string sign" (sharp demarcation along epidermal base) • Irritated seborrheic keratosis (below) • Reticulated seborrheic keratosis (below) • Clonal seborrheic keratoses (below) resemble Borst–Jadassohn phenomenon with intraepidermal nests of basaloid cells

	• Leser–Trelat sign:
	  • Sudden increase in number and size of seborrheic keratoses; pruritic and inflamed (especially trunk area)
	  • Possibly indicates a malignant visceral cancer (GI adenocarcinoma is #1); lymphoproliferative disorder)
	  • May precede onset of cancer symptoms	

Name	Predilection and Clinical Key Features	Histopathology
Dermatosis papulosa nigra (DPN)	• Variant of seborrheic keratosis • Black female adults (10–35% of black race) • Malar area of face, neck • Multiple, small, pigmented papules	• Type of "reticulated-seborrheic keratosis" appearance (hyperkeratosis; elongated and interconnected rete ridges with basal hyperpigmentation)
Melanoacanthoma	• Variant of seborrheic keratosis • Elderly individuals • Head and neck, trunk • Slow-growing, benign, pigmented lesion; may resemble a seborrheic keratosis or a melanoma	• Composed of keratinocytes and melanocytes; features of a seborrheic keratosis but also numerous melanocytes with mature melanosomes and heavy pigment

Name	Predilection and Clinical Key Features	Histopathology
Clear cell acanthoma [PAS+ due to glycogen in cells]	• Middle age to elderly • Legs • Firm, brown–red, dome-shaped papule or nodule; crusted surface with scaly collarette; bleeds easily with trauma • Increased glycogen in cells due to defect in phosphorylase (degrades glycogen) • Multiple clear cell acanthomas are associated with ichthyosis	• Well-demarcated psoriasiform hyperplasia; pale-staining keratinocyte cytoplasm; broad, slender rete pegs; neutrophilic scale-crust on surface; increased vessels in dermal papillae; exocytosis of neutrophils (may form intraepidermal microabscesses)
Clear cell papulosis [Characteristic stain is GCDFP-15, PAS]	• Possibly a benign variant of Paget's • Young women and boys (often Asian or Hispanic descent) • Face, chest, abdomen • Multiple white papules; possibly along milk lines	• Presence of clear cells scattered mainly among basal cells (few in malpighian layer); mild acanthosis • DDx: pagetoid dyskeratosis (contains clear cells higher in epidermis)
Large cell acanthoma	• Possible spectrum of solar lentigo or early seborrheic keratosis • Middle age to elderly • Sun-exposed skin • Sharply demarcated, scaly, lightly pigmented patch	 • Epidermal thickening due to enlarged keratinocyte size of cell and nucleus; sharply demarcated from normal keratinocytes; orthokeratosis; prominent granular layer

Name	Predilection and Clinical Key Features	Histopathology
Epidermal dysplasias • Potential for malignant transformation		
Actinic keratosis (AK)	• "Solar keratosis" • Older individuals • Face, ears, arms (sun-exposed skin) • Hypertrophic AK (pictured above) • Circumscribed, scaly, erythematous papules • 8–20% may transform to SCC (if untreated) • Associated with p53 mutation and chronic sun damage • Possible Tx = cryo (99% cure rate), 5-FU, imiquimod	• Hyperkeratosis; focal parakeratosis overlying atypical keratinocytes; loss of granular layer; loss of orderly stratified arrangement of epidermis; sparing adnexae epidermis and acrosyringium; perivascular/lichenoid lymphocytic infiltrate; solar elastosis • Atrophic actinic keratosis (below) • Hypertrophic actinic keratosis (below)
Actinic cheilitis	• Actinic keratosis of the lip • Vermilion part of lower lip • Dry, whitish–gray, scaly plaques with possible erythema, erosion, or ulceration • Due to chronic sun exposure; also may be associated with smoking and chronic irritation	• Alternating orthokeratosis and parakeratosis; disordered maturation of epidermal cells with increased mitosis and atypia; prominent solar elastosis; moderate infiltrate (including plasma cells below ulcerations)

Name	Predilection and Clinical Key Features	Histopathology
Arsenical keratoses	• Exposure possible through arsenic in drinking water and naturopathic medicines • Palms and soles (keratoses) • Associated with increased risk of NMSC and visceral cancers (GI adenocarcinoma and lung) • Cutaneous, diffuse, or "raindrop-like" hyperpigmentation with keratoses on palms and soles • Associated with Mees' lines on the nail plate (single transverse white bands in multiple nail plates) 	• Prominent hyperkeratosis with papillomatosis, atypical keratinocytes • May resemble a hyperkeratotic seborrheic keratosis, hyperkeratotic actinic keratosis or squamous cell-in-situ
PUVA keratosis	• Non-sun-exposed skin of long-term PUVA patients • Associated with increased risk of NMSC • Warty, raised papule with a broad base and scaly surface	• Variable acanthosis, orthokeratosis, and parakeratosis; papillomatosis possible; few atypical cells, but with absence of solar elastosis (which differs from actinic keratosis)

Name	Predilection and Clinical Key Features	Histopathology
Intraepidermal carcinomas		
SCC-in-situ or Bowen's disease	• 8% progress to SCC • Fair-skinned individuals • Face, legs (sun-exposed areas) • Asymptomatic, well-defined erythematous, scaly plaque that expands centrifugally • Associated with sun exposure, arsenic ingestion, HPV	• Atypical keratinocytes (hyperchromatic, pleomorphic, mitosis) involving full thickness of epidermis; loss of granular layer; parakeratosis; "wind-blown epidermis" (loss of orderly maturation); "flip sign" (superficial epidermis appears like deeper epidermis instead of normal superficial epidermis with larger, mature, eosinophilic cells); perivascular infiltrate; does not spare acrosyringium (as in actinic keratosis) Does not stain S-100 (melanoma) or CEA (Paget's) typically
Erythroplasia of Queyrat	• SCC-in-situ of the penis • 10% progress to invasive SCC • Uncircumcised males • Glans of penis • Circumscribed, asymptomatic, bright red, shiny plaque	• Similar to Bowen's disease (SCC-IS)

Borst–Jadassohn changes	• Borst–Jadassohn phenomenon = discrete clones or nests of squamous, basaloid, or pale keratinocytes within the epidermis
	• DDx:
	  • Clonal seborrheic keratosis, or irritated SK
	  • Hidroacanthoma simplex
	  • Inverted follicular keratosis
	  • Bowen's disease
	  • Actinic keratosis
	  • Epidermal nevi (rarely)
		• Presence of nests of atypical keratinocytes within the epidermis

Name	Predilection and Clinical Key Features	Histopathology
Malignant tumors		

Basal cell carcinoma (BCC)
 	
[bcl-2 and Ber-EP4+ stain extensively (unlike trichoepithelioma and SCC); CD34 negative in stroma, unlike trichoepithelioma]
	• "Trichoblastic carcinoma"
	• #1 skin cancer (70%)
	• Older males
	• Head and neck (80%)
	• Associated with sun exposure (especially UVB burns) and nevus sebaceus
	• Mutations:
	  • p53
	  • PTCH (affects Sonic Hedgehog/SHH signaling): transmembrane protein that inhibits Gli-1
	  • Smoothened (SMO) gene (binds with PTCH)
	
	• Pearly, red macule, papule, or nodule; "rodent eaten-like" ulcer, rolled-up border
	• Risk of metastasis = 0.05%
	• Aggressive subtypes:
	  • Sclerosing/morpheaform
	  • Micronodular
	  • Basosquamous
	  • Infiltrative
	
	• Pigmented BCC (clinical and dermoscopy images above)
		• Variability in morphology of abnormal trichoblasts; nodular variant is most common (70%)
		• Overall, islands of basaloid cells with hyperchromatic nucleus and little cytoplasm, surrounded by a stroma; calcifications; palisading of cells at the periphery and haphazard arrangement in center of islands; stromal retraction/clefting seen; may deposit calcium, amyloid, fibromyxoid stroma; may contain follicular differentiation
		
		Superficial BCC Sclerosing BCC
		
		Pigmented BCC Fibroepithelioma of Pinkus
		
		Micronodular BCC Morpheaform BCC
		
		• Stains:
		  • bcl-2 stains extensively (unlike trichoepithelioma)
		  • Ber-EP4+ (unlike SCC)
		  • Does not stain CD34 in stroma, unlike trichoepithelioma (which is CD34 positive in the stroma)

Name	Predilection and Clinical Key Features	Histopathology
Basal cell syndromes	• Basal cell nevus syndrome (autosomal dominant) = see below Bazex's syndrome (X-linked dominant) = multiple BCC + follicular atrophoderma (dorsa of hands usually) + hypohidrosis (or hyper-) + pili torti + hypotrichosis … but no palmar pits or defective teeth • Rombo syndrome (autosomal dominant) = BCC + atrophoderma vermiculatum (honeycomb, "worm-eaten" cheeks due to perifollicular atrophy following keratosis pilaris); milia + trichoepithelioma + hypotrichosis + peripheral vasodilation with cyanosis • Brooke–Spiegler syndrome (autosomal dominant) = CYLD mutation; BCCs + cylindromas + trichoepitheliomas, spiradenoma • Xeroderma pigmentosum (autosomal recessive) = multiple BCCs + multiple freckles + defective teeth; mutation = nucleotide excision repair	
Nevoid basal cell carcinoma syndrome	• "Gorlin's syndrome" • Autosomal dominant • BCCs when <20 years old • Mutation = PTCH1 gene (tumor suppressor gene encoding Sonic Hedgehog transmembrane receptor protein) • Two or more BCCs; palmoplantar pits (65–80%); jaw cysts (90%); defective teeth; calcification of falx cerebri; hypertelorism; risk of medulloblastomas (may present prior to cutaneous manifestations)	• Basal cell lesions appear similar to typical BCC • Cutaneous cysts usually are epidermal cysts • Palmar/plantar pits with loss of keratin and granular layer: look "superficial BCC-like" • Odontogenic keratocyst: fibrous capsule cyst with corrugated stratified squamous epithelial lining and basaloid cells up into epidermis

Name	Predilection and Clinical Key Features	Histopathology
Squamous cell carcinoma (SCC) [EMA, cytokeratin]	• SCC overall: • Chronic sun-damaged skin (UVB > UVA) • Forehead, face, neck, dorsa of hands • Associated with renal transplant patients, immunosuppressed, and HPV infection (especially HPV-16, -18, -5, or -8); HPV can inactivate *Rb* gene • May develop at sites of chronic injury/scar (Marjolin's ulcer), burns, fistula tracts, hidradenitis suppurativa • Associated with arsenic exposure (i.e. drinking water) • Common mutations = p53 and p16 (tumor suppressors) • Shallow ulcers, often with keratinous crust and elevated, indurated surroundings • Least at risk of metastasis is tumor arising is sun-damaged skin and less than 2 cm in diameter • Usual risk of SCC metastasis is approximately 0.5%, while for SCC in skin not exposed to the sun it is approximately 2–3%. Risk varies by variant and location, too.	• Nests of atypical keratinocytes (hyperchromatic, pleomorphic, mitosis) invading dermis; squamous eddies (keratin pearls); possible perineural invasion with perineural lymphoctyes • [EMA, cytokeratin; S100, desmin, Ber-EP4 negative] • Acantholytic SCC (pictured above)

Name	Predilection and Clinical Key Features	Histopathology
Spindle-cell squamous carcinoma [CK903+]	• Variant of squamous cell carcinoma • Organ transplant patients • Sun-damaged or irradiated skin	• Spindle cells with large, vesicular nucleus and scant, eosinophilic cytoplasm
Adenoid squamous cell carcinoma	Head and neck	• Nests of squamous cells with central acantholysis that appears "gland-like"
Pseudovascular squamous cell carcinoma	• Rare variant of adenoid SCC • Ulcer or crusted nodule on sun-exposed skin; may be mistaken for angiosarcoma	• Pseudovascular structures lined by cords of polygonal or flattened tumor cells • [Stains = cytokeratin, EMA positive, but negative for CD31, CD32, factor VIII]

Name	Predilection and Clinical Key Features	Histopathology
Verrucous carcinoma	• "Wart-gone-wild" = variant of SCC • Plantar lesions ("epithelioma cuniculatum"), oral cavity • Associated with chewing tobacco and HPV-6, -11, -16, -18 • Slow-growing, warty, exophytic, painful tumor • Do not treat with radiation due to HPV association	• Exophytic and endophytic; well-differentiated squamous epithelium; low mitosis; broad, "bulbous" rete ridges with acanthotic down growths
Adenosquamous carcinoma [EMA, cytokeratin; mucin stain with alcian blue at 2.5, PAS]	• Rare, often aggressive, tumor • More commonly a tumor associated with salivary glands • Elderly • Penis • Elevated plaque	• Deeply invasive tumor with islands and strands of SCC admixed with glandular structures with mucin
Carcinosarcoma (metaplastic carcinoma) [Cytokeratin, EMA; not S100]	• Very rare biphasic tumor • Elderly • Face, scalp (sun-exposed areas) • Ulcerated nodule (1–15 cm)	• Biphasic tumor with a mixture of both epithelial (BCC or SCC) and mesenchymal (fibrosarcoma, chondrosarcoma, osteogenic sarcoma) • Squamous, neural, and chondroid differentiation
Lymphoepithelioma-like carcinoma	• Rare tumor • Head and neck • Solitary nodule or papule	• Dermal or subcutis, lobulated, well-differentiated tumor composed of large epithelial cells surrounded by a dense infiltrate of lymphocytes; mitosis frequent

Name	Predilection and Clinical Key Features	Histopathology
Miscellaneous "tumors"		
Cutaneous horn	• Face, ears, dorsa of hands • Solitary, hard, yellowish–brown keratotic "horn" (height > half diameter) • Most commonly overlies an actinic keratosis, seborrheic keratosis, SCC, etc.	• Keratotic material; base of lesion may demonstrate various entities (actinic keratosis, seborrheic keratosis, SCC, verruca vulgaris, etc.)
Stucco keratosis	• Distal legs • Multiple, symmetric, small (1–4-mm), grayish–white keratotic papules	• "Hyperkeratotic seborrheic keratosis-like"; prominent orthokeratosis, papillomatosis; little to no inflammation • No increase in basaloid cells and no horn cysts • HPV-23b and other HPV types often found on PCR

Name	Predilection and Clinical Key Features	Histopathology
Clavus (Corn)	• Feet (areas overlying a bony prominence) • Due to friction or pressure • Painful keratotic lesion with small horny plug	• Thick parakeratotic plug in a "cup-shaped" depression of the epidermis; often loss of granular layer under plug; few telangiectatic vessels
Callus	• Often ball of foot, heel or palm (areas of friction) • Non-painful circumscribed lesion with hyperkeratosis • Due to pressure, foot deformity, or friction	• Similar to clavus, but often thickened granular layer; stratum corneum thickened and compact
Onychomatricoma	• "Onychomatrixoma" • Benign tumor of the nail matrix • Elderly • Fingernails and toenails • Longitudinal yellow, thickened band on nail plate; splinter hemorrhages (proximal nail plate); increased transverse curvature of nail	• Epithelial cell strands originating from the nail matrix and penetrating vertically into the dermis; fibrous stroma sharply delineated from tumor

Name	Predilection and Clinical Key Features	Histopathology
Keratoacanthoma (KA)	• Well-differentiated subtype of SCC • Elderly males • In temperate climates, more common on face; in subtropical climates, usually on extremities, dorsa of hands • Solitary, pink, or flesh-colored dome-shaped nodule with central keratin plug ("volcano-like"); rapid growth (1–2 cm over 1–2 months) • Tendency to involute spontaneously in 3–6 months • Associated with excessive sun exposure, trauma, immunosuppressed, xeroderma pigmentosum, burns, etc.	• Exophytic and endophytic lesion • Keratin-filled crater with "lipping" of lesion edges over the crater; pale, eosinophilic, well-differentiated cells with mild atypia; squamous eddies (keratin pearls); perivascular or lichenoid lymphocytic infiltrate

Name	Predilection and Clinical Key Features	Histopathology
Giant keratoacanthoma	• Tumor >2–3 cm in diameter • Predilection for nose and dorsum of hand	
Keratoacanthoma centrifugum marginatum	• Rare variant • Progressive peripheral growth with coincident central healing • May grow to >20 cm or more in diameter	• Involution and fibrosis in center; "KA-like" at periphery
Subungual keratoacanthoma	• Grows rapidly, often fails to regress • Usually causes pressure erosion of distal phalanx; may invade bone under nail	• More dyskeratotic cells than a typical KA
Multiple keratoacanthomas	*Multiple KAs of Ferguson–Smith:* • "Multiple self-healing squamous epithelioma" • Autosomal dominant • Possible mutation = transforming growth factor beta 1 receptor (TGFβR1) gene • Develop KAs (no more than 12) over time in covered and exposed areas • Starts in adolescence • Regress leaving atrophic scars (possibly disfiguring) *Multiple eruptive KAs of Grzybowski:* • Hundreds of KAs • Form at age 50–60 • May develop on palms/soles and be pruritic *Muir–Torre syndrome* = sebaceous tumors + internal malignancy (especially colon adenocarcinoma) • Lesions may include sebaceous adenomas > sebaceous carcinoma, or KAs • Mutation = MSH-2, MLH-1 (DNA mismatch repair genes): stain for lack of MSH-2 (negative) is diagnostic	

32 Lentigines, Nevi, and Melanomas

Melanoma

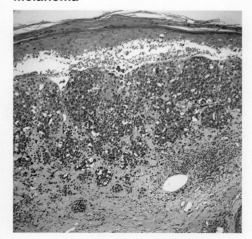

Type of Nevus Cells	Cell Features	Typical Location	Histopathology
Type A	Epithelioid (large, pale nucleus with more cytoplasm); pigmented cytoplasm	Junctional or superficial dermis	
Type B	"Lymphocyte-like" (small, dark nucleus with less cytoplasm); non-pigmented or pigmented	Mid-dermis	
Type C	Small, spindle-shaped (pink cytoplasm) May form neuroid structures	Deeper dermis	

Name	Predilection and Clinical Key Features	Histopathology
Lesions with basal melanocyte proliferation		
Ephelis	• "Freckle" • Appear first 3 years of life • Fair skin (especially if red hair) • Face and shoulders • Related to sun exposure (especially bursts of high intensity) • Multiple, small (1–3-mm), well-circumscribed, red–brown macules • Darken easily with sun 	• Increased basal melanin • No elongation of rete ridges and no nests
Lentigo simplex (simple lentigo)	• Children to young adults • Anywhere including mucosa • Unrelated to sun exposure (or little relationship) • 1–5-mm, brown to black, sharply demarcated macule; may progress to junctional nevus • Associated with Peutz–Jeghers, LEOPARD syndrome, Carney syndrome, etc. Dermoscopy image (above)	• Benign proliferation of melanocytes; variable hyperpigmentation with increased number of melanocytes; regular elongation of rete ridges • No melanocytic nests and no solar elastosis

Name	Predilection and Clinical Key Features	Histopathology

Multiple lentigines	• *LEOPARD syndrome:*
	   • L = lentigines in infancy
	   • E = EKG conduction defects (conduction)
	   • O = ocular hypertelorism (increased width)
	   • P = pulmonary stenosis
	   • A = abnormal genitalia (cryptorchidism)
	   • R = retardation of growth
	   • D = deafness (neural)
	• Autosomal dominant
	• Includes disorders associated with multiple lentigines and systemic findings
	• Mutation = PTPN11 (same in Noonan's)	

	Peutz–Jeghers syndrome: (hereditary intestinal polyposis syndrome) • Hereditary intestinal polyposis syndrome • Autosomal dominant • Average age at diagnosis = 20s • Intussusception (possibly first clinical sign); intestinal hamartomatous polyps; mucocutaneous melanocytic macules • Increased risk of cancers (especially GI, pancreas, liver) • Common mutation = STK11/LKB1 (serine/threonine kinase 11) • Basal hyperpigmentation; possible increase in melanocytes	
	• *Cronkhite–Canada syndrome* = GI polyposis + lentigo simplex macules on face, palms, soles (not lips, possibly buccal mucosa); risk of protein losing enteropathy • *Bandler syndrome* = lentigo simplex + GI bleeds/hemangioma (not polyps)	

	Carney syndrome:
	   • Multiple lentigines, blue nevi, myxomas, psammomatous melanotic schwannoma, and endocrine overactivity
	   • Testicular cancer risk
	   • Mutation = PRKAR1A gene
	   • Carney syndrome = NAME (or LAMB) + endocrine overactivity (i.e. thyroid, Cushing syndrome, etc.)
	   • *"NAME"*:
	      • N = nevi (lentigines, ephelides, blue nevi)
	      • A = atrial myxoma
	      • M = myxoid tumors of skin
	      • E = ephelides
	   • *"LAMB"*:
	      • L = lentigines (mucocutaneous)
	      • A = atrial myxoma
	      • M = mucocutaneous myxomas
	      • B = blue nevi	

Name	Predilection and Clinical Key Features	Histopathology
Laugier–Hunziker syndrome	• Acquired, benign hyperpigmentation disorder with no systemic manifestations • Mucosa macules + skin macules (no intestinal polyp risk); macules are typically brown or black (but are not lentigines) • Multiple hyperpigmented macules on lips, buccal mucosa; also typically longitudinal bands on the nails • Think of LH = "lips and hands" • Do not confuse with syndromes associated with lentigines, such as Cronkhite-Canada syndrome or Peutz-Jeghers syndrome (see p. 530)	• Basal layer hypermelanosis (does not appear like a lentigo histologically); possible pigment incontinence; no increased melanocytes
Labial and genital melanotic macules	• Location dependent: • Lips (especially lower lip vermilion border) • Penis/vulva • Tan-brown to brown-black macule	 • Prominent hyperpigmentation (melanin) in basal layer, accentuated at rete tips; broad rete ridges; slight increase in melanocytes
Melanotic macules of nail bed/matrix	• "Melanonychia striata" • Melanocytes normally in matrix, but usually inactivated • Black individuals • Longitudinal, narrow band of pigmentation of the nail bed and matrix; usually sharply defined and less than 3mm in width	• Increase in melanocytes and hyperpigmentation

Name	Predilection and Clinical Key Features	Histopathology
Solar (senile, actinic) lentigo	• Middle age to elderly • Face, dorsa of hands • Related to sun exposure • Irregular, dark-brown to black macules • May progress to a seborrheic keratosis or lichenoid keratosis	• Hyperpigmented basal layer; increased melanocytes; "dirty feet" elongated, clubbed rete ridges; solar elastosis present; no melanocyte nests
Ink spot lentigo	• Variant of solar lentigo • Black, irregular macule (resembles a "spot-of-ink")	• Increased basal cell hyperpigmentation
Lentiginous nevus	• Evolution of lentigo simplex into a junctional or a compound nevus • Adults • Trunk area • Well-circumscribed tan-brown to black macule or papule	• Advancing edge resembles simple lentigo (lentiginous proliferation of melanocytes) and central area with melanocytic nests (junctional nests, possibly a small number of mature intradermal)

Name	Predilection and Clinical Key Features	Histopathology
Speckled lentiginous nevus (nevus spilus)	• Type of congenital nevus • Birth to childhood • Tan–brown macule with small, dark hyperpigmented speckles • Association with subtypes of phakomatosis pigmentovascularis (congenital syndrome with pigmentary abnormalities + vascular anomalies, such as capillary malformations, Mongolian spots, nevus spilus, etc.)	*"Lentigo simplex + nevus" appearance:* • "Background area" pigmentation resembles lentigo simplex • "Speckled-area" hyperpigmentation resembles lentiginous nevus with areas progressing to a junctional or compound nevus

Name	Predilection and Clinical Key Features	Histopathology
PUVA lentigo	• PUVA patients • Buttocks, palmoplantar (sun-protected areas)	• Varies with similarities to lentigo simplex or may show large, atypical melanocytes in basal layer
Scar lentigo	• Pigmented lesion develops in excised pigmented lesion area	• May show lentiginous hyperplasia, hyperpigmentation with no increase in melanocytes; or may show melanocytic hyperplasia without epidermal hyperplasia
Melanocytic nevi		
Junctional nevus	• Childhood to early adolescence • "Lentigo-like" appearance • Well-circumscribed brown to black macule • May form longitudinal melanonychia if at nail matrix (see p. 531)	• Discrete nests of melanocytes only at DE junction (especially on rete ridges); elongated rete ridges; rare or no mitosis

Name	Predilection and Clinical Key Features	Histopathology
Compound nevus	• Lesion elevates as nests of melanocytes extend ("drop off") into dermis • Children to adolescents • Tan or dark-brown papule, may have minimal elevation to dome-shaped to polypoid	• Both junctional nests (along DE) and intradermal melanocytes; epidermis may be flat to seborrheic keratosis-like with horn cysts • May vary due to location (e.g. genital nevi have enlarged junctional nests with pagetoid spread of melanocytes; flexural nevi show dyshesive pattern)

Name	Predilection and Clinical Key Features	Histopathology
Intradermal nevus	• Most common melanocytic nevi • Maturing nevi with loss of junctional activity and remain only in the dermis, resulting in progressively less pigment with time • Adults • Flesh-colored to light pigmented; dome-shaped, nodular or polypoid lesion; hair may protrude	 • Nests and cords limited to dermis only • Deeper parts may form "neuroid" shape (i.e. "neural nevus" with spindle-shape and Meissner tactile body-like structures)
Osteo-nevus of Nanta	• Secondary change seen in an intradermal nevus, resulting in bone formation (incidental finding)	• Benign nevus with osseous metaplasia (osteoma cutis)

Name	Predilection and Clinical Key Features	Histopathology
Clonal nevi	• Benign variant of a compound nevus with tiny foci of hyperpigmentation ("small tiny dots") 	• Well-circumscribed nodule with foci of atypical epithelioid cells with fine dusty melanin pigment and irregular nuclear contour
Meyerson's nevus	• Nevus surrounded by eczematous halo • Young adults • Eczematous halo around a red, scaling, pruritic junctional, compound, or intradermal nevus; does not regress (unlike halo nevus)	• "Spongiosis + nevus" • Eosinophils usually present and exocytosis

Name	Predilection and Clinical Key Features	Histopathology
Ancient nevus	• Elderly • Face • Dome-shaped, skin-colored or reddish–brown nodule	• Melanocytic nests with two populations (large pleomorphic cells with hyperchromatic nuclei and small monomorphous cells); degenerated hyalinized stroma; often thrombi, hemorrhage
Deep penetrating nevus [S100, HMB-45]	• "Plexiform spindle cell nevus" or "Seab's nevus" • Young adults • Face, upper trunk, proximal extremities • Deeply pigmented nodule	• "Deep-penetrating tongues of nests" • Sharply demarcated nodule in a wedge shape; some pleomorphism; vertically-oriented melanocytes extend to deep dermis, often to fat; usually spindle cells predominant

Name	Predilection and Clinical Key Features	Histopathology
Balloon cell nevus	• Clinically indistinguishable from an ordinary melanocytic nevus • "Ballooning" secondary to improper packaging of melanosomes	• Large, swollen ("ballooned") melanocytes with a clear, pale cytoplasm and central nucleus (>50% balloon cells); often multinucleate balloon cells
Halo nevus [S100]	• "Sutton's nevus" • Teenagers • Trunk • May involve one or more nevi • Depigmented halo around a melanocytic nevus, often preceding lymphocytic destruction and regression	 • Usually compound nevus with dense lichenoid lymphocytic (CD8+) infiltrate; few "surviving" melanocytes; depigmented halo area shows absence of melanin and basal melanocytes

Name	Predilection and Clinical Key Features	Histopathology
Cockarde nevus	• Nevus with a peripheral halo with an intervening non-pigmented zone ("targetoid appearance")	• Central nevus similar to junctional or compound nevus • Non-pigmented zone lacks melanocytes • Peripheral halo contains junctional nests
Eccrine-centered nevus	• Nevus proliferation closely related to eccrine sweat ducts	
Recurrent nevus	• Anywhere on body • Occurs from persistent nevus following a shave biopsy • Pigmented macule/papule within a scar from a biopsy	• Sharply circumscribed; fibrosis and scar (horizontal collagen); junctional melanocytes with possible nests in dermis; no lateral extension of melanocytes (do not extend beyond scar) • Melanocytes may be below the scar; no nuclear atypia

Name	Predilection and Clinical Key Features	Histopathology
Spitz nevus [HMB-45 (less intense deep), S100; Ki-67 (MIB-1) stains only 2–3% of cells, while stains >15% of cells in melanoma]	• Children to young adults • Face, trunk, lower limbs • 75% = pigmented papules; 25% = red, non-pigmented papules • Classic dermoscopy image = "starburst" pattern	• Classical appearance: • Symmetric, sharply demarcated lesion • Hyperkeratotic • Spindle or epithelioid cells (rare or no mitoses seen) • Maturation of cells as become superficial • "Clutching" of nests by rete ridges ("banana-like") • Kamino bodies • Fibroplasia around junctional melanocytes • "Banana-bunches" of melanocytes (below) • Kamino bodies (above) • Major diagnostic criteria: • Symmetry (usually symmetric) • Cell type (epithelioid or spindle): spindle more common • Maturation of cells: smaller, ordinary melanocytes seen deeper • Absent pagetoid spread • Kamino bodies (coalescent eosinophilic globules): • present at DE junction (not specific) • contain laminin, collagen IV, fibronectin

Name	Predilection and Clinical Key Features	Histopathology

Atypical Spitz nevus	• Variant of Spitz nevus
	
	• High risk of metastasis:
	  • Age >10 years old
	  • Diameter >10 cm
	  • Ulceration present
	  • Involving subcutis
	  • Mitotic rate at least 6/mm^2
	• Tx = excision, but also possibly sentinel lymph node biopsy
		• Histological features differ from typical depiction, resulting in uncertain malignant potential

Halo Spitz nevus	• Variant of Spitz nevus • Nevus with depigmented peripheral rim	• Nevus with depigmented rim or nevus with heavy lymphocytic response resembling a halo but sparing of adjacent basal melanocytes with no clinical halo formed

Name	Predilection and Clinical Key Features	Histopathology
Desmoplastic nevus [p16]	• Likely a variant of Spitz nevus • Skin-colored or light-brown papule; may mistake for fibrohistiocytic lesion (i.e. dermatofibroma or epithelioid histiocytoma) clinically	 • Sclerotic dermis; sparse pigment; little or no junctional or nest activity; plexiform arrangement of bundles and lobules of melanocytes
Plexiform Spitz nevus	• Plexiform arrangement of bundles and lobules of enlarged spindle to epithelioid melanocytes	
Malignant Spitz tumor	• Malignant variant of Spitz • Children • Large lesion (>1 cm) • May metastasize to regional lymph nodes, but not any further (benign otherwise with long-term survival)	• Nodule that extends to subcutaneous fat with a high mitotic rate, cellular pleomorphism, less maturation with depth and less cohesion of cells than usual Spitz nevus

Name	Predilection and Clinical Key Features	Histopathology
Pigmented spindle cell nevus	• "Reed nevus" • Variant of Spitz nevus • Female adults • Thighs • Well-circumscribed, deeply pigmented, black papule Clinical image Dermoscopy image	• Symmetric, spindle-shaped cell nests; heavily pigmented; Kamino bodies; symmetric and orderly growth pattern; limited pagetoid cell spread to lower epidermis; vertically oriented nests and pigmented parakeratosis Kamino body (above)

Name	Predilection and Clinical Key Features	Histopathology

Congenital melanocytic nevus	• Birth
	• 1% of newborns
	• Trunk
	
	• Tan–brown papule, patch; may have increased hair in lesion
	• 63% are 1–4 cm in size
	• Association with Carney's syndrome, epidermal nevus syndrome, neurofibromatosis type 1
	• Size classification:
	  • Small <1.5 cm
	  • Medium = 1.5–19.9 cm
	  • Giant = 20+ cm, usually in "bathing suit" area:
	    • risk of melanoma (5%), usually <1 year of age
	    • risk of neurocutaneous involvement
	
		• May be junctional, compound, or intradermal type
		
		• Melanocytes in congenital nevus:
		  • Usually in deeper two-thirds of dermis
		  • Between collagen in single file
		  • Seen in arrector pili muscle
		  • Involve eccrine glands (see below)

Name	Predilection and Clinical Key Features	Histopathology
Dermal melanocytic lesions (May be due to incomplete migration of precursor melanocyte cells during embryogenesis)		
Mongolian spot	• Birth to soon after birth • Oriental race • Sacral region • Bluish–gray patches of discoloration • Tend to disappear with age • Association with phakomatosis pigmentovascularis	• Spindle-shaped melanin-containing melanocytes in lower half of dermis; epidermis appears normal

Name	Predilection and Clinical Key Features	Histopathology
Nevus of Ota	• Birth • Females; pigmented races • Area of ophthalmic and maxillary divisions of trigeminal nerve (CN V) • Diffuse, slightly speckled, macular area of blue to dark-brown pigmentation; may involve conjunctiva/sclera	• Nodular collections of melanocytes resembling a blue nevus; diffuse infiltrate of elongated melanocytes in upper dermis
Nevus of Ito	• Birth • Same as nevus of Ota, but area of supraclavicular and deltoid region (cutaneous branch of brachii lateralis nerve)	• Same as nevus of Ota

Name	Predilection and Clinical Key Features	Histopathology
Blue nevus [S100, Melan-A (MART-1), HMB-45; not CEA]	• After infancy • Females • Extremities • Represents arrested melanocytic migration • Two main variants: 1. Common (dendritic) blue nevus (extremities): • slate-blue or blue–black macule/papule 2. Cellular blue nevus (50% on buttocks, sacrococcygeal): • larger nodule than common blue nevus • more likely to form malignant blue nevus • Other variants: • Epithelioid blue nevus = resembles common blue nevus but has round cells and often associated with Carney complex • Desmoplastic (sclerosing) blue nevus = atrophic variant; dendritic melanocytes and melanophages embedded in a dense, hyalinized stroma ("dermatofibroma-like")	• Common (dendritic) blue nevus (below): • Elongated ("spindle-shaped" with wispy, delicate extensions) dendritic melanocytes in the mid and upper dermis; some melanophages (macrophages with phagocytosed melanin clumps); normal epidermis • Cellular blue nevus (below): • "Dumb-bell-like" with down growth along adnexal structures and bulge-like at the fat; "biphasic pattern" with elongated dendritic cells and pale, plump spindle cells; and have melanophages; normal epidermis

Name	Predilection and Clinical Key Features	Histopathology
Combined nevus	• Presence of two or more different types of melanocytic nevus in a single lesion • "True and blue" nevus = overlying intradermal nevus combined with a blue nevus (photo below): most common type of combined nevus 	• Two melanocytic nevus types in one lesion; most commonly an intradermal nevus and a blue nevus (photos below)
Sclerosing blue nevus	• Variant of blue nevus	• Blue nevus appearance with a dermal fibrosis (sclerosing)

Name	Predilection and Clinical Key Features	Histopathology
Blue nevus with osteoma cutis	• Rare variant of blue nevus associated with bone formation • *Note:* osteo-nevus of Nanta is bone formation in an intradermal nevus (see p. 536)	• Blue nevus with osseous formation
Malignant blue nevus [PCNA (proliferating cell nuclear antigen), Ki-67 (MIB-1)]	• Also known as "variant-of-melanoma" • Exceedingly rare, aggressive tumor • Middle age to elderly • Males (slightly) • Scalp, face, buttocks • Usually arises in cellular blue nevus • Possible nodal and distant metastasis (especially lungs)	• Underlying blue nevus; dense cellular area with atypical mitoses and cytological atypia; necrosis; subcutaneous invasion
Dermal melanocyte hamartoma	• Present at birth (very rare) • Large areas of diffuse gray–blue pigmentation	• Dendritic melanocytes scattered throughout upper and mid-dermis
Phakomatosis pigmentovascularis	• Congenital syndrome with pigmentary abnormalities + vascular anomalies: • Pigmentary abnormalities = nevus spilus, Mongolian spot, nevus depigmentosus, blue nevus, nevus of Ota • Vascular anomalies = all types have a nevus flammeus (i.e. "port-wine stain," capillary malformation) • Variants: • Type I: CM + epidermal nevus • Type II: CM + dermal melanocytosis ± nevus anemicus • Type III: CM + nevus spilus ± nevus anemicus • Type IV: CM + dermal melanocytosis + nevus spilus ± nevus anemicus • Histopathology similar to dermal melanocyte hamartoma	
Cutaneous neurocristic hamartoma	• "Pilar neurocristic hamartoma" • Birth • Neural crest-derived lesion with melanocytes (nevoid), pigmented spindle and dendritic cells and Schwann cells • Clinically, resembles blue nevus or congenital nevus	• Resembles a congenital nevus with neuroid features; mixture of melanocytes, Schwann cells and dendritic blue nevus cells • Pilar neurocristic hamartoma (above) showing folliculocentric lesion with sweat gland involvment

Name	Predilection and Clinical Key Features	Histopathology
Atypical nevomelanocytic lesions		

Dysplastic (atypical, Clark's) nevus	• Older children to young adults
	• Scalp, trunk
	
	• Pigmented macule, papule, or plaque with irregular pigmentation and/or borders
		• Four main features:
		1. Intraepidermal lentiginous hyperplasia of melanocytes:
		  • proliferation of single melanocytes; elongated rete with bridging and poorly circumscribed nests at DE
		2. Random cytological cell atypia:
		  • enlarged hyperchromatic nuclei
		3. Stromal response:
		  • concentric (wrap around rete) and lamellar fibroplasia of papillary dermis
		4. Architectural atypia
		  • "shoulder phenomenon" (peripheral extension of junctional component beyond the dermal component)
		
		• "Shoulder phenomenon" (above)
		
		• "Bridging of rete" (above)
		
		• "Concentric fibroplasia" around rete (above)

Dysplastic nevus syndrome	• Familial or sporadic • Trunk (80 or more nevi) • In childhood, nevi appear normal; then in adolescence to adulthood, nevi appear abnormal • Increased risk of melanoma (10% or more) • Association with intraocular melanomas, oral melanoma in-situ, tumors (especially pancreatic) and endocrine abnormalities	
Lentiginous dysplastic nevus of the elderly	• Elderly (>60 years old) • Back (males); legs (females) • Possible precursor to melanoma (especially superficial spreading type)	• Elongated, uneven rete ridges; extensive junctional nesting; lamellar fibrosis around dermal papillae; variable lymphocytic infiltrate

Name	Predilection and Clinical Key Features	Histopathology
Malignant melanocytic lesions		

Malignant melanoma overall
 	
[S100 most sensitive; HMB-45 and MART-1 more specific; Ki-67 (MIB-1), a proliferation marker]
	• Most common in sun-covered areas
	• Men (on the back) and women (legs)
	• Two-thirds arise in new lesions; one-third arise in pre-existing melanocytic nevi
	
	• Partial regression seen in one-third of melanomas
	• Growth phases:
	  1. Radial growth = typically precedes vertical growth
	  2. Vertical growth:
	    • dermal mitosis, and
	    • dermal nests > junctional nests
	• Risk factors include:
	  • Two or more sunburns before age 15
	  • Intermittent intense sun exposure
	  • Large congenital or atypical nevi
	  • Genetic factors (see below)
	  • Nevi >6 mm
	  • Fair skin or hair color
	  • Tendency to burn easily
	  • Xeroderma pigmentosum
	• Genetic factors:
	  • *CDKN2A* (cyclin-dependent kinase inhibitor), encodes tumor suppressor proteins p16 (part of Rb pathway) and p14^{ARF} (part of p53 pathway)
	  • *B-RAF* gene (60–70%) and NRAS gene, part of cell signaling and growth
	  • PTEN (50%), tumor suppressor gene
	
	• Clinical and dermoscopy images of the same lesion (above)
	• Prognostic and/or staging factors:
	  1. Tumor thickness (Breslow depth) = measured from granular layer to deepest tumor cell
	  2. Ulceration
	  3. Mitoses in primary lesion
	  4. Lymph node involvement (microscopic or macroscopic)
	  5. Distant metastasis and lactate dehydrogenase (LDH) level
		• Proliferation of atypical melanocytes, singly and in nests
		
		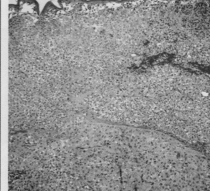

Name	Predilection and Clinical Key Features	Histopathology
Lentigo maligna melanoma (5–15%)	• Elderly • Face, upper extremities • Irregularly pigmented macule that slowly expands; vertical growth of invasive malignancy characterized by elevated plaques or discrete nodules; regression possible • In-situ precursor = lentigo maligna (see p. 558)	• Epidermal atrophy; atypical single and nests of melanocytes in basal layer; pagetoid invasion of epidermis; atypical melanocytes in dermis; solar elastosis; multinucleate melanocytes with prominent dendritic processes ("starburst giant cell"); inflammation • "Starburst" giant cell (pictures below)

In-situ precursor = lentigo maligna (see p. 558)

Name	Predilection and Clinical Key Features	Histopathology
Superficial spreading melanoma (50–75%)	• Any age and anywhere (sun exposed and non-sun exposed) • More common on trunk (males) and legs (females) • Variegated color with an irregular expanding margin; regression possible	• No solar elastosis; "buckshot scatter" of pagetoid melanocyte spread in epidermis; atypical single and poorly formed nests of melanocytes at all levels in the epidermis; often lichenoid infiltrate • Mitotic cells (above)

Name	Predilection and Clinical Key Features	Histopathology
Nodular melanoma (15–35%)	• Any age • Vertical growth with no radial growth phase initially • Dark-brown or blue–black nodular, polypoid, or pedunculated lesion; possible ulceration	• Dermal nodule of atypical melanocytes; no adjacent intraepidermal spread (<3 rete ridges); inflammation

Name	Predilection and Clinical Key Features	Histopathology
Acral lentiginous melanoma (5–10%)	• Elderly male • Black or Asian races • Palmar, plantar, or subungual • Pigmented plaques or nodules; often ulcerate; subungual melanoma may present as longitudinal melanonychia	• Lentiginous elongation of rete ridges with atypical melanocytes in basal layer; epidermal melanocytes may appear misleadingly benign (only slight upward spread)

Name	Predilection and Clinical Key Features	Histopathology
Desmoplastic melanoma [S100; note: HMB-45 and Melan-A/MART-1 often negative!]	• Head and neck • Often found in areas of recurrence or metastasis • Spreading indurated plaque or bulky, firm, swollen lesion; often non-pigmented and high recurrence (but associated with better survival rate)	• "Spindle cells + scar-like stroma" • Strands of elongated spindle-shaped cells in a fibrotic stroma ("scar-like"); infiltrates deep in dermis; often lack pigment; scattered collections of lymphocytes and plasma cells; neural transformation possible ("nerve-like" appearance)

Name	Predilection and Clinical Key Features		Histopathology
Miscellaneous group of melanomas			
Verrucous melanoma	• Rare variant of superficial spreading melanoma • Adult males • Back, limbs		• Marked epidermal hyperplasia; elongation of rete ridges; hyperkeratosis; may be confused with a seborrheic keratosis
Neurotropic melanoma	• Variant of desmoplastic melanoma • If neurotropism, high risk of recurrence		• Spindle-shaped cells with "neuroma-like" pattern (neural transformation); lack pigment; circumferential arrangement around nerves (neurotropism)
Lentigo maligna	• "Hutchinson's melanotic freckle" • Melanoma in-situ of sun-exposed skin with solar elastosis • Head and neck • Pigmented macule on sun-exposed skin • If becomes invasive, then termed a "lentigo maligna melanoma" (see p. 558)		• Solar elastosis; epidermal atrophy; usually spindle-shaped melanocytes and less likely pagetoid cells • Extends down the adnexal structures (above)

Name	Predilection and Clinical Key Features	Histopathology
Balloon cell melanoma	• Occurs in primary and secondary melanomas	• Ballooned melanocytes and atypical melanocytes; show nuclear pleomorphism, mitoses, and cytological atypia (differentiate from balloon cell nevus)
Animal-type melanoma	• Scalp • Blue to jet-black nodule • Heavy melanin production, similar to animal melanomas (especially gray horses where often benign)	• Dermal, heavily pigmented epithelioid and dendritic cells with numerous melanophages • *Note:* called "animal-type" because similar histologically to a melanocytic neoplasm in white and gray horses

Name	Predilection and Clinical Key Features	Histopathology
Nevoid melanoma [S100, HMB-45, Ki-67]	• Variant of melanoma	• Benign-appearing intraepidermal component with possible maturation of cells; presence of deep mitotic activity; cellular atypia deep in the lesion; variable nests and arrangement of small nevus-like cells • May be misdiagnosed as benign, due to symmetry, organized appearance, and cell type superficially; but deep mitosis and atypia help differentiate
Amelanotic melanoma	• Melanoma without any pigment clinically • Clinically, may be misdiagnosed as a BCC or SCC	• Similar histologically to melanoma (i.e. nodular, acral lentiginous, etc.)
Other melanoma variants	• Myxoid melanoma • Signet-ring melanoma • Rhabdoid melanoma • Osteogenic melanoma • Small cell melanoma • Small diameter melanoma • Ganglioneuroblastic melanoma • Angiomatoid melanoma • Bullous melanoma	

Name	Predilection and Clinical Key Features	Histopathology
Clear cell sarcoma [S100, HMB-45, Melan-A]	• "Melanoma of soft parts" • Soft tissue tumor derived from neural crest cells • Adolescents and young adults • Dermal nodule, may become painful ulcer • Translocation (12;22) found in 60% of cases	• Nests and strands of bland oval or elongated cells separated by thin collagenous septa; melanin and glycogen present in two-thirds of cases; multinucleate tumor cells often present

Squamo-melanocytic tumor
[S100, cytokeratin]
	• Middle-aged to elderly
	• Face
	• Purple–black nodule
		• Discrete dermal nodule surrounded by a fibroblastic stroma; no epidermal involvement
		• Two types of cells:
		  1. Epithelial squamous cells (form pearls)
		  2. Atypical epithelioid cells

33 Tumors of Cutaneous Appendages

Name	Predilection and Clinical Key Features	Histopathology
HAIR FOLLICLE TUMORS		
Hamartomas and tumors of hair germ		
(Pilar tumors which form nests, strands, and cords of basaloid cells with varying degrees of differentiation towards a hair follicle)		

Hair follicle nevus	• Head and neck
	• Small nodule or area of hypertrichosis
	• "Faun-tail" clinical variant:
	  • Patch of hair over the lower sacral area
	  • Possibly a cutaneous marker of spinal dysraphism (incomplete closure of neural tube)
		• Closely arranged mature vellus follicles

Trichofolliculoma	• Well-differentiated and structured pilar tumor • Adults • Face, scalp, neck • Small, dome-shaped nodule with small, fine vellus hairs extending from central pore • Associated with activated beta-catenin mutation (CTNNB1 gene); has role in hair follicle development (mutation also may be seen in pilomatricoma)	• Central dilated follicle ("mama hair") and many smaller hair follicles radiating ("baby hairs"); often enveloped in vascular fibrotic stroma • *HP reminder:* looks like ornaments fallen off a Christmas tree, think "fa-la-la-la-liculoma"

Name	Predilection and Clinical Key Features	Histopathology
Sebaceous trichofolliculoma	• Variant of trichofolliculoma (similar to folliculosebaceous cystic hamartoma) • Adults • Nose • Pit-shaped depression with fistulous openings containing hairs	• Large, sebaceous follicles connecting to a central, "comedo-like" cavity lined by stratified squamous epithelium, containing hairs and keratin debris
Trichoadenoma	• Benign pilar tumor with hair follicle-like differentiation (between trichoepithelioma and trichofolliculoma) • Face, buttocks • Solitary, asymptomatic nodule	• Well-defined dermal tumor of epithelial islands with central cystic cavity containing keratinous material; multilayered squamous epithelium lining; no hair shafts present typically and minimal (if any) basaloid islands (verrucous trichoadenoma variant has cysts with some vellus hairs)

Name	Predilection and Clinical Key Features	Histopathology
Trichoepithelioma	<ul><li>Poorly differentiated hamartoma of hair germ</li></ul><ul><li>Three variants:<ol><li>Solitary = skin-colored papule (nose, upper lip, cheeks)</li><li>Multiple (Brooke's disease) = autosomal dominant; onset as child; multiple papules on central face</li><li>Desmoplastic variant</li></ol></li><li>Associated with:<ul><li>ROMBO syndrome (autosomal dominant):<ul><li>trichoepitheliomas, BCCs, atrophoderma vermiculatum (perifollicular atrophy after keratosis pilaris), milia, hypotrichosis, peripheral vasodilation with cyanosis (acrocyanosis)</li></ul></li><li>Brooke–Spiegler syndrome (autosomal dominant):<ul><li>Brooke's disease + cylindromas + spiradenoma</li><li>*CYLD* mutation: increases transcription factor NF-κB</li></ul></li><li>Rasmussen syndrome:<ul><li>cylindroma + milia + trichoepitheliomas</li></ul></li></ul></li></ul>	<ul><li>Dermal tumor with basaloid islands; keratin horn cysts lined with squamous epithelium; hair follicles; papillary mesenchymal bodies (abortive hair follicles with spindle, stromal, fibroblast cells close to basaloid hair bulb); Merkel cells; clefts in stroma (not between aggregates and stroma as in BCC)</li></ul><ul><li>Stains:<ul><li>Ber-EP4 stains focally positive (BCC stains Ber-EP4 diffusely)</li><li>bcl-2 stains basal layer (periphery) only (BCC stains bcl-2 diffusely)</li><li>CK20 due to Merkel cells present (BCC is negative)</li><li>Stroma CD34+ (BCC is CD34 negative)</li><li>CK7 negative (unlike trichoblastoma)</li></ul></li></ul>

Name	Predilection and Clinical Key Features	Histopathology

Desmoplastic trichoepithelioma	• Variant of trichoepithelioma
	• Females, young adults
	• Face
	
	• Asymptomatic, solitary, hard annular lesions with a raised border and depressed center (umbilicated appearance)
		• Well circumscribed tumor in upper and mid-dermis with "central dell"; Merkel cells; horn cysts; cords and small nests of basaloid cells with scant cytoplasm in a fibrous stroma; numerous keratin cysts; foreign body granulomas; eosinophilic rim of collagen; calcifications
		• Positive stains:
		  • Ber-EP4 focally positive (BCC diffusely positive)
		  • bcl-2 stains basal layer (periphery) only (BCC diffuse)
		  • Stroma is CD34+ (negative in BCC)
		  • CK20 due to Merkel cells present (negative in BCC)
		  • Involucrin (negative in syringoma)
		
		• DDx: morpheiform BCC for pseudoclefts and not "syringoma-like" in upper dermis; syringoma usually does not have horn cysts or calcifications; microcystic adnexal carcinoma (MAC) has a deeper component

Name	Predilection and Clinical Key Features	Histopathology
Trichoblastoma [CK7, CK8, and CK19 expressed; trichoepithelioma is CK7 negative]	• Likely on a spectrum with trichoepithelioma (also called immature, solitary, and giant trichoepithelioma) • Rare benign tumor of the hair germ • Scalp, trunk, genital area • Slow-growing, solitary, large (>1 cm) nodule in the deep dermis and subcutis • Similar to odontogenic neoplasms • Associated with nevus sebaceus	• Circumscribed dermal tumor with no epidermal connections and rarely horn cysts; clefting around tumor; fibrotic stroma; irregular nests of basaloid cells; "failed attempt" to form follicular germ/papillae; deeper and larger than trichoepithelioma

Name	Predilection and Clinical Key Features	Histopathology
Cutaneous lymphadenoma	• Trichoblastoma variant • Rare adnexal tumor with a prominent lymphocytic infiltrate inside tumor nests • Face, legs • Small nodule present for months to years	• Multiple, round lobules of basaloid cells with peripheral palisading; fibrous stroma; intense mature lymphocyte infiltrate within lobules • [bcl-2 stains basal layer (periphery) only; stroma CD34+]

Name	Predilection and Clinical Key Features	Histopathology
Panfolliculoma	• Extremely rare tumor • Advanced follicular differentiation towards all elements of the follicle • Overlaps trichoblastoma and matricoma	• Follicular lesion; often cystic containing corneocytes; differentiation towards various elements of the follicle (matrical cells, trichohyalin granules, corneocytes, shadow cells)

Name	Predilection and Clinical Key Features		Histopathology
Follicular hamartoma syndromes	• Generalized hair follicle hamartoma	• Syndrome with papules and plaques on the face, progessive alopecia and myasthenia gravis (also cystic fibrosis)	
	• Basaloid follicular hamartoma	• Numerous variants including solitary, linear, inherited, linear nevoid, generalized forms	• Thin, anastomosed strands and branched cords of basaloid cells with a loose fibrous stroma; affecting majority of pilosebaceous units • No clefting between stroma and aggregates (as in BCC)
	• Linear unilateral basal cell nevus with comedones	• Linear or zosteriform lesions (some with comedone plugs) that present at birth or soon after • Clinically resembles a nevus comedonicus but histologically resembles a basal cell carcinoma	

Name	Predilection and Clinical Key Features	Histopathology
Infundibular and isthmic tumors (Isthmic differentiation has pale cells and small ducts with pink cuticle)		
Tumor of the follicular infundibulum (TFI)	• Actually of isthmic origin • Head, neck, upper chest • Solitary, asymptomatic, smooth or slightly keratotic papule • Associated with: • Cowden's disease • Nevus sebaceus • Schöpf–Schultz–Passarge syndrome: • adult-onset ectodermal dysplasia syndrome with multiple hidrocystomas of eyelid, PPK, hypodontia, hypotrichosis, and nail dystrophy	 • "Plate-like" fenestrated subepidermal tumor with pale or pink-staining glycogen containing cells with a peripheral palisade of basal cells (similar to a superficial BCC); multiple connections to epidermis
Dilated pore of Winer	• Common adnexal lesion • Elderly • Head, neck, upper trunk • Solitary, comedo-like structure with open pore	• Markedly dilated follicular pore; infundibular keratinization with keratohyaline granule formation; acanthosis and finger-like projections into dermis; central horny plug; may have heavy melanin pigmentation in follicular wall

Name	Predilection and Clinical Key Features	Histopathology
Pilar sheath acanthoma	• Rare, benign follicular tumor (isthmic origin) • Upper lip of older individuals • Small lesion (5–10 mm) with a central pore-like opening plugged with keratin	• Central, cystically dilated follicle with keratinous material opening to surface; lobules composed of outer root sheath epithelium (some cells with abundant glycogen) extending from the wall of cystic cavity ("bulbous projections"); no hair present in cavity • More acanthosis than dilated pore of Winer

Name	Predilection and Clinical Key Features	Histopathology
Inverted follicular keratosis (IFK)	• Possible variant of seborrheic keratosis • Males and elderly • Cheek, upper lip, head, and neck • Solitary, flesh-colored nodular or filiform lesion	• "Downward growing seborrheic keratosis" with prominent squamous eddies: endophytic tumor with large lobules or finger-like projections into dermis; both basaloid (periphery) and squamous cells (toward center) present; prominent squamous eddies (concentric layers of squamous cells in a whorled pattern); mild infiltrate

Name	Predilection and Clinical Key Features	Histopathology
Tricholemmal (external sheath) tumors		

Tricholemmoma
[CD34+]
	• Face
	• Small, solitary, asymptomatic, smooth or wart-like papule
	• Associated with:
	  • Cowden's disease
	  • Bannayan–Riley–Ruvalcaba syndrome
		• Sharply circumscribed tumor with downward lobular growth; clear keratinocytes due to glycogen vacuolation; squamous eddies; peripheral layer of palisading columnar cells ("eyeliner" sign)
		• *HP reminder:* looks like pendulous udders and eyeliner, so think of a "trichole-mama" cow (i.e. Cowden's)

Name	Predilection and Clinical Key Features	Histopathology
Desmoplastic tricholemmoma	• Variant of tricholemmoma • Face, neck • Indurated lesion with a central depression and raised border • Associated with nevus sebaceus (not associated with Cowden's disease)	 • Lobulated tricholemmoma pattern + irregular cords into dermis surrounded by hyalinized stroma
Cowden's disease (multiple hamartoma disease)	• Present in adolescence • High risk of breast and thyroid cancer • Mutation = *PTEN* gene (tumor suppressor gene with tyrosine phosphatase and tensin homology) • Multiple tricholemmomas, tumors of the follicular infundibulum, mucosal papillomas; sclerotic fibromas and hamartomas of skin, mucosa, GI, eyes, etc. • Risk of developing Lhermite–Duclos disease (dysplastic gangliocytoma of cerebellum)	
Bannayan–Riley–Ruvalcaba syndrome	• Macrocephaly + multiple tricholemmomas + multiple lipomas + GI polyps • No increased risk of malignancy as in Cowden's disease • Mutation = *PTEN* gene	
Tricholemmal carcinoma	• Rare malignant variant of tricholemmoma • Elderly • Sun-exposed skin on face and extremities • Appears clinically BCC-like	• Multilobular, down growth connected to the epidermis; clear cells with tricholemmal keratinization and peripheral palisading

Name	Predilection and Clinical Key Features	Histopathology
Tumors with matrical differentiation		
Pilomatricoma	<ul><li>"Calcifying epithelioma of Malherbe" or "pilomatrixoma"</li><li>Benign lesion with differentiation toward the matrix of hair follicles</li><li>Children</li><li>Head and neck, extremities</li></ul> <ul><li>Solitary, hard, multilobular papule covered with normal skin; skin-color to bluish color; "tent sign" (stretching of skin shows multiple facets and angles); may discharge calcium through eroded areas</li><li>Multiple lesions associated with myotonic dystrophy, sarcoidosis, Turner's, Gardner's, and Rubinstein–Taybi syndrome</li><li>Mutation = activated beta-catenin (75%), CTNNB-1 gene (catenin, beta-1); role in hair follicle development</li></ul>	<ul><li>Circumscribed, lower dermis nodule similar to a cyst; two cell types present (basophilic cells at periphery and eosinophilic shadow/ghost cells with a pale, empty space instead of nucleus); keratinous debris; calcifications (two-thirds of cases); stroma ossification (13%); foreign body giant cells; mixed inflammatory infiltrate</li></ul> <ul><li>Ghost cells are faulty hair shafts produced by matrical cells</li></ul>

Name	Predilection and Clinical Key Features	Histopathology
Pilomatrix carcinoma	• May arise de novo or in a pilomatricoma • Male adults most common • Scalp, face • Solitary lesion • Local recurrence common, metastasis infrequent • Mutation = CTNNB1 gene (encodes β-catenin)	• Pilomatricoma with high mitotic activity, cytological atypia, locally aggressive behavior; rarely, vascular and lymphatic invasion

Name	Predilection and Clinical Key Features	Histopathology
Melanocytic matricoma	• Face • Small, circumscribed papule	• Well-circumscribed dermal nodule with variable melanized, pleomorphic and mitotically active matrical and supramatrical cells with islands of shadow cells; dendritic cells with melanin pigment
Tumors with prominent perifollicular mesenchyme		
Fibrofolliculoma	• Benign hamartomatous conditions of the mantle epithelium (mantle differentiates into sebaceous duct/gland) • Same tumor as trichofolliculoma, but different stage • Develops in 30s usually • Face • Solitary, skin-colored facial papule • Associated with Birt–Hogg–Dubé syndrome (see p. 579), and nevus lipomatosus (see p. 647)	• Fibrofolliculoma stage: more mantles. Hair follicle with thin cords of epithelium ("antler" or "bat-wing-like"); fibrotic stroma; possible sebaceous ducts

Name	Predilection and Clinical Key Features	Histopathology
Trichodiscoma	• Benign hamartomatous conditions of the mantle epithelium (mantle differentiates into sebaceous duct/gland) • Same tumor as trichofolliculoma, but a different stage • Develops in 30s usually • Face • Numerous skin-colored papules • Associated with Birt–Hogg–Dubé syndrome (see below)	• Trichodiscoma stage: more perifollicular sheath. Well-demarcated, non-encapsulated tumor; fascicles of loose fibrosis in a mucinous stroma without thin follicular extensions; prominent vessels; follicular components "pushed aside"
Birt–Hogg–Dubé syndrome (BHD)	• BHD is associated with fibrofolliculomas and trichodiscoma: • Autosomal dominant genodermatosis • Fibrofolliculoma + Acrochordons + Trichodiscomas ("FAT Hogg") • Risk of renal cell carcinoma, thyroid cancer, colon polyps, and spontaneous pneumothorax • Mutation = FLCN (BHD) gene, which encodes folliculin protein	

Name	Predilection and Clinical Key Features	Histopathology
Neurofollicular hamartoma	• Possibly on a spectrum with trichodiscoma and fibrofolliculoma • Face (especially near nose) • Solitary, pale papule	• Hyperplastic pilosebaceous units with intervening stroma of spindle cells in a broad, haphazard fascicle; stroma has features of an angiofibroma and a neurofibroma (possibly related to folliculosebaceous cystic hamartoma) • Nerve-like cells in the stroma (above)

Name	Predilection and Clinical Key Features	Histopathology
SEBACEOUS TUMORS • See page 322 for general sebaceous gland information		

Ectopic sebaceous glands

Name	Predilection and Clinical Key Features	Histopathology
Fordyce's spots and related ectopias	• Sebaceous glands without an attached follicle, glands empty directly to surface • Upper lip, buccal mucosa (Fordyce's spots), breast areola (Montgomery's tubercles), penis, labia minora 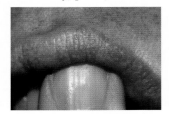 • Tiny yellow papules, especially near mucocutaneous junctions	• Sebaceous glands opening directly to surface without an attached hair follicle 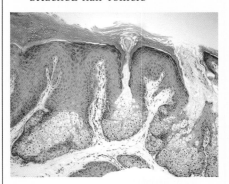 • Fordyce's spot (photo above) 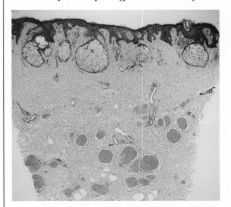 • Montgomery's tubercle (photo above)

Hamartomas and hyperplasias

Name	Predilection and Clinical Key Features	Histopathology
Folliculosebaceous cystic hamartoma	• Rare hamartomatous lesion with follicular, sebaceous, and mesenchymal components • Possible late-stage trichofolliculoma with follicular structure involution • Adults • Central face, nose • Solitary, symmetric papule	• Numerous radiating sebaceous glands; cystic structure or comedo; possible rudimentary hair structures or apocrine glands; fibrosis and spindle-shaped cells in stroma 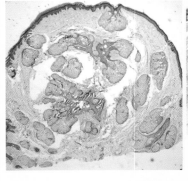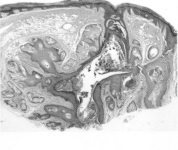 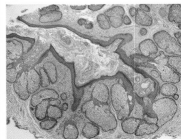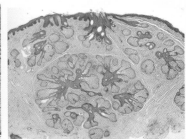

Name	Predilection and Clinical Key Features	Histopathology
Sebaceous hyperplasia	• After age 40 • Forehead, cheeks • Small, cream-colored or yellowish umbilicated papule • Associated with sun exposure, cyclosporine, etc.	• Large, mature sebaceous gland with central, dilated duct (may be filled with debris, bacteria, or vellus hair); often solar elastosis
Juxtaclavicular beaded lines	• Variant of sebaceous hyperplasia • More common in dark-skinned individuals • Supra- and subclavicula area of neck • Tiny papules arranged in closely spaced parallel rows along skin tension lines, likely associated with hair follicle and/or opening	• Similar sebaceous hyperplasia; may also have isolated sebaceous lobules in upper dermis and not obriously connected to hair follicles

Name	Predilection and Clinical Key Features	Histopathology
Steatocystoma	• Young adults • Chest • Multiple yellowish to skin-colored papules/cysts • May be solitary or multiple (multiplex) • Variants: • Simplex (rare) = solitary cyst • Multiplex = numerous cysts; associated with Jackson–Lawler syndrome (pachyonychia congenita, type 2) with keratin 17 mutation	• Empty dermal cyst (oily substance gone) with undulating stratified squamous epithelium; sebaceous glands in wall; eosinophilic cuticle ("red roof"); may have vellus hairs • Reminder: "stea- at the Red Roof Inn" (i.e. red cuticle)

Name	Predilection and Clinical Key Features	Histopathology
Benign sebaceous tumors		
Sebaceous adenoma	• Benign tumor • Elderly • Head and neck • Pink, flesh-colored or yellow papule/nodule; slow growing • May be associated with Muir–Torre syndrome (see below)	• Circumscribed, lobular tumor with peripheral basaloid cells and >50% mature sebaceous cells (sebocytes); openings to surface
Muir–Torre syndrome	• Sebaceous tumors + visceral cancer (usually gastrointestinal carcinomas, most commonly colon adenocarcinoma) • Cutaneous lesion may include sebaceous adenomas, sebaceoma, sebaceous carcinoma, keratoacanthomas or epidermal cysts • Mutation = MSH-2, MLH-1 (DNA mismatch repair genes); lacks MSH-2 stain	• The sebaceous tumors resemble typical sebaceous tumors, but may be difficult to classify. Often they are solid sheets of basaloid cells in some lobules; or intermingled basaloid and sebaceous cells without any orderly maturation. Mucinous and cystic areas may be present; cystic lesions are an important component of this syndrome

Name	Predilection and Clinical Key Features	Histopathology
Sebaceoma	<ul><li>"BCC with sebaceous differentiation" or "sebaceous epithelioma" (old names)</li><li>Face or scalp</li></ul><ul><li>Yellowish papulonodules</li><li>Associated with Muir–Torre syndrome (see p. 584)</li></ul>	<ul><li>Multiple nests of basaloid cells (BCC-like) with <50% mature sebocytes (more basaloid cells present); do not connect to surface</li></ul>
Mantleoma	<ul><li>Benign tumor of the sebaceous mantle which gives rise to the sebaceous gland from undifferentiated sebocytes</li><li>Face</li><li>Small papule</li><li>"Mantle" for "cloak": it appears to cover the hair follicle below the infundibulum–isthmus junction</li></ul>	<ul><li>Cords of undifferentiated basaloid cells "hanging down" from the side of the follicular infundibulum like a "skirt"</li><li>Varying degrees of vacuolization of the cells (sebocyte formation)</li></ul>

Name	Predilection and Clinical Key Features	Histopathology
Folliculocentric basaloid proliferation	• Due to hyperplasia of mantle epithelium • Face • Normal-appearing skin clinically	• Multifocal, multishaped proliferation of uniform basaloid cells which often involves the follicular epithelium (folliculocentric); may form a "pinwheel" appearance or "head of Medusa-like" often vertically oriented; peripheral palisading of cells; lacks direct epidermal attachment; normal stroma; no artificial clefts between the stroma and basaloid cells (Frozen sections pictured below) • *Note:* May be confused with BCC, especially on frozen section in Mohs surgery; however, BCC has artificial clefts between a myxoid stroma and aggregate of cells, with a more reticular and disorganized pattern

Name	Predilection and Clinical Key Features	Histopathology
Malignant sebaceous tumors		
Sebaceous carcinoma [Oil-red-O and Sudan black stain will show lipids in vacuolated cells]	• Slight female preponderance • Two variants: 　1. Periocular (75% of cases): 　　• upper eyelid > lower eyelid 　　• arises from meibomian gland of tarsal plate or gland of Zeiss of the eyelashes 　　• chalazion-like in appearance 　2. Extraocular (25%): 　　• head, neck, trunk 　　• pink to yellow–red nodule • Possible lymph node metastasis (one-third) • May rarely be associated with Muir–Torre syndrome (see p. 584), nevus sebaceous or a rhinophyma	• Lobules or sheets of cells separated by a fibrovascular stroma; extends deep possibly to muscle; variable sebaceous differentiation with foamy or vacuolated clear cells; periocular lesions have pagetoid sebocytes

(see p. 584)

Name	Predilection and Clinical Key Features	Histopathology
APOCRINE TUMORS • See page 325 for general apocrine gland information		
Apocrine cysts and hamartomas		
Apocrine nevus	• Rare tumor (often part of nevus sebaceus) • Upper chest and axilla	• Increased numbers of mature apocrine glands
Apocrine hidrocystoma	• "Apocrine gland cyst" • Cyst arising from apocrine secretory portion (non-proliferative, cystic lesion) • Middle-age to older adults • Head and neck • Solitary, dome-shaped translucent or bluish lesion • May develop from Moll's gland of eyelid • Multiple cysts associated with Schöpf–Schulz–Passarge syndrome (autosomal recessive) = PPK + eyelid apocrine hidrocystomas + hypodontia + hypotrichosis + hypoplastic nails	• Multiloculated, collapsed dermal cyst with columnar cells with decapitation secretion (i.e. "pinch off"); outer layer of elongated, flat myoepithelial cells • *Note:* Hidrocystomas are non-proliferative, cystic lesions (unlike apocrine cystadenomas, which are proliferative and have papillary projections with a fibrous core)

Name	Predilection and Clinical Key Features	Histopathology
Apocrine cystadenoma [Ki-67]	• Cystic proliferation of the apocrine glands • May proliferate, unlike apocrine hidrocystomas • Head and neck • Solitary, dome-shaped translucent or bluish lesion	• Cystic space with papillary projections containing apocrine decapitation

Name	Predilection and Clinical Key Features	Histopathology
Syringo-cystadenoma papilliferum [GCDFP-15, CEA]	• Uncommon benign tumor • Birth to childhood • Scalp and forehead • Raised, crusted, red warty plaque; may be linear (if on scalp, alopecia) • Associated with nevus sebaceus (33%), and possible coexisting BCC (10%)	• Papillomatosis; invaginating cystic spaces open to skin surface; squamous epithelium in upper portion and sweat gland epithelium in lower portion (possible goblet cells), villi present; decapitation secretion; inflammatory infiltrate (plasma cells prominent around tumor) • Abundant plasma cells seen (below)
Benign apocrine tumors		
Hidradenoma papilliferum [PAS, colloidal iron]	• Variant of apocrine adenoma • Women; middle age • Vulva, perianal area • Solitary, asymmetric papule or nodule (<1 cm); often central ulceration	• Circumscribed dermal tumor with "maze-like" glandular spaces; papillary folds; apocrine decapitation; often no connection to epidermis; thin myoepithelial layer • *Remember:* hidradenoma "hides" from the epidermis (not connected) and from sight (groin)

Name	Predilection and Clinical Key Features	Histopathology
Apocrine adenoma	• "Tubular adenoma" or "apocrine fibroadenoma" • Axilla, scalp • Slow-growing, solitary nodule • May be associated with nevus sebaceus	• Circumscribed dermal tumor with lobules of well-differentiated tubules; apocrine decapitation; papillae without stroma project into tubule's lumina (like "stacked-cells")
Apocrine adenoma		

Name	Predilection and Clinical Key Features	Histopathology
Apocrine hidradenoma [S100, CAM 5.2, CEA]	• Previously many were reported as eccrine hidradenoma and eccrine acrospiroma (see p. 605) • Females, any age • No body site predilection • Solitary nodule (2–3 cm), indistinguishable from eccrine variant	• Circumscribed, non-encapsulated multilobular tumor; centered on dermis; may connect to epidermis; duct-like structures; fibrous tissue to hyalinized collagen stroma between lobules • Polygonal, clear, and mucinous cells noted (which are not present in eccrine variant, see p. 605) • Biphasic cytoplasm in tumor cells with either clear or eosinophilic cytoplasm • *Note:* Clear cell variant should be differentiated from metastatic renal cell carcinoma

Name	Predilection and Clinical Key Features	Histopathology
Apocrine mixed tumor [CEA, cytokeratin; outer layer S100, vimentin+]	• "Chondroid syringoma, apocrine type" • Male; middle age to elderly • Solitary, slow-growing nodule on the head and neck • Eccrine variant of mixed tumor also (see p. 603)	• Circumscribed dermal tumors with an epithelial component in a myxoid, chondroid and fibrous stroma; focal calcification; hyaline epithelial cells; apocrine ducts in continuity with tumor

Myoepithelioma
 	
[Vimentin, S100, Smooth muscle actin, EMA]
	• Benign tumor
	• Derived from myoepithelial cells around eccrine/apocrine glands (aid in contraction)
	• Any age
	• Face, extremities, trunk
	• Dome-shaped, exophytic nodules
	• May occur in salivary glands, deep soft tissue or other organs
		• Circumscribed, non-encapsulated dermal or subcutis tumor
		• Three cell types:
		  1. Spindle-shaped cells
		  2. Epithelioid cells
		  3. Plasmacytoid (hyaline) cells with pale eosinophlic cytoplasm and monomorphous ovoid nuclei

Name	Predilection and Clinical Key Features	Histopathology
Apocrine poroma	• Poroid neoplasm with apocrine features	Anastomosing lobules of small uniform basaloid cells forming small ductal structures with eosinophilic cuticles; often hair follicle and sebaceous differentiation
Cylindroma [CK7, CK8, CK18, CEA]	• May be neoplasm variant of eccrine spiradenoma • Middle age to elderly females • Head and neck • Usually solitary, smooth, red nodules • Multiple scalp tumors = "turban tumor"	• Basaloid cell islands in a "jigsaw puzzle" arrangement in dermis; two basaloid cells (one larger and paler than the other); "islands" surrounded by hyaline material and contain sweat ducts • Hyalinized basement membrane cylinders contain collagen type IV and are PAS positive

	• Brooke–Spiegler syndrome (autosomal dominant):
	  • Cylindroma + multiple trichoepithelioma + spiradenoma
	  • *CYLD* mutation (increases transcription factor NF-κB)
	• Rasmussen syndrome:
	  • Cylindroma + trichoepitheliomas + milia	

Name	Predilection and Clinical Key Features	Histopathology
Spiradenoma [CEA]	• May be variant of cylindroma • Young adults • Head, neck, trunk • Solitary, painful, gray–pink nodule • Associated with Brooke–Spiegler syndrome (see p. 565 and 594)	• Sharply demarcated, round basophilic dermal nodule ("blue balls in dermis"); two basaloid cell types (dark, basaloid cells and larger, pale nucleus cells in center), often arranged in a rosette; duct-like structures; vascular stroma
Malignant apocrine tumors		
Apocrine adenocarcinoma [GCDFP-15, CEA, PAS, S100]	• Axilla, anogenital region • May metastasize (40%) to regional lymph nodes and visceral organs • Single or multinodular mass (2–8 cm)	• Variation; non-encapsulated tumors in lower dermis and subcutaneous tissue; complex, variable glandular arrangement; cells with eosinophilic cytoplasm

Name	Predilection and Clinical Key Features	Histopathology

Extramammary Paget's disease
 	
[CK7, mucicarmine, alcian blue at pH 2.5, CEA, GCDFP-15]
	• Elderly female
	• Vulva, anogenital, axilla (areas of dense apocrine glands)
	
	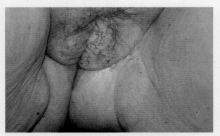
	
	• Erythematous, eczematous, slow-spreading plaque; intractable pruritus
	• Typically, no underlying carcinoma (as in mammary Paget's), but possible (especially perianal extramammary Paget's may be associated with visceral or adnexal carcinoma)
		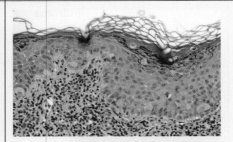
		
		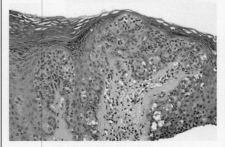
		
		• Abundant pale cytoplasm in cells and large pleomorphic nuclei; possible signet ring-appearing cells; mitoses present; chronic inflammatory infiltrate; abundant mucin (unlike Paget's)
		
		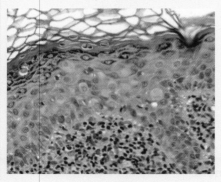
		
		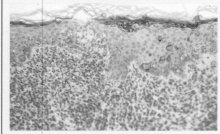
		
		• Primary extra-mammary Paget's:
		  • CK7, GCDFP-15+
		  • Negative CK20
		• Secondary extramammary Paget's:
		  • Associated with visceral cancer
		  • CK 7, CK20, GCDFP-15+
		
		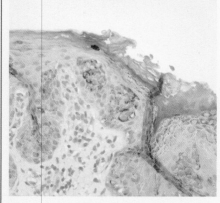
		
		• CK7 stain (above)

Name	Predilection and Clinical Key Features	Histopathology
Adenoid cystic carcinoma [EMA, CEA]	• Rare cutaneous tumor, usually arises in salivary glands • Scalp, chest	• Islands and cords of basaloid cells with cribriform and tubular areas; abundant basophilic mucin in cysts; mitoses uncommon; perineural invasion often
Mucinous carcinoma [CK7; mucin is PAS+; CK20 negative]	• Middle age to elderly • Eyelids (most common location), face, scalp • Slow-growing, red, painless nodule • 15% metastasize	• "Islands in sea of mucin" • Dermal tumors with large pools of basophilic mucin divided by fibrovascular septa; "floating nests" or small islands of epithelial cells in pool of mucin • CK7 positive (same as breast cancer); CK20 negative (unlike colon cancer); as a result, may be difficult to differentiate from breast cancer metastasis
Endocrine mucin-producing sweat gland carcinoma	• Extremely rare • Eyelids	• Solid and cystic dermal nodule with some containing mucin pools similar to mucinous carcinoma
Malignant mixed tumor [Chondroid areas express S100]	• "Malignant chondroid syringoma" • Very rare • Trunk and extremities • May metastasize to lymph nodes or distant	• Lobular appearance with an epithelial component at periphery and a mesenchymal component more abundant toward the center; ossification; more atypia, necrosis, and invasion than benign variant

Name	Predilection and Clinical Key Features	Histopathology
Hidradeno-carcinoma	• Elderly • Face and extremities • Ulcerated, reddish nodule • Clear cell variant often called "clear cell eccrine carcinoma"	• Sheets of cells with glycogen-containing pale cytoplasm and distinct cell membranes; focal necrosis; cytoplasmic vacuoles (important feature)
Malignant cylindroma	• Arises in long-standing cylindroma • Patients with multiple cylindromas • Scalp • Multiple smooth, red nodules	• Nests and cords of basaloid cells with frequent mitoses, focal necrosis
Malignant spiradenoma [Cytokeratins, EMA, p53]	• "Spiradenocarcinoma" • Trunk, elbow, digits • Often fatal metastasis (20%) • Clinically = rapid enlargement of a longstanding, cutaneous nodule	• Solid islands of tumor cells with a benign spiradenoma component (possibly abrupt transition) • May be side-by-side with benign variant and transition to nodule of carcinoma

Name	Predilection and Clinical Key Features	Histopathology
Tumors of modified apocrine glands		
Adenocarcinoma of Moll's glands	• Moll's gland is a modified apocrine gland on the eyelid • Resembles apocrine adenocarcinoma with architecture and cytology resembling malignancy; possibly iron granules in cytoplasm	
Erosive adenomatosis of the nipple	• Benign tumor of nipple • "Nipple papilloma" • Females • Nipple with erosion; later a crusted papule/plaque • May mimic Paget's disease	• Well-circumscribed, non-encapsulated dermal tumor with papillary projections into lumen; apocrine decapitation with a backing of myoepithelial cells; infiltrate with possible plasma cells; often connects to epidermis surface
Ceruminous adenoma and adenocarcinoma	• Rare tumor • Cerumen gland is a modified apocrine gland • Pedunculated nodule or cystic lesion in the external auditory canal	• Circumscribed nodules with an inner layer of cuboidal to columnar epithelium with decapitation secretion and an outer layer of myoepithelial cells
ECCRINE TUMORS		
• See page 326 for general information on eccrine glands		
Hamartomas and benign eccrine tumors		
Eccrine nevus	• Variant of eccrine hamartomas • Childhood to adolescence • Upper extremities • Localized areas of hyperhidrosis	• Increased size and number/size of normal-appearing eccrine coils

Name	Predilection and Clinical Key Features	Histopathology
Eccrine angiomatous hamartoma	• Variant of eccrine hamartomas (benign) • Extremities (especially legs) • Slow-growing nodule with blue–purple color; often pain, hyperhidrosis	Increase in eccrine glands and small vessels, possibly increased nerve fibers, mucin, or fat
Acrosyringeal nevus [PAS]	• Similar to "eccrine syringofibroadenoma" (see p. 604), but acrosyringeal nevus is PAS+ and has abundant plasma cells	
Porokeratotic eccrine ostial nevus	• "Comedo nevus of the palm" • Variant of eccrine hamartomas • Birth to early childhood • Hands and feet • Multiple punctate pits/papules with comedo-like plugging	• Parakeratotic cornoid lamellae overlying a dilated eccrine duct

Name	Predilection and Clinical Key Features	Histopathology
Eccrine hidrocystoma [CK7, CK8, CK19]	• Adult females • Periorbital area, face, trunk • Translucent or blue, dome-shaped, cystic papule • May fluctuate in size with sweating or ambient temperature • Rarely, develops to SCC • Associated with Schöpf–Schulz–Passarge syndrome = adult-onset focal ectodermal hypoplasia with multiple hidrocystomas of eyelid, PPK, hypodontia, hypotrichosis, nail dystrophy	• Unilocular cyst with wall containing two layers of cuboidal epithelium with eosinophilic cytoplasm; often close to eccrine gland; often unilocular dilated duct or gland; no "decapitation" secretion
Papillary eccrine adenoma [CEA, S100, CK8, CK14]	• Black women • Extremities • Small, slow-growing, firm nodule	• Circumscribed dermal tumor of dilated duct-like structures; papillary projections into dilated lumen; fibrous stroma; hyalinized collagen

Name	Predilection and Clinical Key Features	Histopathology
Syringoma [CEA, ferritin, EKH-6]	• Females • Periorbital (lower eyelids, cheeks), genitals • Associated with 1 in 5 Down syndrome patients • Multiple, small papules • Different variants, such as: • Disseminated syringomas • Clear-cell syringomas: associated with diabetes • Solitary syringomas • Eruptive syringomas (picture below): may be associated with Nicolau–Balus syndrome (eruptive syringomas + milia + atrophoderma vermiculata) 	• Multiple, small, irregular islands with central "tadpole" cysts ("comma-like"); fibrotic stroma • Histology differential = syringoma, microcystic adnexal carcinoma (MAC), desmoplastic trichoepithelioma, sclerosing BCC • Clear cell syringoma (pictured above)

Name	Predilection and Clinical Key Features	Histopathology
Eccrine mixed tumor [CEA]	• "Chondroid syringoma, eccrine type" • Epithelial (eccrine, apocrine) + stromal (mucin, chondroid or fibrous) components • Middle age to elderly • Face, extremities • Solitary, slow-growing nodule • Apocrine variant of mixed tumor also (see p. 593)	• Well-circumscribed, small, non-branching ducts (resemble a syringoma) in a mucinous and cartilaginous stroma

Poroma group

Name	Predilection and Clinical Key Features	Histopathology
Eccrine poroma [PAS+, diastase sensitive, K1, K10]	• Derived from acrosyringium • Middle age • Palms and soles, scalp • Eroded, firm, rubbery, friable pink or red exophytic nodule; pyogenic granuloma-like clinically	• Circumscribed tumor with cords and broad columns of basaloid "poroid" cells extending into dermis from the acanthotic epidermis; melanin pigment; sweat ducts and small cysts; often necrosis; vascular stroma (causes red color clinically)

Name	Predilection and Clinical Key Features	Histopathology
Dermal duct tumor [PAS]	• "Dermal eccrine poroma" • Originates from intradermal portion of eccrine sweat duct • Middle age to elderly • Lower legs, head/neck • Firm nodule	• Islands of basaloid cuboidal cells within dermis (not connected to epidermis); numerous ducts
Hidroacanthoma simplex	• "Intraepidermal poroma" • Extremities, trunk • Solitary plaque	• Cuboidal/oval basaloid or clear cells and ductal openings totally within epidermis; some glycogen; few ductal structures in islands • Histologically, may resemble clonal seborrheic keratosis (lacks glycogen) or BCC in appearance

Eccrine syringofibro-adenoma	• "Acrosyringeal nevus"
	 • Extremities
	 • Five clinical variations
	 • Solitary, hyperkeratotic nodule (or multiple)
	 • Associated with hidrotic ectodermal dysplasia variants:
	   1. Clouston's syndrome = autosomal dominant, connexin 30 mutation; palmoplantar keratoderma (PPK) with transgradiens, nail dystrophy with micronychia, sparse hair, and tufted terminal phalanges
	   2. Schöpf-Schulz-Passarge syndrome = multiple syringofibroadenomas, PPK, ectodermal dysplasia (hypodontia, nail hypoplasia), hypotrichosis, eyelid hidrocystoma; present in adolescence
		• Anastomosing epithelial cords and strands forming a "lattice" and connecting to the epidermis; sweat ducts; fibrovascular stroma; chronic inflammatory infiltrate

Name	Predilection and Clinical Key Features	Histopathology
Hidradenomas		
Hidradenoma	• In past, also called "eccrine acrospironma," "solid-cystic hidradenoma," "clear cell hidradenoma," "eccrine sweat gland adenoma," or "poroid hidradenoma" • Eccrine hidradenoma variant • Usually middle-aged females • No body site predilection • Solitary, solid, or partially cystic, blue–gray nodule (eccrine and apocrine variants are indistinguishable clinically) • Confusion currently on classification of hidradenoma, variants, and eccrine vs. apocrine groups (see p. 592)	• Circumscribed, encapsulated dermal tumor with poroid and cuticular cells; ductal structures in zones of cuticular cells; keratinous cysts (lacks polygonal, clear and mucinous cells like apocrine variant; see p. 592)
Malignant eccrine tumors		
Microcystic adnexal carcinoma (MAC) [CEA, EMA, keratin (especially CK7); sclerosing BCC does not stain the same]	• "Syringoma-gone-wild" • Upper lip, nasolabial fold (perioral area) • Indurated, firm plaque or nodule; slow growing • Locally aggressive; recurrence (50%)	• Islands and strands of squamous and basaloid epithelium with variable ductal differentiation; horn cysts; perineural invasion; deep and infiltrating and involves dermis and subcutis ("bottom-heavy"); varying size/shape of cysts • DDx includes sclerosing BCC (see p. 519)

Name	Predilection and Clinical Key Features	Histopathology
Eccrine carcinoma	• "Syringoid carcinoma" • Middle-aged females • Scalp, extremities, trunk • Slow-growing infiltrating plaque • Tendency for local recurrence, but metastases rare	• Mid-dermis tumor; irregular, narrow tubular strands (atypical basaloid cells) in a dense, hyalinized, fibrous stroma; may have "tadpole" appearance; perineural invasion
Squamoid eccrine ductal carcinoma	• "Ductal eccrine carcinoma with squamous differentiation" • Nodule on head, neck, extremities	• Eccrine ductal differentiation + squamous proliferation (atypia, keratin cysts, squamous eddies)
Polymorphous sweat gland carcinoma	• Extremities • Large, slow-growing dermal nodule	• Highly cellular proliferations with variety of growth patterns, including solid, trabecular, tubular, pseudopapillary and cylindromatous

Name	Predilection and Clinical Key Features	Histopathology
Digital papillary adenocarcinoma [S100, CEA, cytokeratin]	• "Aggressive digital papillary adenocarcinoma" • Fingers and toes • Solitary, painless nodule; grossly cystic (90%) • Metastases may occur	• Dermal and subcutis tumor; poorly circumscribed; mitoses; tubuloalveolar and ductal structures with papillary projections into lumina; may be poor glandular differentiation; glandular lumina may contain eosinophilic secretory material

Name	Predilection and Clinical Key Features	Histopathology
Porocarcinoma or malignant eccrine poroma [PAS, CEA, PCNA, EMA]	• Elderly • Lower extremities • Verrucous plaque or polypoid growth; may bleed with minor trauma • Possible recurrence and metastases (especially regional nodes) • Often seen in association with eccrine poroma	• Intraepidermal nests and islands of small basaloid cells; broad, anastomosing cords, solid columns and nests of large cells extending into dermis; ductal structures; clear cell areas in dermal nests; similar to eccrine poroma, but necrosis, irregular shape, and cellular atypia

Name	Predilection and Clinical Key Features	Histopathology
Complex adnexal tumors (Hamartomas with differentiation toward > 1 adnexal structure)		
Organoid nevus	• "Nevus sebaceus of Jadassohn" • Present at birth (congenital lesion) • Near scalp on head or neck • Yellowish, verrucous, linear plaque; alopecia in involved area • Birth = macular shape (below) • Puberty = enlarges to cerebriform plaque due to androgens (below) • May develop trichoblastoma, syringocystadenoma papilliferum, BCC, or other adnexal tumor in lesion	• Papillomatosis; hyperplasia; sebaceous glands (often not associated with mature hair shaft); mature hair follicles; numerous apocrine glands; basaloid hyperplasia • Key features = epidermal hyperplasia + immature pilosebaceous units
Adnexal polyp of neonatal skin	• Neonate • Areola of nipple • Solitary nodule • Falls off the neonate in the first week of life	• Contains hair follicles, eccrine glands, and vestigial sebaceous glands
Combined adnexal tumor	• Differentiation towards sebaceous glands + pilar and sweat duct structures	

Review of common tumors of cutaneous appendages

Germ cell origin ("basaloid" appearance)

Trichofolliculoma

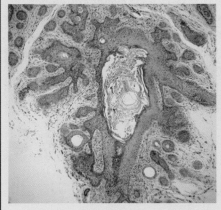

- Hair follicles projecting outwards
- Looks like ornaments fallen off Christmas tree; think "fa-la-la-la- liculoma"

Trichoadenoma

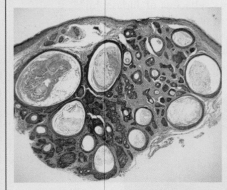

- Lots of horn cysts with minimal basaloid islands

Basaloid follicular hamartoma

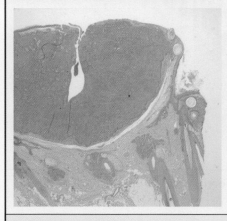

Trichoepithelioma

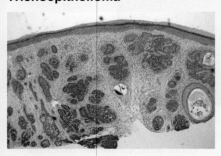

- CD34+ stroma, CK20+ and periphery of islands are bcl-2+
- Associated with Brooke–Spiegler and Rombo syndromes

Trichoblastoma

- Fibrotic stroma; cribriform blue clusters

[CK7, 8 positive]

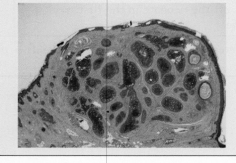

Infundibular origin

Dilated pore of Winer

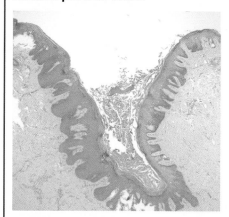

- No hair follicle

Inverted follicular keratosis (IFK)

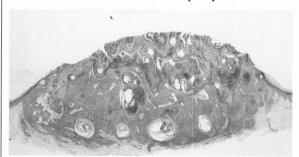

- "Downward growing seborrheic keratosis" with prominent squamous eddies

Isthmus origin
(Pale cells and small ducts with pink cuticles)

Pilar sheath acanthoma

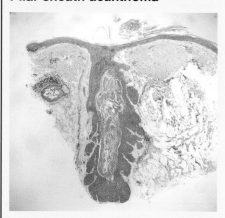

- "Bulbous projections" and more acanthosis than dilated pore of Winer

Tumor of follicular infundibulum (TFI)

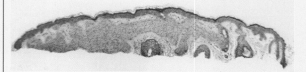

- "Plate-like" with multiple epidermal connections and slightly pale cells
- Associated with Cowden's disease and Schöpf-Schulz-Passarge syndrome

Tricholemmal (outer sheath) origin

Tricholemmoma
[CD34+]
- Multiple lobules with clear cells, wart-like, "eyeliner sign" with rim of basaloid cells
- Associated with Cowden's disease ("Le-mama" cow with pendulous udders)

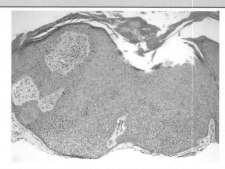

Matrix origin

Pilomatricoma

- Basaloid cells + shadow/ghost cells + possible calcifications

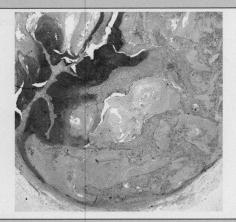

Mesenchymal origin

Trichodiscoma

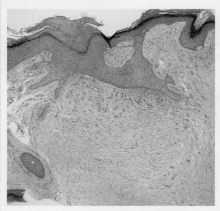

- Lacks follicular extensions; follicular units "pushed aside"; fibrosis
- Associated with Birt–Hogg–Dubé syndrome

Fibrofolliculoma

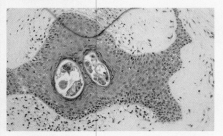

- "Antler-like" or "batwing-like" follicular cells radiating out; fibrotic stroma
- Associated with Birt–Hogg–Dubé syndrome

Hamartomas and hyperplasias

Folliculosebaceous cystic hamartoma

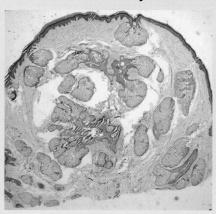

- Sebaceous glands radiating outwards, fibrosis, no connection to epidermis

Sebaceous hyperplasia

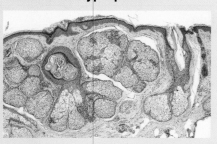

- Thin layer of basaloid cells in glands; i.e. epithelial layer "squashed"
- Associated with Sun exposure, cyclosporine

Sebaceous tumors (associated with Muir–Torre syndrome)

Sebaceous adenoma

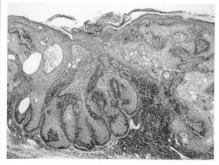

- Basal cells surround, lobular down growth, opens to surface with >50% mature sebocytes

Sebaceoma

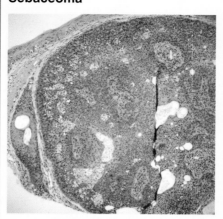

- No lobular down growth, <50% mature sebocytes

Apocrine tumors

Apocrine hidrocystoma

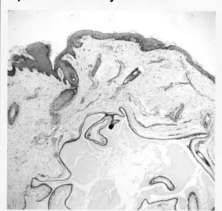

- "Decapitation" secretion
- Associated with Schöpf–Schulz–Passarge syndrome

Syringocystadenoma papilliferum

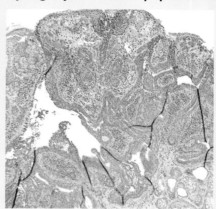

- Cyst open to surface; "decapitation" secretion; plasma cells; epithelial layers of squamous epithelium in upper portion and glandular epitheliun in lower

Cylindroma

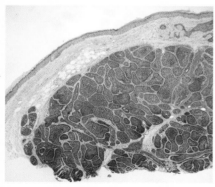

- "Jigsaw puzzle" with two basaloid cells; one larger and paler
- Associated with Brooke–Spiegler syndrome

Spiradenoma

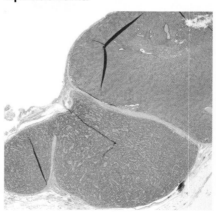

- "Blue balls" in dermis with two cell types
- Associated with Brooke–Spiegler and Schöpf syndromes

Hidradenoma papilliferum

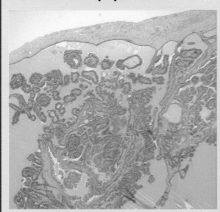

- "Maze-like" glands; papillary folds; "hides" from epidermis

Apocrine adenoma (tubular adenoma)

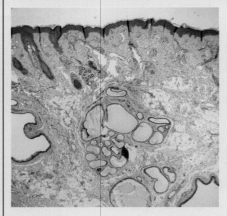

- Papillary projections without stroma, "stacked-cells"

Mucinous carcinoma

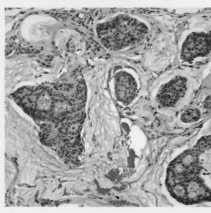

"Islands in sea of mucin"

Extramammary Paget's disease

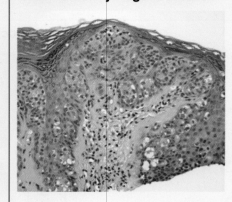

Eccrine tumors

Eccrine hidrocystoma

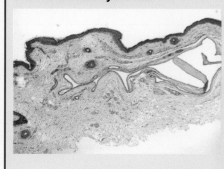 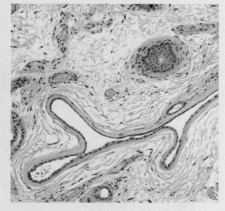

- Associated with Schöpf–Schulz–Passarge syndrome

Syringoma

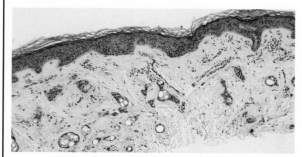

- DIF = syringoma, microcystic adnexal carcinoma, desmoplastic trichoepithelioma, sclerosing BCC
- "Tadpole" cysts
- Associated with Down syndrome

Chondroid syringoma or eccrine mixed tumor

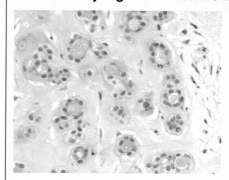

- Eccrine variant (photo above)

Poroma group

Hidroacanthoma simplex

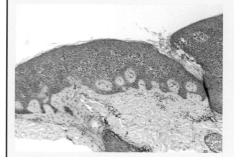

- "Intraepidermal poroma"

Eccrine poroma

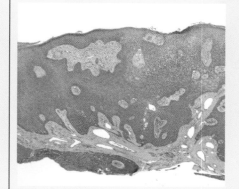

- Acanthotic epidermis with "poroid" cells in lower portion + ducts

Dermal duct tumor

- "Dermal poroma" with no epidermal connection

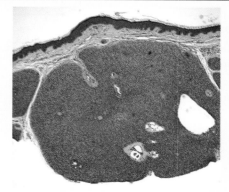

Malignant eccrine tumors

Microcystic adnexal carcinoma

- "Syringoma-gone-wild"
- Deep, "bottom-heavy," infiltrating lesion; perineural invasion; varying size/shape cysts

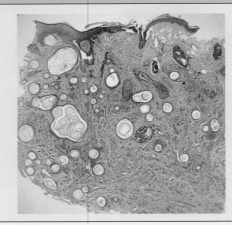

Eccrine carcinoma or syringoid carcinoma

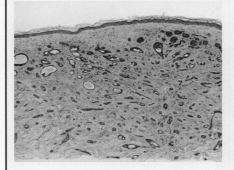

Malignant eccrine poroma (porocarcinoma)

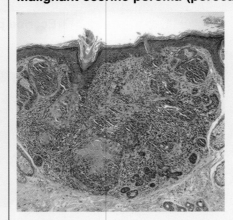

- Necrosis, more invasion and atypia than eccrine poroma

Complex adnexal tumors

Nevus sebaceous or organoid nevus

- Hyperplasia + immature pilosebaceous units
- Papillomatosis; apocrine glands, sebaceous glands, mature hair follicles

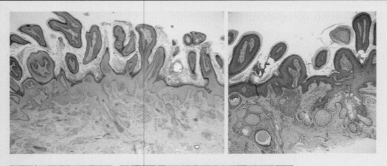

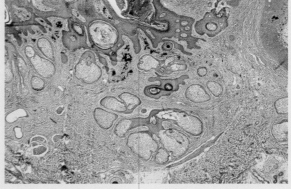

Fibrous Tumors and Tumor-like Proliferations

34

Dermatofibrosarcoma protuberans (DFSP)

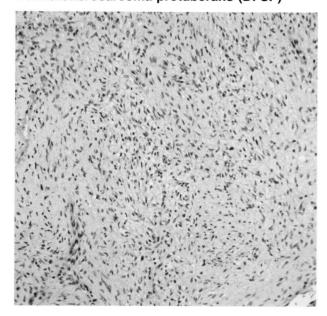

Name	Predilection and Clinical Key Features	Histopathology
Acral angiofibromas (fibrous papule)		
<ul><li>Collagen oriented in vertical axis or concentric around follicles; few vessels; plump fibroblasts</li><li>Dermal dendrocytes may stain with factor XIIIa or CD34</li><li>Clinically = small, red, or skin-colored papules</li><li>Several conditions related: adenoma sebaceum; acral fibrokeratoma; fibrous papule of face; pearly penile papules (see below)</li></ul>		
Facial angiofibromas [Factor XIIIa and due to vascularity also CD31+]	<ul><li>"Adenoma sebaceum"</li><li>Butterfly area of face, especially nasolabial groove</li><li>Childhood</li></ul> <ul><li>Pink to yellow–brown papules/nodules (usually accompanied by scalp/ungual fibroma and "shagreen patch")</li><li>May see facial angiofibromas in tuberous sclerosis, neurofibromatosis 2, and MEN I</li></ul>	<ul><li>Elevated growths; flattened rete ridges with patchy melanocytic hyperplasia; hyperkeratosis; increased blood vessels</li></ul> <ul><li>"Onion-skin" arrangement around follicles and vessels common</li></ul>
Fibrous papule of the face	<ul><li>Nose</li><li>Middle-aged adults</li><li>Solitary, dome-shaped papules (3–5 mm)</li></ul> 	<ul><li>Similar to adenoma sebaceum, but ectatic vessels and less concentric fibrosis</li></ul>

Name	Predilection and Clinical Key Features	Histopathology
Pearly penile papules	• Coronal margin and sulcus of penis • Asymptomatic, small (1–3 mm) pearly-white papules in a group or row 	• Papule with fibroblasts, rich vascularity, dense connective tissue

Acral fibrokeratoma
[Factor XIIIa]
	• Middle-aged adults
	• Often areas of trauma
	
	• Solitary, dome-shaped or thin horns
	• Variants:
	  • Acquired digital fibrokeratoma (pictured above)
	  • Acquired periungual fibrokeratoma
	  • "Garlic clove" fibroma
	  • Subungual and periungual fibromas of tuberous sclerosis (often in clusters; develop after puberty; 50% TS patients); also called Koenen's tumor (photo below)
	
		• Massive orthokeratosis; core of thick collagen bundles oriented in vertical axis; small vessels in dermal papillae; no nerves, eccrine ducts, or cartilage
		
		• Acquired digital fibrokeratoma (pictured above)

Name	Predilection and Clinical Key Features	Histopathology
Fibrous overgrowths, fibromatoses, etc.		
Peyronie's disease	• "Penile fibromatosis" • Males, more often in diabetics • Shaft of penis (often dorsum side) • Fibrous plaque; causes curvature of the penis with erection; may be painful	• Diffuse fibrous proliferation

Acrochordons (skin tags)	• Most common fibrous tumor of the skin
	• Obese females
	• Axilla, neck, groin, eyelids
	• Clinical variants:
	  • Furrowed papule
	  • Filiform lesion
	  • Large bag-like protuberance
	
	• May be associated with diabetes, abnormal lipids, colonic polyps
	• Associated with Birt–Hogg–Dubé syndrome (see p. 579)
		• Varies histologically on clinical type
		• Polypoid with loose fibrous stroma, lacks adnexal structures
		• Fibrovascular core may be replaced by adipose tissue

Name	Predilection and Clinical Key Features	Histopathology
Pleomorphic fibroma [CD34; does not express S-100 (melanoma), CD68 (DF), or desmin]	• Adult • Trunk extremities • Appears clinically as a polypoid skin tag (slow-groming)	• Dome-shaped nodule with dermal hypocellular, spindle cells containing nuclear pleomorphism; rare mitoses; histiocytes and plump, stellate, irregularly-shaped multinucleated giant cells (may be "floret-like")
Sclerotic fibroma [Vimentin, actin > CD34]	• "Storiform collagenoma" or "plywood" fibroma • Solitary lesion or multifocal, flesh-colored papules/nodules (0.5–3 cm) • Associated with Cowden's disease (autosomal dominant, multiple hamartoma syndrome, PTEN mutation; risk of breast, GI, thyroid cancer)	• "Plywood-like," circumscribed, unencapsulated dermal nodules; eosinophilic collagen bundles in laminated fashion ("plywood" or "storiform" pattern); low cellularity

Name	Predilection and Clinical Key Features	Histopathology
Collagenous fibroma	• "Desmoplastic fibroblastoma" • Adult males • Firm, non-tender nodules (2–3 cm)	• Appears similar to a "deep" pleomorphic fibroma • Well-demarcated in the subcutaneous tissue and muscle (dermis location rare)
Knuckle pads	• Variant of superficial fascial fibromatosis • Multiple, well-formed skin-colored nodules on hands over IP and MCP • Bart–Pumphrey syndrome: knuckle pads + white nails (leukonychia) + deafness	• Prominent hyperkeratosis and epidermal acanthosis
Pachydermo-dactyly	• Localized form of superficial fibromatosis, likely due to trauma, rubbing • Males • Fibrous thickening of lateral aspects of PIP joints; spares thumbs and fifth fingers	• Dermis thickening with coarse collagen bundles; mucin deposits; no inflammation
Bite fibroma	• Lips • Due to biting of mucosal surface • Firm, whitish nodule	 • Thickened squamous mucosa with submucosal fibroplasia and angioplasia

Name	Predilection and Clinical Key Features	Histopathology

Nodular fasciitis [Actin, vimentin, CD68, factor XIIIa; these stains are negative in fibrosarcoma]	• Reactive proliferation of myofibroblast cells with "pseudosarcomatous" reaction process
	• Young to middle-aged adults
	• Upper extremities
	
	• Rapid growth to median diameter of 1.5 cm, but self-limiting; possibly due to trauma to area (20%)
	• Variants:
	  • Cranial fasciitis (child, involves scalp and cranium)
	  • Intravascular fasciitis (vessels involved)
	  • Ossifying fasciitis (osteoid or bone present)
	  • Proliferative fasciitis (ganglion-like cells)
		• Spindle-shaped to plump fibroblasts in haphazard array ("tissue culture appearance") or bundles forming "S-shaped" curves; extravasated RBCs
		
		• "Tissue culture appearance" (below)

Atypical decubital fibroplasia	• "Ischemic fasciitis" • Immobilized or debilitated patients • Subcutaneous mass over bony prominences	• Atypical fibroblasts with necrosis, reactive fibrosis, neovascularization involving deep dermis, subcutis, and deep fascia
Postoperative spindle-cell nodule	• Genital skin or GU system following surgical procedure	• Spindle-shaped cells in an interlacing fascicle pattern

Name	Predilection and Clinical Key Features	Histopathology
Solitary fibrous tumor [CD34, vimentin]	• Rare mesenchymal typically involving the pleura • Head and neck • Circumscribed nodule (may appear cyst-like)	• Circumscribed; alternating hypercellular and less cellular areas ("pattern-less" growth pattern appearance); spindle cells in fascicular, haphazard, or storiform pattern; keloidal hyalinization

Name	Predilection and Clinical Key Features	Histopathology
Fibrous hamartoma of infancy [Vimentin, desmin, actin]	• Birth to 2 years old • Males (3:1) • Axilla, upper arm • Benign, skin-colored, subcutaneous nodule	• Poorly defined margins in subcutis • Three components: 1. Fascicles of bland spindle cells 2. Islands of small, round cells in a myxoid matrix 3. Mature fat

Name	Predilection and Clinical Key Features	Histopathology
Digital fibromatosis of childhood [Actin, vimentin]	• "Infantile digital fibromatosis" • Birth to 1 year old • Dorsal and lateral aspects of digits (spares thumb and big toe) • Benign, dome-shaped, firm nodule • Regression usually in 2–3 years	 • Non-encapsulated, extends beneath epidermis to subcutis; spindle-shaped cells with small, eosinophilic, "RBC-like," cytoplasmic inclusion bodies [Inclusions stain "red" with Masson's trichrome and "purple" with PTAH, and are actin positive] • More cellular and not polypoid clinically as compared to an acquired digital fibrokeratoma (see p. 619)

Name	Predilection and Clinical Key Features	Histopathology
Angiomyofibro-blastoma of the vulva [Stroma cells are actin, vimentin]	• Vulva • Solitary dermal nodule	• Edematous stroma with abundant capillary vessels irregularly distributed; spindle cells (some plump) often aggregated around vessels

Name	Predilection and Clinical Key Features	Histopathology
Dermatomyo-fibroma [Actin, vimentin; negative CD34, S100, factor XIIIa]	• Young female adults • Shoulder area, axilla, abdomen • Skin-colored to red–brown, asymptomatic plaque	• Non-encapsulated, fascicles of bland spindle cells oriented parallel to skin; resembles keloid in appearance; dermis contains small, round, "muscle-bundle-like" structures; spares adnexa; no collagen trapping or epidermal involvement like in dermatofibromas (see p. 636)

Name	Predilection and Clinical Key Features	Histopathology
Infantile myofibromatosis	• Birth to 2 years old • Male • Head, neck, trunk • May involve bone (lytic) or internal organs (GI, kidney, lung, heart) • Firm-to-rubbery, skin-colored to purple-colored nodule(s)	• "Disordered-smooth-muscle-bundle" appearance • Well circumscribed, grouped short fascicles, delicate collagen bundles; spindle cells with myofibroblast features and rounder, smaller cells; "stag-horn" pattern of vessels; vascular in center area
Myopericytoma [Actin, h-caldesmon]	• Variant of "perivascular myxoma" • Middle-aged males • Distal extremities • Dermal or soft tissue tumor	• Thin-walled vessels and concentric perivascular arrangement of ovoid, plump, spindled-to-round myoid cells

Name	Predilection and Clinical Key Features	Histopathology
Inflammatory myofibroblastic tumor	• "Inflammatory fibrosarcoma" • Usually lungs, mesentery; but may involve head, neck, extremities • Mean age of presentation = 13 years	• "Multinodular" appearance with a mixture of myofibroblasts and fibroblasts arranged in short interwoven fascicles
Fibromyxoid sarcoma (low grade) [Vimentin]	• "Myxoid fibrosarcoma" • Young adults • Develops in deep soft tissues • 50% may metastasize (especially lung)	• Bland spindle cells with whorled or focally linear arrangement; alternating fibrous or myxoid stroma
Myxofibrosarcoma [Vimentin, some cells may stain with CD34]	• Previously a variant of malignant fibrous histiocytoma (MFH) • Elderly • Extremities • Subcutaneous nodule	• Myxoid appearance with low-grade areas of vacuolated, myxoid matrix with scattered spindled fibroblast-like cells and stellate cells; more high-grade tumors resemble pleomorphic MFH • Negative staining for S100, desmin, EMA, or keratin

Name	Predilection and Clinical Key Features	Histopathology
Myxoinflammatory fibroblastic sarcoma	• Low-grade sarcoma • Hands and feet	• Similar to myxofibrosarcoma, but with numerous inflammatory cells; three types of tumor cells (spindle cells, large bizarre ganglion-like cells, and multivacuolated cells resembling lipoblasts in the myxoid areas)
Fibrosarcoma	• Deep soft tissue malignant tumor of fibroblasts, rarely develops in skin • Adults • Usually lower extremities	• Uniform, spindle cells in "herringbone" fascicles; mitoses common

Name	Predilection and Clinical Key Features	Histopathology
Myofibroblastic sarcoma	• Low-grade, spindle-cell sarcoma • Adults • Extremities • More common in the bone than skin	• Myofibroblastic differentiation; myxoid stroma

Name	Predilection and Clinical Key Features	Histopathology
Fibrohistiocytic tumors		
Dermatofibroma (DF) [Factor XIIIa, stromelysin-3, metallothionein and tenascin (DE junction); negative CD34, unlike DFSP]	• "Benign fibrous histiocytoma" • Young adults • Lower extremities 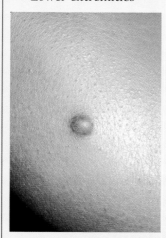 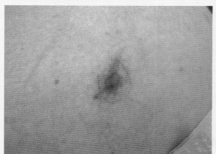 • Round, ovoid, firm dermal nodules; often central white scar; "dimple sign" • Multiple eruptive DF variant associated with autoimmune disorders (i.e. SLE), leukemia, atopic dermatitis; immunosuppression (HIV) ; initiation of HAART medications 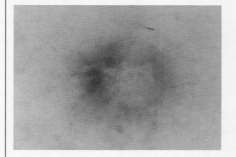 • Classically, dermoscopy shows central white, scar-like area and delicate pigment network at periphery (picture above)	• Poorly demarcated; centered on dermis; grenz zone; epidermal hyperplasia ("dirty fingers"); spindled, heterogeneous fibroblasts ("boomerang"); giant cells; hemosiderin 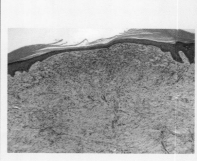 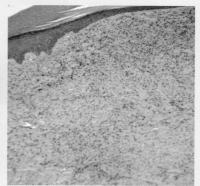 • (Numerous variants histologically) • Myofibroblasts parallel epidermis; "collagen trapping" at edges May be pigmented (below left) or cause basaloid induction (below right) 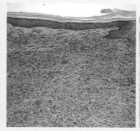 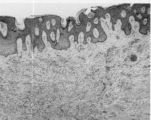 • Factor XIIIa stain (below) 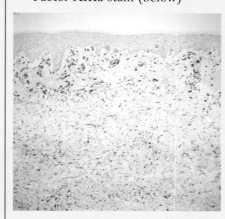 • Collagen trapping (below) 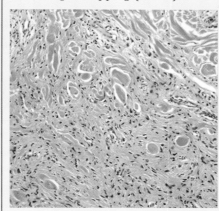

Name	Predilection and Clinical Key Features	Histopathology
Hemosideric dermatofibroma	• Variant of DF • Possible early stage development of an aneurysmal variant • Lesion more red in color than normal DF and may reach 10 cm in diameter	• DF-like but with increased vessels and hemosiderin deposition
Dermatofibroma with monster cells [Ki-M1p]	• "Atypical fibrous histiocytoma" • Variant of DF • Rare development of distant metastasis	• Large, bizarre cells with abundant foamy cytoplasm and hyperchromatic nuclei; may have atypical mitoses

Name	Predilection and Clinical Key Features	Histopathology
Epithelioid cell histiocytoma	• Variant of DF (fibrous histiocytoma) • Adults • Extremities • Elevated nodule	• Epidermal collarette; sharply circumscribed; sheets of angulated epithelioid cells with abundant eosinophilic cytoplasm; numerous blood vessels

Plexiform fibrohistiocytic tumor
 	
[Vimentin, actin; negative CD34, unlike DFSP]
	• Soft tissue tumor
	• Infants to children
	• Upper limbs
	• Possible metastasis
		• Dermal–subcutaneous junction nodule with dual population of:
		  1. Fascicles of fibroblastic cells
		  2. Aggregates of histiocyte-like cells in nodules
		• Also "osteoclast-like" giant cells with 3–10 nuclei
		• "Plexiform" appearance (intricate network or web-like)

Name	Predilection and Clinical Key Features	Histopathology
Giant cell fibroblastoma [CD34, vimentin]	• "Juvenile variant of DFSP" • Soft tissue tumor • Young males • Neck, trunk • Solitary, slow-growing, skin-colored nodule • May recur or transform to DFSP (see below) • Associated with t(17:22) translocation which fuses PDGF and collagen type I genes	• Poorly circumscribed dermis–subcutis nodule; infiltrating spindle-cell tumor in loose mxyoid matrix; uninucleate and multinucleate giant cells • Characteristic finding = branching sinusoidal spaces ("pseudovascular") lined by giant cells with hyperchromatic nuclei
Dermato-fibrosarcoma protuberans (DFSP) [CD34, CD99; negative Factor XIIIa, stromelysin-3, tenascin, unlike DF; negative S100 unlike melanoma]	• Young to middle-aged men • Trunk and proximal extremities (possibly in area of previous trauma) • Associated with translocation t(17;22)(q22;q13) involving PDGF and collagen I genes • Slow-growing nodules; red color or flesh colored • Often "Infected keloid" appearance • May metastasize (<5%), possibly to lungs • Possible Tx = Mohs (preferred option), wide local excision (WLE) of 3-cm, and possibly imatinib, which is a platelet-derived growth factor (PDGF) inhibitor	• Dermis–subcutis nodule; infiltrates around small groups of fat cells; grenz zone; uniform, small spindle cells with plump nuclei; may extend into fat and cause "honeycomb" appearance

Name	Predilection and Clinical Key Features	Histopathology
Bednar tumor [CD34]	• Pigmented variant of DFSP • 1–5% of DFSP cases • Young women • Trunk and proximal extremities • Pigmented nodule • No metastasis reported • Melanin likely due to colonization of a DFSP by melanocytes	• Same as DFSP but dendritic cells contain melanin (not hemosiderin) • May stain with S-100

Name	Predilection and Clinical Key Features	Histopathology
Atypical fibroxanthoma (AFX) [CD10, CD68, α₁-antitrypsin, α₁-antichymotrypsin, procollagen I, CD99, vimentin, CD74; negative S100 (melanoma) and keratin (SCC)]	• Superficial form of pleomorphic undifferentiated sarcoma (previous name was malignant fibrous histiocytoma or MFH); see p. 639 • Elderly • Head and neck (sun-exposed skin) 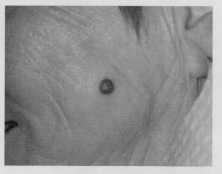 • Solitary, gray to pink to red dome-shaped nodule • May recur or regress (low-grade sarcoma)	• Well-circumscribed, non-encapsulated, highly cellular tumor in upper dermis • Mixture of three cells: 1. Plump spindle-shaped cells 2. Large polyhedral cells 3. Multinucleate, giant cells 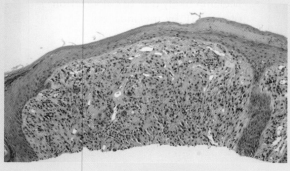 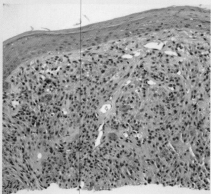 • If see multinucleate giant cells and spindle cells, then consider AFX! • Undifferentiated pleomorphic sarcoma (or MFH) is deeper and "uglier" (see p. 639) 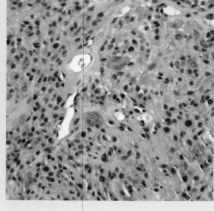 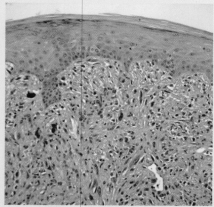

Name	Predilection and Clinical Key Features	Histopathology
Pleomorphic undifferentiated sarcoma [CD10, CD68, CD74, procollagen I; <50% are CD99+]	• Old name was "malignant fibrous histiocytoma" (MFH) • Most common soft tissue sarcoma of elderly adults • 50–70 years old • Lower extremities (especially thighs) • Painless enlarging nodule • Involves deep soft tissue or striated muscle of proximal extremities (rarely cutaneous tumors) • High recurrence rate (Possible treatment includes amputation, WLE with radiation, etc.)	• Similar to AFX (see p. 638), but deeper and "uglier" looking nuclei and cells; infiltrative margin; hemorrhage; necrosis; inflammatory cells

Name	Predilection and Clinical Key Features	Histopathology
Presumptive synovial and tendon sheath tumors		
Fibroma of tendon sheath	• Middle-aged males • Fingers, wrists • Solitary, slow-growing subcutaneous tumor, usually attached to a tendon	• Sparse, spindle/stellate cells embedded in dense fibrocollagenous stroma in subcutis; hyalinization • Characteristic features = slit-like or dilated vascular channels
Giant cell tumor of tendon sheath [CD68, vimentin]	• Most common tumor of the hand • Young to middle-aged female • Hands and fingers (dorsal aspect) • Slow-growing, asymptomatic, firm, fixed nodule • Benign, but local recurrence of 30%	• "DF-like + giant cells" attached to a tendon • Multilobulated with eosinophilic collagenous stroma; lipid-laden histiocytes; hemosiderin; multinucleate giant cells with 60+ nuclei possible! Usually attached to a tendon

Name	Predilection and Clinical Key Features	Histopathology
Epithelioid sarcoma [Characteristic triad of + stains = keratin, EMA and vimentin; negative S100, HMB45, and CD31]	• Most common soft tissue sarcoma of hand/wrist • Young adult males • Extremities (especially hands and fingers) • Slow-growing tan-white nodule; ulceration • May appear "sporotrichoid-like" clinically as spreads up the extremity • Usually involves deep subcutis and underlying soft tissue • Risk of metastases (lymph nodes and lungs) • 5-year survival = 50%	• Low-power appearance resembles a necrobiotic or granulomatous process • Ill-defined cellular lesion with vague nodules in dermis/subcutis; oval-polygonal cells and plump spindle cells; hemosiderin; central "geographic" necrosis and fibrosis; may appear palisading "granuloma-like" • Distinction from other tumors requires immunohistochemical stains

Synovial sarcoma
 	
[Cytokeratins, EMA]
	• Soft tissue sarcoma (rare skin involvement)
	• 90% show a chromosomal translocation t(X;18)
	• Young to middle-aged adults
	• Extremities
		• Two main patterns:
		  1. Monophasic form with spindle cells in a fascicular pattern
		  2. Biphasic form with spindle cells with glandular structures

Name	Predilection and Clinical Key Features	Histopathology
Miscellaneous entities		
Ossifying fibromyxoid tumor [Vimentin, S100]	• Males • Upper and lower extremities • Soft tissue tumor (median 4 cm)	• Circumscribed tumor with fibrous capsule and incomplete peripheral shell of new bone (bone may be central rather than peripheral); cords, nests, and sheets of round and spindle-shaped cells with a well-vascularized stroma
Juvenile hyaline fibromatosis [Actin, cytokeratin, vimentin]	• Infancy to childhood • Autosomal recessive disorder • Scalp, ears, face • White, firm, cutaneous nodules • Condition is characterized by large tumors (especially scalp); white cutaneous nodules; hypertrophy of gingiva; flexural contractures; osteolytic bone erosion • Recurrent infections may lead to death • Mutation = CMG2 (capillary morphogenesis protein 2)	• Thickened dermis with a "chondroid-appearance;" fibroblast-like cells with abundant granular cytoplasm embedded in an amorphous, hyaline-like, eosinophilic ground substance [PAS+]

Name	Predilection and Clinical Key Features	Histopathology
Pleomorphic hyalinizing angiectatic tumor (PHAT) [CD34, vimentin]	• Mesenchymal tumor • Distal extremities • Soft tissue nodule	• Some resemblance to malignant fibrous histiocytoma and neurilemmoma; ectatic, fibrin-containing vessels with prominent circumferential hyalinization; spindled and pleomorphic stromal cells with intranuclear inclusions and variable inflammatory component

Name	Predilection and Clinical Key Features	Histopathology
Cutaneous myxoma	• Benign cutaneous mass • Eyelids, nipples, buttocks • May not be associated with any systemic abnormalities • 50% of Carney complex patients have cutaneous myxomas	• Similar to focal mucinosis (p. 271), but prominent capillaries and deep in dermis; sharply circumscribed, non-encapsulated lesion; prominent mucin; variable fibroblasts
Superficial acral fibromyxoma [CD34, EMA, CD99]	• Fingers and toes; tendency to involve the nail region • Solitary mass • Recurrence may exceed 20%	• Spindle- and stellate-shaped cells with random loose storiform and fascicular growth pattern in the dermis and subcutis; myxoid or collagenous stroma; often with accentuated vascularity and increased mast cells

Name	Predilection and Clinical Key Features	Histopathology
Superficial angiomyxoma [Stromal cells stain with vimentin, focally positive for actin]	• Variant of myxoma with epithelial elements • Any part of body • Slow-growing, painless nodules	• Usually centered on subcutis, with extension into dermis invariable; spindle-shaped and stellate cells in a copious, well-vascularized basophilic matrix; presence of an epithelial component (epithelial strands or keratin-filled cyst)

35 Tumors of Fat

Angiolipoma

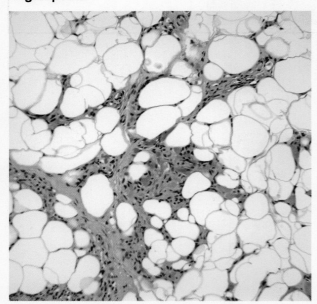

Name	Predilection Clinical Key Features	Histopathology
Nevus lipomatosus superficialis	• Rare connective tissue nevus • Present at birth to 20s • Pelvic girdle and trunk, usually unilateral • Plaque-type flesh-colored or yellow papules; may have linear or zosteriform arrangement • Usually solitary lesions, but may be generalized	• "Fatty-skin tag" • Mature fat cells in dermis that extend to epidermal undersurface; thickening of the collagen bundles; increased vessels in the papillary dermis • May be difficult to distinguish histologically from focal dermal hypoplasia, but it has attenuated collagen and differs clinically
Piezogenic pedal papules	• Pressure-induced herniations of subcutaneous fat through acquired or inherited defects in connective tissue of the heel • Heels • Painless or asymptomatic, multiple small papules/nodules that disappear when pressure is relieved to the heel • Associated with Ehlers–Danlos syndrome (one-third of patients) and Prader–Willi syndrome • Similar lesions may form on the wrist (piezogenic wrist papules)	• Protrusion of fat into the dermis; mucin deposits often at the periphery of the lesion and within fat lobules

Name	Predilection Clinical Key Features	Histopathology
Infantile pedal papules	• Similar to piezogenic pedal papules • Birth to infancy • Medial aspect of heel • Painless, symmetric nodules	• Well-defined lobules of mature fat in the mid and deep dermis, mostly in a periadnexal distribution
Lipoblastoma	• Benign tumor arising from fetal white fat • Infants to children • Proximal extremities, trunk, head, and neck • Light-yellow to tan-yellow tumor (average 5 cm)	• Lobulated, thin, well-vascularized connective tissue septa; mature fat cells with spindle-shaped mesenchymal cells and lipoblasts; often plexiform capillary pattern in the lobules and patchy myxoid stroma; no mitoses or atypia (as in liposarcoma)
Lipofibromatosis	• Pediatric neoplasm • Present at birth to childhood • Hands and feet • Subcutis and deep soft tissue nodule	• Adipose tissue (>50% of tumor) and spindled fibroblastic element in thickened septa
Hemosiderotic fibrolipomatous tumor	• Middle age to elderly (unlike age of lipofibromatosis) • Ankle and feet area • Subcutis, "lipoma-like" tumors (1–13 cm)	• Varying proportions of mature adipocytes and fibroblastic spindle cells; associated with abundant hemosiderin deposits in macrophages within the spindle cell component; inflammatory cells scattered through lesion • [Spindle-cell component stain CD34]

Name	Predilection Clinical Key Features	Histopathology
Lipoma	• 50–60 years old • Upper trunk, upper extremities, thighs, neck • Asymptomatic, subcutaneous tumor • Possible mutation = HMBA2 gene (regulates transcription) • Multiple lipomas associated with Fröhlich syndrome and PTEN (phosphatase and tensin) mutation syndromes, such as Bannayan–Riley–Ruvalcaba syndrome (lipomas + hemangiomas), Cowden's disease and Proteus syndrome	• Sheets of mature fat dissected by thin, incomplete fibrous septa with few blood vessels; fibrous capsule present

Name	Predilection Clinical Key Features	Histopathology
Clinical lipoma syndromes	• *Madelung's disease (benign symmetric lipomatosis):* • Middle-aged men: alcohol-related liver disease, metabolic abnormalities • Neck, back, upper trunk • Misdiagnosis as obesity (a "sight diagnosis") • HP = non-capsulated fatty masses; symmetric • *Familial multiple lipomatosis:* • Autosomal dominant • Develops in 30s • Forearms, trunk, and thighs • *Dercum's disease (adiposis dolorosa):* • Lower extremities, abdomen, buttocks • Painful fatty deposits on lower extremities • Mental disturbances • *Diffuse lipomatosis:* • Onset before 2 years • Limb or trunk: associated with tuberous sclerosis • HP = infiltrating masses of mature adipose tissue • *Encephalocraniocutaneous lipomatosis:* • Cutaneous component = "nevus psiloliparus" • Subcutaneous lipomas on scalp with alopecia • Cranial and ocular abnormalities • *Lipedematous scalp:* • Thick and soft scalp; alopecia • HP = thick subcutaneous scalp fat	

Name	Predilection Clinical Key Features	Histopathology
Angiolipoma	• Puberty (young adults) • Forearms • Subcutaneous, firm, circumscribed tumor with mild pain (often when pressure applied) • Normal karyotype (not associated with cytogenetic changes)	• Thin fibrous capsule with incomplete fibrous septa (lobules); both fatty tissue and many small blood vessels (vessels compose >5% of tumor); fibrin thrombi often noted in vessels

Name	Predilection Clinical Key Features	Histopathology
Angiomyxolipoma	• "Vascular myxolipoma" • Likely a variant of dendritic fibromyxolipoma • Shares cytogenetic changes with lipoma, spindle-cell/pleomorphic lipoma, and myxoma (unlike angiolipoma which has a normal karyotype)	• Resembles a spindle-cell lipoma (see p. 653) with a myxoid stroma
Adenolipoma	• Thigh • Soft, lobulated nodule	• Lobules of mature adipose tissue admixed with normal-appearing eccrine glands

Name	Predilection Clinical Key Features	Histopathology
Chondroid lipoma [Vimentin, S100]	• Females • Lower extremities • Deep-seated, firm tumor (average 3–5 cm)	• Lobulated, thin capsule, multivacuolated cells in a chondromyxoid matrix; mature adipocytes
Sclerotic (fibroma-like) lipoma	• Variant of lipoma • Males • Fingers and distal extremities	• Circumscribed nodules in the subcutis with a prominent sclerotic stroma (sometimes storiform appearance) and varying amounts of fat
Spindle-cell lipoma [CD34, factor XIIIa, vimentin]	• Benign tumor of subcutis • Men (50s–70s) • Upper back and neck • Slow-growing; painless, soft, oval, lobular mass • Mutation = often involves loss of 16q or monosomy 16	• "Rope-like" collagen + myxoid stroma + spindle-cells + mast cells + mature fat • Circumscribed, unencapsulated; no lipoblasts present or significant nuclear atypia (unlike liposarcoma); thick trabeculated area with fat; "ropy" collagen

Name	Predilection Clinical Key Features	Histopathology
Pleomorphic (giant-cell) lipoma [CD34, factor XIIIa]	• Benign tumor • Middle-aged to elderly men • Shoulder, back of neck • Soft subcutaneous mass (average 5 cm) • Mutation = often involves loss of 16q	• Similar to spindle-cell lipoma + pleomorphic "floret" cells (giant cells with marginally-placed, overlapping nuclei)
Hibernoma	• Benign, rare tumor from brown fat (brown fat used for warmth) • Adults (30's) • Scapula, axilla, neck • Tan-brown lobulated tumor (average 10 cm); possibly increased warmth in area • Mutation = loss of MEN1 gene (chromosome 11)	• Deep, thinly encapsulated and divided lobules with a thin septum; prominent blood vessels; prominent nucleolus but no mitosis • "Mulberry cells" (central nucleus and multivacuolated cells that are filled with mitochondria); look like vacuolated cells with "ping-pong" balls inside

Name	Predilection Clinical Key Features	Histopathology
Liposarcoma		
Liposarcoma overall	<ul><li>Most common soft tissue tumor</li><li>Older adults</li><li>Thighs and buttocks</li><li>Usually presents as a deep subcutaneous mass</li></ul>	
Well-differentiated liposarcoma	<ul><li>Good prognosis</li><li>Resembles normal fat; nuclear pleomorphism</li><li>Lipoblasts = immature, multivacuolated fat cells with hyperchromatic, scalloped nuclei</li></ul>	
Spindle-cell liposarcoma	<ul><li>Spindle-cell proliferation in fascicles and whorls in a myxoid stroma</li></ul>	

Name	Predilection Clinical Key Features and Histopathology
Myxoid liposarcoma	• Lower extremities • Metastasizes to extrapulmonary sites • Fusiform or stellate cells with abundant mucoid stroma; delicate plexiform network of capillaries ("crow's foot" or "chicken wire" vessels)
Round cell liposarcoma	• Poorly differentiated form of myxoid liposarcoma • Diffuse sheets of round/oval cells with a single cytoplasmic vacuole; mitoses abundant • High-grade liposarcoma and risk of metastasis to skin
Pleomorphic liposarcoma	• Highly cellular, numerous mitoses, bizarre/pleomorphic multivacuolated lipoblasts with one or more nuclei • "Dedifferentiated liposarcoma" = histological variant of pleomorphic liposarcoma: Contains a well-differentiated portion + dedifferentiated areas resembling malignant fibrous histiocytoma or myxofibrosarcoma

Tumors of Muscle, Cartilage, and Bone

Leiomyoma
(Benign cells with cigar-shaped nuclei)

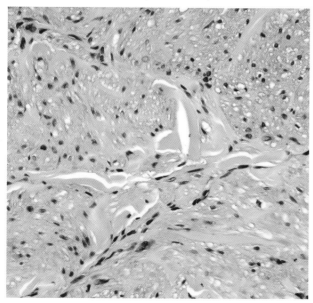

Leiomyosarcoma
(Bizarre cells with dark nuclei)

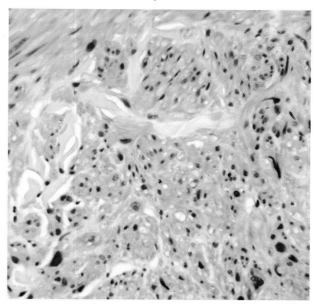

Name	Predilection and Clinical Key Features	Histopathology
Tumors of smooth muscle		

Leiomyoma or piloleiomyoma
 	
[Desmin, actin]
	• Pilar leiomyoma
	• Lesion derived from arrector pili muscle
	• Age = 20s–30s
	• Trunk and extensor surface of extremities
	
	• Solitary or multiple, firm, painful (especially in cold weather), reddish-brown papulonodular lesions
	• Multiple leiomyomas area associated with:
	  • CLL
	  • HIV
	  • Reed syndrome (see below)
		
		• Circumscribed non-encapsulated tumor centered on dermis; uninvolved epidermis separated by "grenz zone"; whorled pattern; elongated nuclei with blunt ends ("cigar-shaped" nuclei); perinuclear vacuoles
		
		• Trichrome stain (above)

Scrotal (vulval) leiomyoma	• Scrotum (vulvar variant is on labia majora) • Firm solitary asymptomatic nodules 1–14 cm • Vulvar lesion = 1–5-cm nodule (expresses estrogen and progesterone receptors, unlike piloleiomyoma)	• Ill-defined infiltrative margins, more cellular than pilo-variant (vulvar is usually spindle-cell type)
Cutaneous and uterine leiomyomas	• "Reed syndrome" • Autosomal dominant disorder • Multiple cutaneous + uterine leiomyomas • Mutation = fumarate hydratase (enzyme in mitochondria Krebs cycle) • Associated with papillary renal cell cancer	• Same as cutaneous leiomyomas

Name	Predilection and Clinical Key Features	Histopathology
Angioleiomyoma [Vimentin, desmin, actin]	• Middle age • Lower leg • Solitary, slow-growing, asymptomatic, firm gray–white round/oval nodule	• Well circumscribed, round, deep nodule with a fibrous capsule; smooth muscle > vascular vessels • Three variants: 1. Solid type 2. Cavernous type 3. Venous type • Perinuclear vacuoles and cigar-shaped nucleus (deep dermis)

Name	Predilection and Clinical Key Features	Histopathology
Angiomyolipoma	• Variant of cutaneous angioleiomyoma	• Angioleiomyoma + fat cells (mixture of blood vessels, smooth muscle, and adipocytes)

Name	Predilection and Clinical Key Features	Histopathology
Smooth muscle hamartoma [CD-34]	• Infants (usually congenital) • Extremities and trunk • Trunk, proximal extremities (does not involve scrotum) • Flesh-colored or lightly pigmented plaque (<10 cm); pseudo-Darier sign seen clinically	• Scattered smooth muscle bundles in dermis plus normal number of hair follicles (similar to Becker's nevus; see p. 230)
Leiomyosarcoma overall	• Histopathology = elongated spindle-shaped cells with cigar-shaped nuclei; pleomorphic nuclei; vacuoles in cell cross-sections • "Leiomyoma-like" + "ugly" mitotic cells • Stains = vimentin, desmin (70%), actin, and Masson trichrome stains (show myofilaments)	

Name	Predilection and Clinical Key Features	Histopathology
Dermal leiomyosarcoma	• Men in 60s • Extensor surface of extremities, head, and neck • Erythematous or hyperpigmented solitary nodule • May recur (30%), but rarely metastasizes (better prognosis than subcutaneous leiomyosarcoma)	• Irregular outline, majority in dermis, flattening of rete ridges • Actin stain (above)
Subcutaneous leiomyosarcoma	• Painful, well-circumscribed, deep tumor • May recur (50–70%) • Risk of metastases to lung, liver, bone (one-third of cases)	• Similar dermal leiomyosarcoma, but extends to lower dermis, prominent vascular pattern, areas of necrosis, and possible vascular invasion
Secondary leiomyosarcoma	• Arises from retroperitoneal and uterine primary lesions • Scalp and back • Multiple spheroidal tumors	• Often multiple, spheroidal in outline, and sometimes present in vascular lumina
Tumors of striated muscle		
Striated muscle hamartoma	• Neonates • Head and neck • Polypoid lesion in midline location	• Multiple bundles of striated muscle surrounded by fibrofatty tissue with telangiectatic vessels
Rhabdomyoma (adult type) [Myoglobulin, desmin]	• Benign tumor • Head and neck • Well circumscribed, soft reddish-brown	• Large polygonal cells with granular, eosinophilic cytoplasm, "spider-web" cells and cells with cross-striations ("jack-straw," rod-like striations)

Name	Predilection and Clinical Key Features	Histopathology
Rhabdomyo-sarcoma [Myogen, myoglobulin, MyoD1, desmin]	• #1 soft tissue sarcoma of childhood • Head and neck, GU tract, retroperitoneum • Rarely presents as dermal nodule	• Three subtypes histologically: 1. Embryonal 2. Alveolar 3. Pleomorphic
Malignant rhabdoid tumor [Vimentin, cytokeratins]	• Present at birth • Papulonodular skin lesions • Average survival <6 weeks	• Sheets of polygonal cells with abundant hyaline eosinophilic cytoplasm and a peripherally displaced vesicular nucleus; prominent mitotic activity

Name	Predilection and Clinical Key Features	Histopathology
Tumors of cartilage		
Chondroma [S100]	• Cutaneous chondromas are without bony connections and are extremely rare • Fingers • Firm, round nodule	• Well-circumscribed expansile tumor composed of chondrocytes in cartilaginous matrix; effacement of rete ridges
Subungual osteochondroma	• Subungual exostosis is a common benign proliferation of the bone that often causes a nail abnormality due to the predilection for the distal phalanx • Young and adult males • Distal phalanx (especially big toe) • Painful tumor; diagnosis can be confirmed by x-ray 	• Mature trabecular bone with a proliferating cap of mature cartilage; osteogenesis occurs by endochondral ossification
Parachordoma [S100, cytokeratin 8/18, CK1/10, 7, 20]	• Slow-growing, soft tissue neoplasm • Extremities adjacent to tendon, synovium, or bone • Skin nodule may develop by direct extension from underlying tumor or distant metastasis • Not related but similar to chordoma, which has an axial body location and is a sacrococcygeal tumor from the neural tube remnant	• Strands and cords of vacuolated cells (physaliphorous) in myxoid stroma

Name	Predilection and Clinical Key Features	Histopathology
Tumors of bone		
Osteosarcoma [Vimentin; negative for S100 and cytokeratin]	• Primary lesion may be in the bone • Elderly • Legs and areas of prior radiation • Deep nodule with ulcerations • May recur locally and spread to lungs or other organs	• Dermis or subcutis tumor; spindle cells with scant eosinophilic cytoplasm and elongated nuclei; ulceration often occurs

Schwannoma

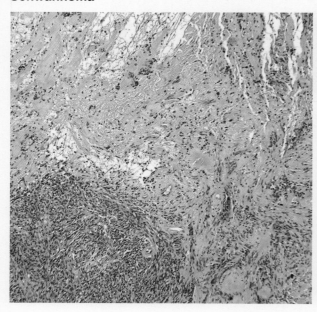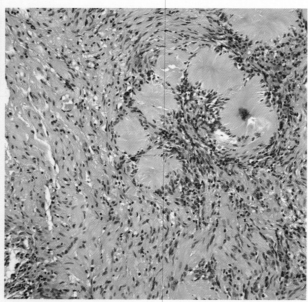

Three Main Cells in Peripheral Nerve Sheath	Stain	EM	Tumor
Perineurial cells	EMA, vimentin (not S100)	No basement membrane	Perineurioma
Schwann cells	S100, vimentin (not EMA)	Basement membrane (type IV)	Neuroma, schwannoma, neurofibroma (differ by proportion and arrangements)
Fibroblast	Vimentin		

Name	Predilection and Clinical Key Features	Histopathology
Nerve sheath tumors		
Neuromas (Axons:Schwann cell fascicles ratio = 1:1)		
Traumatic neuroma [S100, MBP, Bodian stain]	• Site of trauma, scar or amputation (often acral skin) • Firm, skin-colored or reddish, oval, pea-sized nodule	• "Scar + nerve" • Well-circumscribed, irregular arrangement of nerve fascicles in a fibrous scar/sheath; perineural cells surround each fascicle

Name	Predilection and Clinical Key Features	Histopathology
Rudimentary polydactyly	• "Rudimentary supernumerary digit" • Birth to childhood • Base of fifth finger on ulnar border • Small flesh-colored papule or nodule	• Numerous nerve fiber bundles in connective tissue in upper dermis; oval corpuscles present (resembles Meissner corpuscles) Oval, Meissner-like corpuscles (above)

Name	Predilection and Clinical Key Features	Histopathology
Palisaded and encapsulated neuroma [S100]	• "Solitary circumscribed neuroma" • Middle-aged adults • Face • Slow-growing, single, painless nodule on face (average 0.5 cm) • Possible response to trauma	• Well-developed, circumscribed fascicles in loose matrix; perineural tissue capsule surrounds tumor (pseudocapsule); clefting around tumor (unlike neurofibroma); no fibrous tissue sheath around fascicles (unlike traumatic neuroma)

Multiple mucosal neuromas and possible syndrome	• MEN syndrome, type IIB (Sipple) or multiple endocrine neoplasia:
	   • Autosomal dominant
	   • Mutation = RET proto-oncogene mutation
	   • Marfanoid habitus; multiple mucosal neuromas
	   • High risk for medullary carcinoma of thyroid: lab = calcitonin
	   • Risk of pheochromocytoma:
	     • adrenal gland, high blood pressure
	     • lab = urinary vanillylmandelic acid (VMA)	

Name	Predilection and Clinical Key Features	Histopathology
Ganglioneuroma	• Rare primary tumor • H/O neuroblastoma and neurofibromatosis	• Neurofibroma + mature ganglion cells in spindle cell fascicles (typically a ganglion cell is trapped by a neurofibroma)
Epithelial sheath neuroma	• Elderly • Upper back • Papule or nodule	• Enlarged nerve fibers in upper dermis ensheathed in squamous epithelium
Perineurioma [EMA, vimentin; not S100, CD34, enolase]	• Tumor of only perineural cell • Middle-aged adults • Trunk and extremities • Firm nodule • Associated with NF-1 and NF-2 (see pp. 672 and 673)	• Firm, circumscribed non-encapsulated lesion; "storiform pattern" and spindle cells with elongated, bipolar cytoplasmic processes; concentric "onion bulb" whorls

Name	Predilection and Clinical Key Features	Histopathology
Sclerosing perineurioma [EMA, vimentin]	• Young adults • Fingers and palms • Associated with aberrations to chromosome 10 and NF-2 gene (chromosome 22)	• Abundant dense collagen with small epithelioid and spindle cells with cord, trabecular, and "onion skin" patterns (may be confused with fibroma of tendon sheath or sclerotic fibroma of Cowden's disease)
Schwannoma (neurilemmoma) [S100, vimentin, EMA and type IV collagen in basement membrane; negative myelin basic protein]	• Benign neoplasm of nerve sheath (not neural cells) • Adults • Limbs • Solitary, pink-to-yellow, slow-growing tumor; possibly pain and paresthesia 90% solitary with no associated syndrome • Associates with neurofibromatosis (especially NF-2) and familial syndrome of schwannomatosis • Variants: • Cellular schwannoma • Neuroblastoma-like • Epithelioid schwannoma • Psammomatous melanotic schwannoma: associated with Carney's complex	• Circumscribed, encapsulated, deep dermal tumor • Deep dermis/subcutaneous; encapsulated in perineurium; nerve of origin is along border (pushed to the side) • Two tissue types seen: 1. Antoni A (hypercellular) = spindle-shaped Schwann cells in interlacing fascicles, Verocay bodies (eosinophilic masses formed by cell processes and rows of nuclei) 2. Antoni B (hypocellular) = loose meshwork of gelatinous tissue with widely separated Schwann cells • Verocay bodies (above)

Name	Predilection and Clinical Key Features	Histopathology
Plexiform schwannoma	• Benign variant of schwannoma	• Plexiform appearance with multiple interlacing and interconnecting fascicles and nodules; predominantly Antoni A-type tissue
Psammomatous melanotic schwannoma [S100, HMB-45, MART-1, vimentin]	• Component of Carney's complex (disorder with myxomas, spotty pigmentation, and endocrinopathy) • Located at posterior spinal nerve roots, GI tract, bone and soft tissue • Skin is uncommon site	• Well circumscribed, partially encapsulated, psammoma bodies, pigmented melanocytes

Neurofibroma and neurofibromatosis

| Neurofibromatosis overall | • NF-1 = 85–90% cases; chromosome 17; autosomal dominant:
   • NF1 gene mutation; encodes neurofibromin protein (tumor-suppressor function)
 • NF-2 = chromosome 22; autosomal dominant:
   • Acoustic neuromas, schwannomas, intracranial tumors, juvenile posterior subcapsular lenticular opacity
   • NF2 gene mutation; encodes merlin/neurofibromin 2
 • NF-3 = mix of NF-1 and NF-2
 • NF-4 = diffuse neurofibromas and café-au-lait pigmentation
 • NF-5 = Segmental form (unilateral or bilateral localization):
   • Possible mutation = postzygotic NF-1 gene
 • NF-6 = only have café-au-lait pigmentation
 • NF-7 = late onset
 • NF-8 = miscellaneous group
 • Additional disorders related to NF-1 gene mutations:
   • Watson syndrome (autosomal dominant) = NF-1 mutation: pulmonic valve stenosis, café-au-lait macules, short stature, neurofibromas, Lisch nodules, axillary freckling
   • Noonan syndrome (autosomal dominant) = usually has PTPN11 mutation, but possible NF-Noonan overlap syndrome (NF-1 mutation): characteristic facies, short stature, cardiac defects (especially pulmonic valve stenosis), nevi | | |

Name	Predilection and Clinical Key Features	Histopathology
Classic neurofibromatosis (NF-1)	• "von Recklinghausen disease" • Autosomal dominant • Birth or early childhood • If six or more café-au-lait lesions in an infant, then suspect NF-1 • Clinical features may include: • Neurofibromas (during puberty and pregnancy) • Plexiform neurofibroma • >Six café-au-lait macules (99% of patients) • Axillary freckles ("Crowe's sign"): most specific sign and pathognomonic • Lisch nodules (pigmented hamartoma of iris) • Macrocephaly • Mental retardation • Kyphoscoliosis • Bone hypertrophy • Risk of hypertension: may be due to renal stenosis or pheochromocytoma • Mutation = neurofibromin protein defect (chromosome 17, tumor suppressor function) • Patients with NF-1 + juvenile xanthogranuloma (JXG) have reported 20-fold increased risk of juvenile myelomonocytic leukemia (JMML)	*Clinical images* • Café-au-lait macules (above) • Neurofibromas (above) • Axillary freckling or "Crowe's sign" (most specific cardinal criterion for NF-1), photos above
"NF-1-like" syndrome	• "Legius syndrome" • Café-au-lait macules, axillary freckling • Mutation = SPRED1 gene (loss-of-function)	• Appears like a café-au-lait macule histologically

Name	Predilection and Clinical Key Features	Histopathology
Neurofibroma [S100, myelin basic protein; Bodian stain shows axons]	• Neoplasm of entire peripheral nerve • Upper trunk • Soft, flesh-colored papule • "Buttonhole" sign = invaginates with pressure on lesion • Associated with NF-1	• Non-encapsulated, loosely textured tumor centered in dermis; grenz zone; thin fascicles of cells with a "wavy," spindle, "S-shaped" nucleus with sharp pointed ends; mitoses rare; "bubblegum" stroma; mast cells

Name	Predilection and Clinical Key Features	Histopathology
Plexiform neurofibroma	• Due to irregular cylindrical or fusiform enlargement of subcutaneous or deep nerve • Soft, enlarged, "bag-of-worms" tumor; often hyperpigmented • Lesion is specific for NF-1	• Similar to neurofibroma histologically • Numerous large nerve fascicles embedded in a cellular matrix with mucin; cells with spindle, "S-shaped" nucleus and sharp pointed ends
Pacinioma	• Sacral region (associated with spina bifida occulta) • Painful nodule • Rare association with NF-1	• Hamartomatous overgrowth of mature Vater–Pacini corpuscles
Pacinian neurofibroma/ neuroma	• Hands and feet • Multiple nodules	• Round/ovoid corpuscles with multiple concentric lamellae (close resemblance to Vater–Pacini corpuscles)

Name	Predilection and Clinical Key Features	Histopathology
Nerve sheath myxoma [S100, vimentin]	• Peripheral nerve sheath tumor of Schwann cells • Middle-aged females (40s) • Hands, knees, and extremities • Solitary, painless, slow-growing multinodular masses • Recurrences common, especially if incompletely removed	• Well-defined fascicles; multilobulated, non-encapsulated with spindle cells in whirling, lamellar, concentric patterns in a hypocellular myxoid stroma (mainly chondroitin-4 or chondroitin-6 sulfate present); peripheral fibrous border

Name	Predilection and Clinical Key Features	Histopathology
Neurothekeoma [NK1/C3, PGP 9.5, vimentin]	• "Cellular neurothekeoma" • Unknown histogenesis (no longer considered of nerve sheath differentiation) • Young females (20s) • Face, extremities • Asymptomatic, dome-shaped nodules • Lesion is not associated with NF	• Ill-defined multilobular fascicles of mainly epithelioid cells and spindle cells with a "whorl" appearance; possible dystrophic calcification and ossification • Stains with NK1/C3 • Does not stain with S100 or desmin

Name	Predilection and Clinical Key Features	Histopathology

Granular cell tumor
 	
[S100 (unlike xanthoma); CD68; granules, PAS/diastase resistant +; myelin basic protein +]
	• Benign tumor
	• Females and black skin
	• Age 40s–50s
	• Tongue, head, and neck area
	
	• Asymptomatic, solitary, skin-colored, firm nodule (<2 cm)
	• Tumor from neural origin (Schwann cells)
	• Multiple granular cell tumors are associated with neurofibromatosis and Hodgkin's disease
	• *Note:* Congenital epulis (gingival giant cell tumor) is a morphologically similar lesion:
	  • Often found on the anterior alveolar ridge of female neonates
	  • Not as common as the acquired epulis
	  • Often regress spontaneously
		• Superficial, non-encapsulated, irregularly arranged sheets of large polyhedral cells with central hyperchromatic nucleus and coarse granular eosinophilic cytoplasm; round nuclei; induces pseudoepitheliomatous hyperplasia above tumor; large cytoplasmic granules (lysosomes) are surrounded by a clear halo ("pustulo-ovoid bodies of Milan")

Name	Predilection and Clinical Key Features	Histopathology
Malignant granular cell tumor	• 1–3% of granular cell tumors • May metastasize to regional lymph nodes	• Granular cell tumor, similar to larger size (>5 cm), vascular invasion, necrosis, and rapid growth; mitoses and pleomorphic nuclei may be present

Name	Predilection and Clinical Key Features	Histopathology
Malignant peripheral nerve sheath tumor (MPNST) [S100, enolase, MBP, neurofilament]	• Majority arise from a malignant transformation of neurofibroma (10% risk in NF-1) • Neurofibromatosis patients (50% of cases); young and middle-aged adults • Predilection for proximal extremities (deep, soft tissue) • Soft tissue mass • Mean survival = 2–3 years	• Usually spindle-cell growth with cells arranged in tight wavy or interlacing bundles; sometimes dense cellular areas alternating with more loosely textured areas; mitoses present

Name	Predilection and Clinical Key Features	Histopathology
Herniations and ectopias		
Nasal glioma and neural heterotopias [S100 and GFAP (glial fibrillary acid protein)]	• Hamartomas from sequestration of heterotopic neural (brain) tissue during embryogenesis • Birth to early infancy • Nose and scalp • Red–blue, firm smooth tumor near bridge of nose or on scalp; "hair collar sign" (dark, coarse hair circle around congenital scalp lesion and may indicate ectopic neural tissue)	• Islands of neural (astrocytes) and fibrovascular tissue in the subcutis; "brain-like" stroma • May have intracranial connection (consider MRI imaging prior to biopsy or removal)
Cutaneous meningioma [S100, vimentin and EMA]	• Scalp, forehead, and paravertebral area • Hemorrhagic cyst, nodule or plaque; possibly associated with underlying bone defect • Type I lesions: • Birth (ectopic arachnoid cells) • Scalp, forehead, paravertebral • Neural tube closure problem • Type II lesions: • Adults • Around sensory organs: follow cranial nerves • Type III lesions: • Direct cutaneous or metastasis of intracranial tumor	• Psammoma bodies often seen; other histology depends on type • Type I: • Confined to subcutis • Irregular strands of meningothelial cells in collagenous stroma • Type II and III: • May also involve dermis • Circumscribed and more cellular than type I

Name	Predilection and Clinical Key Features	Histopathology
Neuroendocrine carcinomas		
Merkel cell carcinoma [CK20, EMA, enolase and cytokeratin show paranuclear dots or globules; negative S100 and thyroid transcription factor (differs from lung small cell cancer)]	• Elderly • Sun-exposed head, neck, and extremities • Associated with polyomavirus • Rapid growing, red-to-violaceous nodule (average 2 cm) • 50% of Merkel cell carcinomas exhibit trisomy 6 • May have neuropeptides (i.e. VIP, calcitonin, ACTH, gastrin, and somatostatin) • Possible Tx = Wide local excision (3-cm margins), LN dissection, XRT and/or chemotherapy	• "Blue tumor" • Small, round-oval cells of uniform size with vesicular nucleus and multiple small nucleoli; mitoses; "salt-n-pepper" nuclei • "Salt-n-pepper" nuclei in uniform cells • CK20 stain (below)

Name	Predilection and Clinical Key Features	Histopathology
Malignant primitive neuroectodermal tumor (MPNET) [CD99, enolase]	• Small-cell skin malignancy which is highly aggressive and eventually metastasizes • Peak incidence in 20s, slight male predilection • Trunk and lower extremities • Deep soft tissue mass • Considered on a spectrum with extraskeletal Ewing's sarcoma; both have a chromosomal translocation 11:22	• Numerous hyperchromatic, small blue cells with small amount of cytoplasm (similar to Merkel cell); Homer Wright rosettes (cells in "rose petal-like" pattern); may contain glycogen • Does not stain for epithelial membrane antigen (EMA) or CK20 (like Merkel cell carcinoma)
Extraskeletal Ewing's sarcoma [CD99 stain in membranous pattern]	• Peak incidence in 20s, slight male predilection • Trunk and lower extremities • Deep soft tissue mass • Considered on a spectrum with malignant primitive neuroectodermal tumor; both have a chromosomal translocation 11:22	• Sheets of hyperchromatic, small blue cells with small amount of cytoplasm (similar to Merkel cell); Homer Wright rosettes ("rose petal-like" pattern of cells around a lumen); cells often contain glycogen • Does not stain for epithelial membrane antigen (EMA) or CK20 (like Merkel cell carcinoma) and negative S100 • Homer Wright rosettes (photos below)

38 Vascular Tumors

Glomangioma

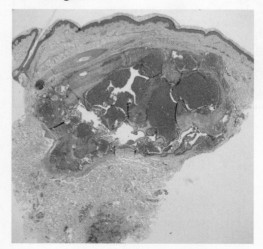

	Vascular/Lymphatic Endothelium	Lymphatic Only Tumors
Stains	CD31; CD34; PAL-E; factor VIII; Ulex	VEGFR-3 (vascular endothelial cell growth factor); poloplanin; LYVE-1; Prox-1; D2-40; thrombomodulin
Electron microscopy	Weibel–Palade bodies in endothelium cell: • "Rod-shaped" organelles • Storage organelle with vWF, P-selectin, endothelin-1, TPA, etc.	

Name	Predilection and Clinical Key Features	Histopathology
Hamartomas and vascular malformations		
Eccrine angiomatous hamartoma	• Rare malformation with increased number of small blood vessels and increased number of eccrine glands	

Phakomatosis pigmentovascularis	• Coexistence of a vascular hamartoma (in form of nevus flammeus) and a melanocytic lesion:
	  • Usually mongolian spot or nevus spilus
	  • Genetic model explanation = "twin spotting" (two different clones of neighboring cells in a background of normalcells)	

Nevus flammeus	• Often called "capillary malformation" or "port wine stain"
	• Congenital malformation (newborns)
	• Forehead, face, neck
	
	• Salmon-red colored patch
	• Associated with Sturge–Weber (leptomeninges, V1 branch involvement, risk of glaucoma); Klippel–Trenaunay–Weber (limb); and Cobb's syndrome (lower back)
	• Does not fade with time (permanent)
	• Variants:
	  • "Port wine" stain (unilateral along V1/V2)
	  • "Salmon" patch (posterior neck, eyelids, and glabella)
	  • "Stork bite" (glabellar lesions with lesions on nape of neck)
		• Variable dilation of thin-walled vessels; progressive ectasia; erythrocyte stasis; grows proportional to child; does not spontaneously involute

Name	Predilection and Clinical Key Features	Histopathology
Venous malformations	<ul><li>"Cavernous hemangiomas"</li><li>Congenital</li><li>Infants</li><li>Blue–purple papule, nodule</li></ul><ul><li>Lacks proliferative phase and does not typically regress over time (like capillary hemangiomas)</li><li>Associated with:<ul><li>"Blue rubber bleb" nevus = multiple compressible blue, rubbery hemangiomas (venous) on skin and GI tract; areas of hyperhidrosis</li><li>Maffucci's syndromes = enchondromas of bone; chondrosarcoma risk; spindle-cell hemangioendothelioma: may be due to parathyroid receptor mutation in some cases</li></ul></li></ul>	<ul><li>Large dilated vascular channels lined by flat endothelium in deep dermis/subcutis; thrombosis; calcifications of walls</li></ul>
Cutis marmorata telangiectatica congenita (CMTC)	<ul><li>Congenital (sporadic, autosomal dominant)</li><li>Neonate</li><li>Trunk and extremities</li></ul><ul><li>Reticulated vascular pattern with dermal atrophy in segmental pattern; dark violet–blue vessels; spider nevus-like telangiectases; risk of glaucoma with periocular involvement</li><li>Often improves by 2 years of age</li><li>May be associated with:</li><li>Adams–Oliver syndrome (CMTC + cutis aplasia congenita)</li><li>Type V phakomatosis pigmentovascularis</li><li>Cornelia de Lange syndrome:<ul><li>mutation (50%) often in NIPBL gene</li><li>short stature, retardation, synophrys (confluent eyebrows), trichomegaly (long eyelashes), hirsutism, microcephaly, low-pitch cry</li></ul></li></ul>	<ul><li>Various changes, including dilated capillaries and veins in the dermis and subcutis</li><li>DIF: neonatal lupus may present with a CMTC-like appearance; consider lupus serology work-up in infants with CMTC</li></ul>

Name	Predilection and Clinical Key Features	Histopathology
Glomulovenous malformation [Smooth muscle actin, vimentin]	• "Glomangioma" • In past, it was considered a glomus tumor variant • Sporadic or familial (glomulin gene mutation) • Extremities and trunk • Painless, blue, or violaceous macules, nodules, or plaques	• "Lots of vessels + few glomus" • Poorly circumscribed/encapsulated; prominent vessels surrounded by a few layers of glomus cells (round, monotonous cells)

Name	Predilection and Clinical Key Features	Histopathology
Lymphangioma circumscriptum	• Cutaneous type of cystic lymphatic malformation • Birth to infancy • Proximal limbs, girdle • Clusters of vesicles/papulovesicles with red–purple areas ("frogspawn-like") • May develop SCC at site; epidermis elevated with ectatic lymphatics in papillary dermis	• Multiple lymph vessels in upper dermis; flat endothelium

Deep lymphangiomas	Variants:
	• Cavernous lymphangioma
	• Cystic hygroma:
	  • neck and axilla area
	  • associated with Turner's syndrome (45, XO), Down syndrome, Noonan's syndrome
	  • soft swellings in skin, epidermis normal
		• Dilated lymph vessels deeper in dermis

Lymphan-giomatosis	• Child • Primarily bone, parenchymal, soft tissue involvement, but may have skin lesions	• Dilated lymphatic channels in dermis/subcutis with single layer of flat endothelium lining
Verrucous hemangioma	• Birth to childhood • Legs • Bluish–red soft papules, plaques, or nodules that become wart-like; may develop satellite lesions • Recurrence frequent after removal due to deep component	• Numerous small and large vessels in dermis and subcutis; irregular papillomatosis; overlying a verrucous hyperplasia of epidermis

Name	Predilection and Clinical Key Features	Histopathology
Vascular dilatations (telangiectases)		
Hereditary hemorrhagic telangiectasia	• "Osler–Rendu–Weber disease" • Puberty or childhood • Mutations: • HHT1 (endoglin): TGF-β binding protein • HHT2 (ALK-1): activin receptor-like kinase • Multiple punctate telangiectases in skin and mucosa of lips, nose; epistasis (often clinical presentation); increase with age and pregnancy • May involve respiratory, GI or GU tracts • Associated with pulmonary (HHT1 mutation), liver (HHT2 mutation), and cerebral AV fistulas	• Dilated thin-walled vessels lined by a single endothelium layer in the dermal papillae

Name	Predilection and Clinical Key Features	Histopathology
Generalized essential telangiectasia	• Childhood • Females • Lower extremities then trunk and arms • Telangiectatic macules and diffuse erythematous areas composed of a fine meshwork of ectatic vessels	• Thin-walled vascular channels in upper dermis due to a dilation of postcapillary venules of the upper horizontal plexus
Hereditary benign telangiectasia	• Autosomal dominant trait • Appears in childhood • Widespread cutaneous telangiectases; more prominent during pregnancy	• Dilation of the horizontal subpapillary venous plexus
Unilateral nevoid telangiectasia	• "Unilateral dermatomal superficial telangiectasia" • Females • May present at birth or acquired later (especially duing puberty and pregnancy) • Face and upper trunk (i.e. trigeminal area or third and fourth cervical dermatome) • Unilateral cluster of telangiectases • May be associated with excess estrogen (puberty, pregnancy), chronic liver disease	• Dilated vessels in superficial dermis; may have increased number of estrogen and progesterone receptors in area

Name	Predilection and Clinical Key Features	Histopathology
Ataxia–telangiectasia	• "Louis–Bar syndrome" • Autosomal recessive • Childhood • Bulbar conjunctiva, face, pinnae, neck, limb • Chromosome 11 (ATM gene) • Telangiectases • Ataxia is usually first presenting sign; risk of leukemia and lymphoma	• Progressive cerebellar ataxia (cerebellar cortical atrophy); cell-mediated and humoral immunity dysfunction; thymic aplasia or hypoplasia
"Spider" angioma	• 10–15% normal adults (increased number in chronic liver disease and pregnancy) • Face, neck, upper trunk, arms (i.e. above umbilicus); in children, often on hands, fingers • Central punctum with circular erythema and fine radiating "legs"	• Central ascending spiral thick-walled arteriole that ends in a thin-walled ampulla below epidermis; branching vessels off main arteriole

Name	Predilection and Clinical Key Features	Histopathology
Venous lake	• Elderly • Ear, face, lip, neck • Dark blue, multiple papules; bleed with minor trauma	• Single large dilated vascular channel in upper dermis; thin fibrous wall and flat endothelial lining; thrombus; sun-damaged skin

Name	Predilection and Clinical Key Features	Histopathology
Mibelli variant of angiokeratoma	• Females, childhood to adolescence • Warty lesions on bony prominences of hands, feet, elbows, knees	• Dilation of papillary dermal vessels to form large cavernous channels; irregular acanthosis of epidermis with elongation of rete ridges that enclose channels ("clutching rete"); looks like "small papule in epidermis" • Angiokeratoma vessels do not express CD34
Fordyce (scrotal) variant of angiokeratoma	• Most commonly elderly men (may develop in the 20s and 30s) • Red–black papules along superficial scrotum vessel (vulva also)	
Solitary or multiple angiokeratoma	• Lower extremities or anywhere 	
Angiokeratoma circumscriptum variant of angiokeratoma	• Child • Unilateral plaque with small discrete or hyperkeratotic papules	
Angiokeratoma corporis diffusum variant of angiokeratoma	• Bathing-trunk distribution • Multiple papules, often clusters • Associated with Anderson–Fabry disease (deficiency of lysosomal enzyme–galactosidase A causes accumulation of lysosomes; X-linked recessive disorder), fucosidosis, and other enzyme disorders	• Dermoscopy = demonstrates dark lacunae
Costal fringe	• Acquired lesion in elderly men • Band-like pattern of telangiectasis across anterior aspect of thorax	• Band-like pattern of telangiectasis
Milroy disease	• Congenital lymphedema (autosomal dominant) form of primary lymphedema • Present at birth (75% females) • Swelling of one or more limbs, or other body parts • Failure of lymphatics to form • Mutation = VEGFR3 mutation (a lymphatic-specific tyrosine kinase receptor)	• Lymphangiectasia and/or little-to-poor lymphatic formation

Name	Predilection and Clinical Key Features	Histopathology
Meige disease	• "Lymphedema praecox" • Primary lymphedema which occurs after birth to age 35	• Similar to Milroy disease
Lymphedema tarda	• Occurs after age 35 • Swelling of limbs	• Similar to Milroy disease
Elephantiasis nostra verrucosa	• "Mossy foot" • Due to chronic obstruction of lymphatics • Lower extremities • Enlarged limb with non-pitting edema; malodorous hyperkeratosis with generalized lichenification; cobblestoned papules; verrucous changes • Associated with surgery, overweight, lymphedema	• Pseudoepitheliomatous hyperplasia with dilated lymphatic spaces; chronic inflammation and fibroblast proliferation

Name	Predilection and Clinical Key Features	Histopathology
Vascular proliferations (hyperplasia and benign neoplasms)		
Infantile hemangioma [GLUT1]	• Most common tumor of infancy • "Hemangioma of infancy" or "strawberry nevus" • First few weeks of life (2% newborns); common in premature infants • Females • Head, neck, trunk, over parotid gland • Bright-red, raised papule or plaque • Majority of lesions regress by 5–7 years of age	• Highly cellular; vascular lumina slit-like and small with plump endothelial cells; central draining lumen may be evident in each lobule
Diffuse neonatal hemangiomatosis	• Birth to infancy • Usually fatal – often die due to high output cardiac failure (due to AV shunts, especially in liver), CNS involvement or bleeding associated with Kasabach–Merritt syndrome • Multiple cutaneous capillary hemangiomas and visceral hemangiomas • Associated with PHACES syndrome (posterior fossa malformations, hemangiomas, arterial anomalies, coarctation of the aorta and cardiac defects, eye abnormalities, sternal clefting)	
Sinusoidal hemangioma	• Acquired, benign lesion in adults • Adult females • Trunk, breast, limbs • Nodule involving subcutis and dermis	• Lobular architecture with thin-walled interconnecting vascular channels forming a sinusoidal pattern located in the subcutis and dermis; little stroma

Name	Predilection and Clinical Key Features	Histopathology
"Cherry" angioma	• After puberty (40s) • Trunk and proximal limbs 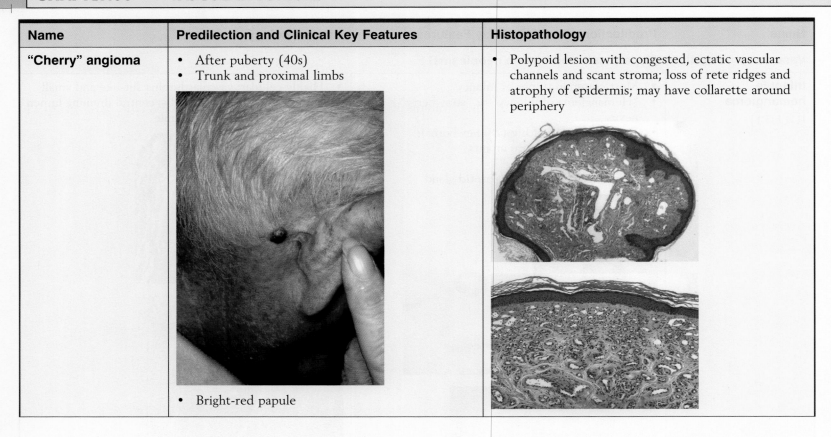 • Bright-red papule	• Polypoid lesion with congested, ectatic vascular channels and scant stroma; loss of rete ridges and atrophy of epidermis; may have collarette around periphery

Name	Predilection and Clinical Key Features	Histopathology
Glomeruloid hemangioma	<ul><li>Japanese race</li><li>Trunk and limbs</li><li>Eruptive, multiple, red/purple papules</li><li>Marker for POEMS syndrome or multicentric Castleman's disease (giant lymph node hyperplasia)</li><li>POEMS syndrome:<ul><li>P = polyneuropathy</li><li>O = organomegaly (hepatomegaly, spleen)</li><li>E = endocrinopathy (hypothyroid)</li><li>M = monoclonal gammopathy (paraproteinemia due to plasmacytoma or multiple myeloma)</li><li>S = skin changes (hyperpigmentation is most common skin finding)</li></ul></li></ul>	<ul><li>Dilated (sinusoidal) dermal vascular spaces with grape-like aggregates of small capillary vessels ("glomeruloid-like" appearance)</li><li>Plump endothelial cells (PAS+ eosinophilic granules)</li></ul>

Name	Predilection and Clinical Key Features	Histopathology
Arteriovenous (AV) hemangioma	<ul><li>"Acral arteriovenous tumor"</li><li>Middle-aged to elderly men</li><li>Predilection for lips, the perioral skin, nose and eyelids</li><li>Solitary, red/purple papule</li><li>Associated with chronic liver disease, epidermal nevus syndrome and other vascular malformations</li></ul>	<ul><li>Well-circumscribed, non-encapsulated collection of large, thick-walled vessels in upper/mid-dermis; myxoid stroma</li></ul><ul><li>Acral AV hemangioma (below)</li></ul>
Arteriovenous (AV) hemangioma	<ul><li>"Acral arteriovenous tumor"</li></ul>	

Name	Predilection and Clinical Key Features	Histopathology
Microvenular hemangioma [Factor VIII, CD34, CD31, Ulex europaeus-1 lectin]	• Acquired vascular tumor • Young to middle-aged adults • Forearms, trunk, limbs • Single, slow-growing purple/red papule or nodule	• Thin, uniform branching collapsed-looking vessels with inconspicuous lumina in dermis; myxoid stroma; endothelial cells plumper than normal, but not atypical

Name	Predilection and Clinical Key Features	Histopathology
Targetoid hemosiderotic hemangioma	• "Hobnail" hemangioma • Young to middle-aged men • Trunk and limbs • "Targetoid" violaceous central papule with area of palor and brown ring	• Dilated superficial dermal vessels with plump, "hobnail" endothelial cells (protrude lumen); fibrin thrombi; hemosiderin • Differential of "hobnailing" ("DR HAPpy"): D = Dabska's tumor R = retiform hemangioendothelioma H = hobnail hemangioma (targetoid hemosideric) A = angiolymphoid hyperplasia with eosinophilia P = PILA (papillary intralymphatic angioendothelioma)

Name	Predilection and Clinical Key Features	Histopathology
Spindle-cell hemangio-endothelioma [CD31, factor VIII]	• "Spindle-cell hemangioma" • Benign lesion • Children to young adults • Hands and feet • Possibly a reactive vascular process arising in association with a local, abnormal blood flow • Multiple, firm, red–blue, hemorrhagic nodules • May be seen in Maffucci's syndrome and Klippel–Trenaunay syndrome • 60% tend to recur after excision	• Three components in dermis/subcutis: 1. Vascular = thin-walled cavernous channels 2. Solid area of spindle cells with slit-like vascular spaces 3. Plump endothelial cells
Angioma serpiginosum	• Before puberty (females) • Extremities (not palms/soles/mucous membranes) • Multiple, pin-size puncta, often expand with age	• Ectatic, congested, thin-walled capillaries in the papillary dermis

Name	Predilection and Clinical Key Features	Histopathology
Angiolymphoid hyperplasia with eosinophilia	• Young to middle-aged adults • Around ears, forehead, scalp • Pink to red–brown papules/nodules; painful, pruritic, or pulsatile • May recur after excision (one-third) • Possibly associated with arteriovenous shunts	• Plump, partly vacuolated endothelial cells (may look "hobnail-like" or "cobblestone-like"); circumscribed collection of vessels and inflammatory cells including lymphocytes and eosinophils (and mast cells, plasma cells); often edematous stroma around the vessels

Name	Predilection and Clinical Key Features	Histopathology
Kimura's disease	<ul><li>"Eosinophilic lymphogranuloma"</li><li>Young Asian males</li><li>Close to ears or in parotid gland</li><li>Large subcutaneous mass</li></ul>	<ul><li>Reactive lymphoid follicles with a dense infiltrate of eosinophils; may form eosinophilic abscesses; mast cells increased; vessels increased with flat endothelial cells</li></ul>

Name	Predilection and Clinical Key Features	Histopathology
Pyogenic granuloma [CD31, CD34, factor VIII]	• Variant of lobular capillary hemangioma • Any age; 3:2 male preponderance • Gingiva, lips, fingers, face • Red or red–brown polypoid and pedunculated lesion that typically evolves over weeks • Associated with trauma, drugs (retinoids, indinavir, OCP), and pregnancy ("pregnancy tumor," especially occurs on gingiva or oral mucosa)	 • Well-developed collarette from elongated rete ridges; pale edematous stroma (granulation-like); collarette • DDx: bacillary angiomatosis appears similar, but has neutrophil infiltrate without ulceration (see p. 430).

Name	Predilection and Clinical Key Features	Histopathology
Intravenous pyogenic granuloma	• Variant of lobular capillary hemangioma that occurs inside veins • Neck, arms, and hands • Slow-growing, subcutaneous nodule	• Lobular proliferation of capillaries in a fibromyxoid stroma; fibrovascular stalk usually connects the lesion to the vein intima

Name	Predilection and Clinical Key Features	Histopathology
Tufted angioma	• "Angioblastoma of Nakagawa" • Variant of lobular capillary hemangioma • Usually acquired, but can be congenital • Children to young adults • Neck and upper trunk • Slowly spreading erythematous macules, papules; may be painful • Platelet trapping may produce Kasabach–Merritt syndrome	• "Cannonball" appearance of cell tufts that compress vessels; multiple, separated cellular lobules; semilunar vessel appearance; spindle-shaped and polygonal cells

Name	Predilection and Clinical Key Features	Histopathology
Glomus tumor [Smooth muscle actin, vimentin, CD34]	• Adults • Extremities (fingers and toes); subungual • Painful, solitary, purple dermal nodule • *Glomus function:* controls arteriovenous anastomosis, called the Sucquet–Hoyer canal	• "Lots of glomus + few vessels" • Well-circumscribed/encapsulated dermal tumor; few blood vessels surrounded by sheets of glomus cells (round, monotonous cells with eosinophilic cytoplasm and round/oval nuclei) • Smooth muscle actin (SMA) stain (below)

Name	Predilection and Clinical Key Features	Histopathology
Multinucleate cell angiohistiocytoma [Vimentin]	• Females >40 years old • Legs (especially calves and thighs); hands • Slow-growing, grouped, red-to-violet papules • Resemble Kaposi's sarcoma (p. 712), but not associated with HHV-8	• Two components: 1. Increased narrow dermal vessels 2. Large angulated multinucleate giant cells with palisading nuclei and eosinophilic cytoplasm (characteristic feature) • Multinucleate giant cell with palisading nuclei and eosinophilic cytoplasm (above)

Name	Predilection and Clinical Key Features	Histopathology
Reactive angioendo-theliomatosis [CD31, CD34, factor VIII]	• May be due to some type of vessel "blockage" • Any site on body • Red-to-blue patches/plaques; necrosis and ulceration may develop • Associated with DIC, infections, hemodialysis AV fistulae • Usually resolves after removal or cure of initiation process	• Benign intraluminal proliferation of endothelial cells which may occlude the lumina; vessels are dilated; endothelial cells may be large and mildly atypical, but are not malignant; minimal inflammation

Name	Predilection and Clinical Key Features	Histopathology
Acroangio-dermatitis [CD34]	• "Pseudo-Kaposi sarcoma" • Males • Lower extremities (prominent on first and second toes) • Purple papules/nodules with variable scale; stasis dermatitis • Associated with chronic venous insufficiency, limb paralysis, amputation, congenital AV malformation	• Proliferation of small vessels in edematous dermis; increased fibroblasts; plump endothelium; hemosiderin

Name	Predilection and Clinical Key Features	Histopathology
Intravascular papillary endothelial hyperplasia [CD34]	• "Masson's tumor" • Adult females • Veins in fingers, head, neck • Firm, blue/purple nodule; sometimes painful	 • Regarded as an unusual pattern of organization of a thrombus within a vein • Vascular channels present within the lumen of dilated vessels; thrombus; proliferation of papillary processes in the lumen; single layer of plump endothelial cells covering each papillary frond • Differs from angiosarcoma, which has anastomosing vessels, mitoses, and is not within a vessel lumen; see p. 714
Bacillary angiomatosis [Warthin–Starry, or GMS stain to see organisms]	• Exposure to cats (64%); HIV/organ transplant individuals • Multiple dusky-red, pedunculated lesions that bleed/are tender	• "Pyogenic granuloma-like + neutrophils" (see p. 430)
Verruga peruana ("Peruvian wart") [Romanowsky-Giemsa stain = red granules in endothelial cells, organism in phagosome]	• Eruptive phase of Carrion's disease (bartonellosis) caused by *Bartonella bacilliformis* • South America at altitudes 800–2500 meters • Multiple, miliary hemangioma-like lesions • Transmitted by sandflies	• Proliferation of capillary-like vessels in papillary dermis with formation of collarette; inflammatory infiltrate (plasma cells/lymphocytes) • Rocha–Lima inclusions (conglomerates of intracellular cytoplasmic granules within endothelial cells; color red with Romanowsky–Giemsa stain); mitotic figures frequent
Acquired progressive lymphangioma	• "Benign lymphangioendothelioma" • Adults • Occurs anywhere on body • Erythematous patch/plaque that enlarges over years	• Thin-walled interconnecting vascular channels in dermis/subcutis arranged horizontally; chronic inflammatory cells; possible "promontory sign" (similar patch stage of Kaposi's Sarcoma; see p. 712)

Name	Predilection and Clinical Key Features	Histopathology
Tumors with variable or uncertain behavior		

Kaposi's sarcoma (KS)
 	
[HHV-8 by PCR, CD31, PAS+]
	Variants:
	
	1. Classic:
	   • 50–60-year-old men
	   • Jews, Eastern European, Mediterranean
	   • Extremities
	   • Edema first?
	
	2. African (endemic):
	   • Tropical Africa
	   • Associated with EBV and HHV-8 (encode IL6 homolog, possible growth factor)
	
	3. Immunosuppressive Tx:
	   • Renal transplants; chemotherapy; long-term corticosteroids
	
	4. Epidemic (HIV-associated):
	   • Mucosa, trunk, head, neck, arms
	   • May have internal organs (GI, lungs) involved with no skin lesions
	
	• Early lesions are brown–red macules/papules then bluish–purple in color
		• Groups of perivascular lymphocytes and plasma cells; extravasated blood; eosinophilic hyaline granules; vessels often in horizontal direction; spindle cells in parallel array trapping red cells ("school of fish")
		• "Promontory sign" (jagged, vascular channels with plump endothelial cells surrounding existing vessels, especially patch stage); may see "Dorf balls" (pink amorphous globules in vessels)
		• Stages:
		  1. Patch ("promontory sign")
		  2. Plaque ("slit-like vessels")
		  3. Nodular

Name	Predilection and Clinical Key Features	Histopathology
Hemangio-pericytoma	• Some classify as a "solitary fibrous tumor" *Two forms:* 1. Congenital or infantile: • Birth to first year of life; boys • Head and neck, extremities, trunk • Now considered same as infantile myofibromatosis 2. Adult type (more common): • Adults • Arises in deep soft tissue • Lower extremities, pelvis	1. Congenital form is similar to adult form, but is multilobulated with perivascular and intravascular tumor outside of the main tumor mass 2. Adult type has tightly packed cellular area surrounding endothelium-lined ramifying vessels; nuclei are round/oval tumor cells separated from endothelial cells by a basement membrane and are surrounded by a reticuline fiber meshwork
Kaposiform hemangio-endothelioma	• Children (<2 years old) • Single lesion involving deep soft tissue of upper extremities, chest wall, scalp, neck • Associated with Kasabach–Merritt syndrome or lymphangiomatosis • Photos of patient with history of Kasabach–Merritt syndrome as an infant that was associated with a kaposiform hemangioendothelioma	• Nodules/fascicles of spindled endothelial cells lining slit-like or crescent-shaped vessels • Differs from Kasposi's sarcoma by: • Fascicles shorter/narrower • Hemosiderin present • No HHV-8 detected • Deeper tissue involvement
Papillary intralymphatic angioendothelioma (PILA) or Dabska tumor	• "Endovascular papillary angioendothelioma of childhood" • Low-grade variant of angiosarcoma (likely a lymphatic differentiated neoplasm) • Infants to children (4 months to 15 years of age) • Diffuse swelling of skin or intradermal tumor • Low metastatic risk	• Irregular vascular channels in dermis/subcutis; lined by varying endothelial cells ("hobnails") forming intraluminal papillary projections with a "rosette-like" or "matchstick-like" pattern

Name	Predilection and Clinical Key Features	Histopathology
Malignant tumors		

Angiosarcoma
 	
[CD31, CD34, factor VIII, cytokeratin, 30% are EMA+]
	Variants:
	1. *Idiopathic cutaneous AS:*
	   • Males
	   • Face/scalp
	   • Bluish–violaceous nodules/plaques ("rosacea-like" or "bruise that won't resolve"); metastasis risk
	2. *AS complicating lymphedema (Stewart–Treves):*
	   • Associated with post-mastectomy lymphedema: 12.5 years after surgery
	   • Purplish–red macular or polypoid tumor
	3. *Post-irradiation AS:*
	   • Associated with radiotherapy for benign/malignant conditions: 12–21 years after treatment
	4. *Miscellaneous:*
	   • Pre-existing benign vascular tumor, port wine stain or lymphangioma, etc.
	
	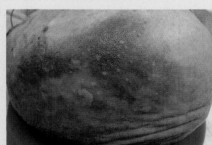
		• Blood + busy dermis + vessels (vessel cells "pile-up" on each other and arch or bridge vessel)
		• Poorly circumscribed dermal tumors; irregular dissecting vessels lined with crowded, varying endothelial cells; mast cells increased; papillary processes extend into lumen; vessels often with a downward orientation
		
		• Stains:
		   • Negative mitogen-activated protein kinase (MAPK), or caveolin which differs from benign vascular tumors
		   • Negative antibody AE1 stain which differs from carcinoma
		   • Negative CEA unlike Paget's or metastatic adenocarcinoma

Name	Predilection and Clinical Key Features	Histopathology
Lymphangio-sarcoma	Difficult to differentiate from angiosarcoma: • Use VEGFR3 (vascular endothelial cell growth factor receptor type 3) = lymphatic endothelium only • Stains = VEGFR3, poloplanin, LYVE-1, D2-40	
Epithelioid hemangio-endothelioma	• Most in soft tissue/organs; but skin lesions occur • Associated with underlying bone lesions	• Proliferation of nests and cords of plump endothelial cells in a fibro-myxoid stroma; intracytoplasmic vacuoles with RBCs
Retiform hemangio-endothelioma	• Slow-growing, exophytic or plaque-like tumors • Limbs and trunk of young to middle-aged adults	• Arborizing vessels that resemble the rete testis and lined by "hobnail" endothelial cells; prominent lymphocytic infiltrate
Malignant and atypical glomus tumors	• Differences between malignant and atypical/benign glomus tumor: • Size >2 cm • High mitotic rate • Nuclear atypia • Increased cellularity	
Tumors with significant vascular components		
Angiofibromas	• Clinically diverse group that includes fibrous papules of the face, adenoma sebaceum, pearly penile papules, acral fibrokeratoma • See p. 618 for more information	• Elevated growth; flattened rete ridges with patchy melanocytic hyperplasia; hyperkeratosis; increased blood vessels
Angioleiomyoma	• Lower extremities • Solitary nodule • See p. 659 for more information	• Well-circumscribed lesions of interlacing bundles of smooth muscle around and between vascular channels
Angiolipoma	• Extremities, especially forearm • Painful nodule • See p. 651 for more information	• Subcutaneous tumor with lobules of fat with capillaries comprising 5–50% of the lesion
Spindle-cell lipoma (angiomatoid variant)	• Elderly men • Upper back and neck • Painless, soft, oval nodule • See p. 653 for more information	• Circumscribed unencapsulated tumor with adipose tissue and elongated and haphazardly-arranged spindle cells
Angiomyxoma	• Benign, myxomatous tumor with blood vessels • Vulva, penis • May recur • See p. 645 for more information	• Myxoma + vessels • Spindle cells in a myxomatous stroma with vessels
Other vascular-component tumors	• Angiomyofibroblastoma • Dermatofibroma (aneurysmal variant) • Angioplasmocellular hyperplasia	

39 Cutaneous Metastases

Metastatic lobular breast carcinoma
("Indian file" or "stack-of-pennies")

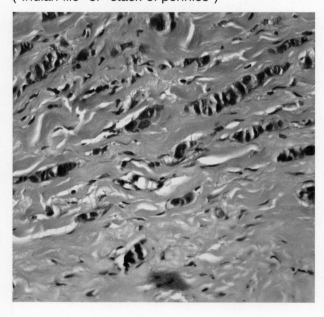

Markers for undifferentiated neoplasms

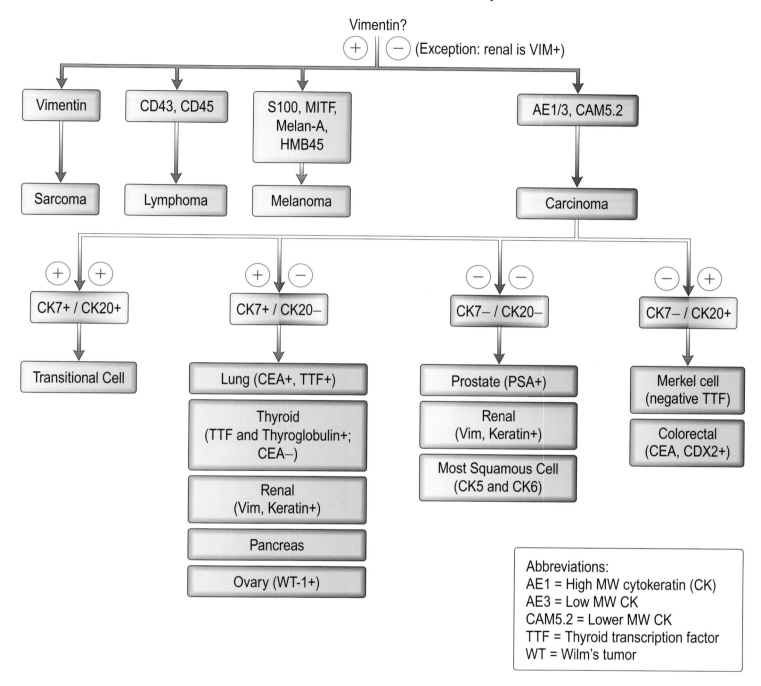

Precocious metastases = cutaneous metastases are the first indication of visceral cancer (especially kidney, lung, thyroid, ovary)

Metachronous metastases = cutaneous metastases develop months or years after primary cancer diagnosed (especially breast, kidney, and melanoma)

Synchronous metastases = primary tumor and cutaneous metastases diagnosed simultaneously (especially breast and oral cavity)

	Men	Women
Primary tumor frequency	1. Lung (24%) 2. Colon (19%) 3. Melanoma (13%) 4. Squamous cell, oral cavity (12%)	1. Breast (69%) 2. Colon (9%) 3. Melanoma (5%) 4. Ovary (4%)

Name	Common Metastasis Site	Histopathology
Specific metastases		
Breast [CK7, GCDFP-15, estrogen and progesterone receptors]	• Anterior chest wall (#1) and scalp 	• Lobular breast carcinoma = "Indian-file" pattern or "stack-of-pennies"(due to E-cadherins in cells) • Ductal breast carcinoma: poorly differentiated; possible "signet-ring" cells; attempt to form ducts (lack E-cadherins, so no "Indian-filing")

Name	Common Metastasis Site	Histopathology
Lung [CK7, CEA, TTF]	• Chest wall, abdomen; or in oat-cell, the back *Note:* Merkel cell similar, but TTF negative	• Most commonly squamous cell type (40%); adenocarcinoma (20%), or undifferentiated (40%)
Oral cavity squamous cell [CK 5, 6]	• Face or neck; also direct extension 	• Eosinophilic keratinization; keratinizing cells • SCC metastasizes to lymph node (below)

Name	Common Metastasis Site	Histopathology
Colorectal [CK20. CDX2, CEA]	• Abdominal wall or perineal region • May have Sister Mary Joseph nodule 	• Usually well-differentiated adenocarcinoma; columnar cells forming glands • "Goblet cells" or "signet-ring" (mucin vacuoles in cells pushing nuclei over to side) • "Dirty" mucin material in lumina of glands • Sister Mary Joseph nodule (photo below) is due to a primary tumor of adenocarcinoma of the stomach, large bowel, ovary, pancreas gall bladder, endometrium, or breast, metastasizing to the unbilicus

Name	Common Metastasis Site	Histopathology
Renal [Vimentin, keratin]	• Scalp/head; nephrectomy scars; external genitalia 	• Clear cells in clusters (cohesive cells); vascular with hemorrhages
Bladder [CK7, CK29, CK20]	• Rare occurrence • Upper extremities, trunk, penis • Usually multiple at a single site (zosteriform or herpetiform in distribution)	• Transitional cell carcinoma or anaplastic carcinomas which may show areas of squamous differentiation

Name	Common Metastasis Site	Histopathology
Prostate [PSA]	• Inguinal region • Firm, violaceous nodule	• Firm, violaceous nodules; usually adenocarcinoma
Ovary [CK7]	• Chest or abdomen • Usually multiple nodules at a single site • Usually late complication (poor prognosis)	• Well-differentiated adenocarcinoma; sometimes papillary configuration with psammoma bodies • [CK20 negative, except mucinous variant may be CK20 positive]
Thyroid [CK 7, TTF]	• Scalp	• Cuboidal epithelium around eosinophilic material (follicles); multiple, well-circumscribed clusters; psammoma bodies
Carcinoid tumor [Neuron-specific enolase]	• Trunk • Multiple nodules	• Solid islands and nests of uniform cells; thin collagenous septa extend between the tumor nests • [Negative staining for CK5/6, CK7, CK20, p63]

Name	Common Metastasis Site	Histopathology
Neuroblastoma [Neuron-specific enolase]	• Most common tumor of childhood • Adrenal origin • Neonate variant more commonly has cutaneous metastases • Cutaneous, blanching nodule • May resemble "blueberry muffin baby" in a neonate	• Small cells with hyperchromatic nuclei and rosette formation
Melanoma [S100, MITF, melan-A, HMB45]	• Skin, subcutaneous tissue (develop nodules in regional lymph nodes) 	• Invasion of cells between collagen bundles in reticular dermis; inflammatory infiltrate

Name	Common Metastasis Site	Histopathology
Oncocytoma	• Rare skin involvement • Most common benign kidney tumor • May develop in salivary gland and thyroid gland	• Tumor of oncocytes (eosinophilic, large cells with round nuclei)
Osteosarcoma	• Extremities, scalp (primary skin possible) • More commonly to lungs, bones; kidneys	• Non-mineralized bone (pink material) surrounds osteocytes • Lacunar cells (osteocytes) = cells surrounded by white halo

Cutaneous Non-lymphoid Infiltrates

40

Wells' syndrome flame figures

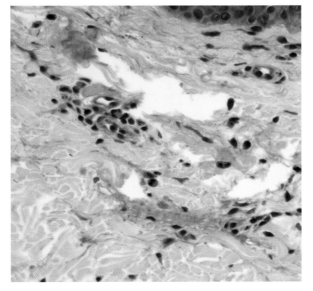

Note: flame figures may be seen in other disorders with eosinophils (i.e. arthropod bites, parasitic infections, BP, internal cancers)

Name	Predilection and Clinical Key Features	Histopathology
Neutrophil infiltrates		
<td colspan="3"><ul><li>Bone marrow origin:<ul><li>Maturation of 7–10 days</li><li>Functional in tissue for 1–2 days</li></ul></li><li>Primary function is phagocytosis and release of various enzymes stored in cytoplasmic granules</li><li>Two to five distinct nuclear lobes and cytoplasm contains two distinct types of granules:<ul><li>Larger granules = azurophilic and contain myeloperoxidase, bactericidal substances, elastase</li><li>Smaller granules = contain lactoferrin, lysozyme, collagenase, alkaline phosphatase</li></ul></li></ul></td>		

Epidermal neutrophilic infiltrates	• Conditions such as:
	  • Impetigo and toxic shock syndrome
	  • Orf
	  • Pustular psoriasis and acute generalized pustulosis
	  • Glucagonoma
	  • Verruciform xanthoma	

Dermal neutrophilic infiltrates	Conditions such as:
	• Infections and infestations:
	  • ecthyma
	  • chancroid and granuloma inguinale
	  • actinomycosis and mycetoma
	• Neutrophilic dermatoses:
	  • Sweet's syndrome
	  • bowel-associated dermatosis–arthritis syndrome
	• Acute generalized pustulosis:
	  • Behçet's syndrome
	  • pyoderma gangrenosum
	• Subepidermal blistering diseases:
	  • dermatitis herpetiformis
	  • cicatricial pemphigoid
	• Folliculitides:
	  • bacterial and fungal folliculitis
	  • secondary syphilis
	• Miscellaneous conditions:
	  • neutrophilic urticaria
	  • polymorphic light eruption	

Subcutaneous neutrophilic infiltrates	• Conditions such as:
	  • Infective panniculitis
	  • α1-Antitrypsin deficiency	

Name	Predilection and Clinical Key Features	Histopathology
Eosinophil infiltrates		
• Bone marrow origin • Contain major basic protein (cause histamine release from basophils) and other granules which are potent toxins (especially to parasites coated with IgE) • Stimulated by IL-5, GM-CSF, and IL-3		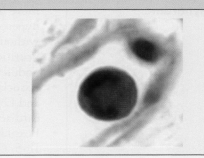
Wells' syndrome	• "Eosinophilic cellulitis" • Any age • Extremities and trunk 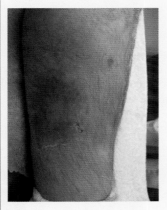 • "Cellulitis-like" • Edematous infiltrated plaques, often blisters/bullae; deep urticaria; followed by development of slate-gray morphea-like induration which resolves (4–8 weeks) • Usually idiopathic, but may be associated with arthropod bite, parasite, drug, tetanus vaccine	• Granular eosinophilic material produces "flame figures" (partly surrounded by palisading histiocytes and maybe giant cells); dermal edema, numerous eosinophils 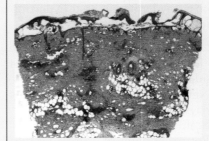 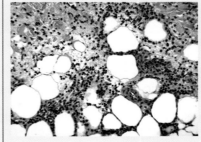 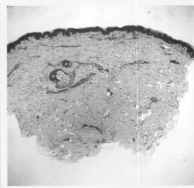 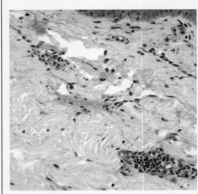 • Flame figure due to eosinophil granule major basic protein encrusting on collagen (non-specific sign and flame figures seen in other conditions, such as arthropod bites, parasitic infections, BP, internal cancers)

Name	Predilection and Clinical Key Features	Histopathology
Hypereosinophilic syndrome	• Idiopathic systemic disorder of one or more organs and persistent hypereosinophilia ($>1.5 \times 10^9$/I) without an identifiable cause • Pruritic erythematous papules/nodules; mucosal ulcerations • Associated with eosinophilic leukemia and Löffler's syndrome; possible cardiac involvement • Possibly due to dysregulation of IL-3, IL-5, GM-CSF	• Perivascular eosinophils; dermal edema
Pachydermatous eosinophilic dermatitis	• Possible variant of hypereosinophilic syndrome • Generalized pruritic papular eruption on pachydermatous base, hypertrophic lesions in the genital area and peripheral blood eosinophilia	• Eosinophil-rich lymphohistiocytic infiltrate and variable dermal fibrosis
Eosinophilic pustulosis	• "Eosinophilic pustular folliculitis of infancy" • Newborn infants (birth to first few days) • Scalp and face • Recurrent crops of pruritic pustules	• Heavy dermal infiltrate of lymphocytes, neutrophils, and numerous eosinophils around follicles and interstitium; no primary folliculitis

Plasma cell infiltrates

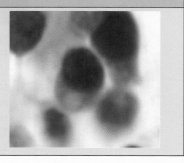

- Derived from stimulated B lymphocytes
- Life span of 2–3 days
- Produce and secrete antibodies for a specific antigen
- Appear basophilic with an eccentric-located nucleus and have coarse chromatin granules in the cytoplasm
- Russell bodies = round, eosinophilic, intracytoplasmic inclusions (accumulation of immunoglobulins/glycoproteins) that may displace the nucleus

Name	Predilection and Clinical Key Features	Histopathology
Plasmacytoma [Plasma cell Ab PC-1, CD79a, methyl green pyronin (stains plasma cell cytoplasm red)]	• May be primary cutaneous variant or secondary plasmacytoma • Rare monoclonal proliferations of plasma cells usually associated with multiple myeloma, extramedullary plasmacytoma, or plasma cell leukemia • Trunk • Dusky red or violaceous dome-shaped nodules (1–5 cm)	• Circumscribed, non-encapsulated dense infiltrate of plasma cells in reticular dermis; Russell bodies (pink globules that displace plasma cell's nucleus); stretched epidermis

Name	Predilection and Clinical Key Features	Histopathology

Cutaneous disorders associated with paraproteinemias	*Includes conditions such as:*
	• Necrobiotic xanthogranuloma
	• POEMS syndrome:
	  • polyneuropathy, organomegaly, endocrinopathy, M-protein, and skin lesions
	  • associated with glomeruloid hemangiomas (see Ch. 38, Vascular Tumors)
	• Schnitzler's syndrome:
	  • Chronic urticaria associated with macroglobulinemia	

Waldenström's macroglobulinemia [IgM]	• Lymphoproliferative disorder (IgM-producing lymphoplasmacytoid cells) • Elderly • Face, trunk, or proximal extremities; also weight loss, weakness, anemia (bleeding) • Translucent papules and violaceous plaques/nodules (blood hyperviscosity and bleeding tendency)	• Eosinophilic hyaline deposits filling dermis; artificial clefts
Zoon's balanitis	• "Plasmacytosis mucosae" • Glans penis of elderly = "Zoon's balanitis" (vulva = Zoon's vulvitis) • Solitary, asymptomatic, sharply defined red–brown glistening patch (1–3 cm) • Possible Tx = circumcision, topical steroids, and other topical regimens	• Dense, band-like infiltrate of inflammatory cells in upper dermis, mostly polyclonal plasma cells; blood vessels prominent; ulceration

Name	Predilection and Clinical Key Features	Histopathology
Castleman's disease	• "Giant lymph node hyperplasia" • Lymph node disease • Mediastinum of young to middle-aged person • Non-specific (xanthomas and vasculitis) • Associated with IL-6 and HHV-8	• "Onion-skin" appearance by a mantle of lymphocytes and transversed by hyalinized capillary-sized vessels; circumscribed nodule

Mastocytosis/mast cell infiltrates

• Derived from bone marrow stem cells
• Release histamine, leukotrienes, prostaglandin D_2, and mast cell growth factor (stimulates melanocytes and causes pigmentation)
• Mutation = c-kit proto-oncogene (CD117), encodes KIT (tyrosine kinase and receptor for mast cell growth factor)
• Labs = tryptase serum level; urinary histamine, urinary *N*-methylhistamine (NMH), urinary *N*-methylimidazoleacetic acid levels
• Stains = tryptase, CD117 (c-kit receptor), Giemsa stain (grains stain metachromatic), toluidine blue

Name	Predilection and Clinical Key Features	Histopathology
Urticaria pigmentosa (UP)	• Most common cutaneous variant of mastocytosis (80%) • Onset first 4 years of life (75% cases) • Trunk area • Generalized eruption of multiple red–brown macules • Darier's sign (wheal and flare when rubbed) • Adult-onset disease is associated with persistence of lesions and development of systemic disease (40%)	• Upper one-third of dermis involved with variable number of mast cells; eosinophils; no epidermotropism (as in histiocytosis); basal hyperpigmentation • Mast cells do not enter epidermis (above) • Giemsa stain (above)

Name	Predilection and Clinical Key Features	Histopathology
Solitary mastocytoma	• 10% of childhood cutaneous mastocytosis • Childhood • Trunk and wrists • Small solitary red nodule; involutes spontaneously • "Mast cell nevi" = smaller lesions • "Mastocytoma" = lesions >3 cm • May be associated with extralesional symptoms including pruritus, flushing, headaches	• Dense aggregate of mast cells in the dermis; similar to UP histology

Name	Predilection and Clinical Key Features	Histopathology
Diffuse cutaneous mastocytosis	• Rare cutaneous variant of mastocytosis • Early infancy • Thickening of skin; pruritus and blistering common • Systemic involvement common	• Similar histology as other mastocytosis • May have loosely arranged mast cells throughout the dermis; fibrosis may be present
Telangiectasia macularis eruptiva perstans (TMEP)	• Adult form with high systemic involvement • Trunk, proximal extremities • Erythema and telangiectasia in faintly pigmented, tan-brown macules, usually without Darier's sign • Rare association with multiple myeloma • Dermoscopy image (above)	• Mast cells with increased telangiectasias; increase in mast cell number may be subtle: mast cells tend to be fusiform and loosely arranged around dilated vessels of the superficial plexus
Systemic mastocytosis	• Proliferations of mast cells in various tissues besides the skin; bone marrow is most common (then liver, spleen, GI, lymph nodes); may progress to malignant mastocytosis [anti-tryptase antibody G3] or mast cell leukemia	

Name	Predilection and Clinical Key Features	Histopathology

Brachioradial pruritus	• Tropical dermatosis
	• Caucasians living in tropical climates
	• Chronic intermittent intense pruritus on elbows by brachioradialis muscle
	  • Often accompanied by burning sensation, worsens toward evening
	  • Application of ice pack provides relief	

Histiocytic infiltrates (non-Langerhans cell)

(No Birbeck granules present)

Name	Predilection and Clinical Key Features	Histopathology
Juvenile xanthogranuloma (JXG) [CD68, factor XIIIa, HAM-56, HHF35; negative Mac387, S100 and CD1a]	• Most common histiocytosis • 6–9 months old (two-thirds of cases) • Male • Head and neck, upper trunk, proximal limbs • Unknown cause 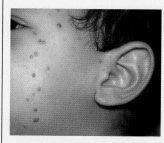 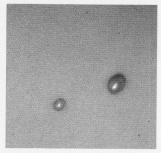 • Solitary, dome-shaped, red–brown papules/nodules (1–10 mm+); spontaneously involute • Also often have café-au-lait macules, possible blindness with ocular lesions (eyes are most common extracutaneous involvement) • Most common cause in children of spontaneous hyphema (blood in anterior chamber of eye) • Associated with neurofibromatosis type I and CML • If JXG and NF-1 present, then 20-fold increased risk of juvenile myelomonocytic leukemia (JMML)	• Nodular, poorly demarcated dense infiltrate of small foamy histiocytes in dermis; plump cells; giant Touton cells; eosinophils 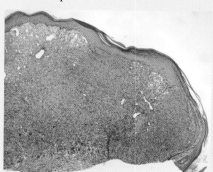 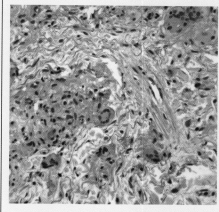 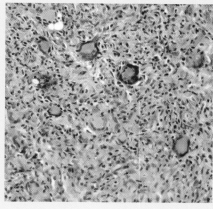

Name	Predilection and Clinical Key Features	Histopathology
Adult xanthogranuloma [CD68, factor XIIIa, HAM-56, HHF35]	• Adolescence to adults • Similar to JXG, but does not occur in first 6–9 months of age • Spontaneously resolves in months to years • Red-brown nodule • Dermoscopy image (above)	• Similar to JXG (see p. 735)

Name	Predilection and Clinical Key Features	Histopathology
Benign cephalic histiocytosis [CD68, factor XIIIa, CD11b, HAM-56; negative CD1a, S100]	• Non-lipid, non-X histiocytic proliferation • Infants <1 year old • Head and neck • Asymptomatic red–brown maculopapule (2–5 mm+); self-limited; may resolve into atrophic pigmented macules	• Diffuse infiltrate histiocytes in upper dermis; oval vesicular nucleus; no cytoplasmic lipid or Touton cells (as seen in JXG) • EM = "comma-shaped" bodies with no Birbeck granules

Name	Predilection and Clinical Key Features	Histopathology
Progressive nodular histiocytosis [Factor XIIIa, CD68, HAM-56; negative S100, CD1a]	• Skin, mucous membranes • Multiple yellowish-brown papules (dermatofibroma-like)	• Histiocytes, foam cells, spindle-shaped cells, delicate matrix; usually no inflammatory cells such as eosinophils/plasma cells
Xanthoma disseminatum [Factor XIIIa, CD68, CD11b; negative S100, CD1a]	• All ages • Normolipemic patients • Flexural areas, proximal extremities, trunk • Cutaneous and mucosal xanthomas + diabetes insipidus • Red–brown papule/nodule then yellow color; mucous membrane lesions; rarely, bone lesions (which are common in Langerhans cell histiocytosis) • Mucous involvement and diabetes insipidus help differentiate from JXG	• Similar to JXG histologically (see p. 735) • Histiocytes, foam cells, spindle-shaped cells, Touton cells, inflammatory cells (differs from papular xanthoma); may have intercellular accumulation of iron (siderosis) • EM = no Birbeck granules present

Sea-blue histiocyte syndrome
 	
[Giemsa, CD68]
	• Inherited systemic histiocytosis characterized by histiocytes with deep blue azure granules in the cytoplasm on Giemsa, toluidine blue and May–Gruenwald staining:
	  • Secondary forms associated with storage disease, such as Niemann–Pick disease (type B)
	  • Possibly due to partial deficiency of sphingomyelinase
	• Cutaneous lesions rare: nodular lesions and brown pigmented macules on the face	

Generalized eruptive histiocytoma [Factor XIIIa, CD68, CD11b; Negative S100, CD1a]	• Adults > children • Symmetric on trunk, extensors of extremities • Recurrent crops of hundreds of small red papules (symmetric) • Resolves spontaneously, often with hyperpigmentation	• Histiocyte-like cells in upper/mid-dermis; nests around blood vessels; pale cytoplasm and oval nucleus • No Touton cells (as seen in JXG) • EM = no Birbeck granules; may see "comma-shaped" bodies
Progressive mucinous histiocytosis	• Autosomal dominant • Face and extremities • Eruption of red–brown papules	• Dermal infiltrate of epithelioid and spindle-shaped histiocytes; numerous mast cells • EM = zebra and myeloid bodies in cytoplasm

Name	Predilection and Clinical Key Features	Histopathology
Multicentric reticulohistio-cytosis [CD68, CD11b, CD45, HAM-56; Negative S100, Mac387]	• Interphalangeal joints of hand, face, mucosa (oral, nasal, and pharyngeal) 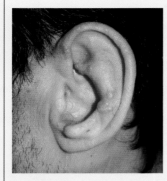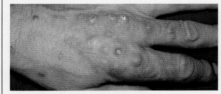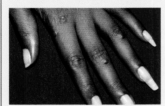 • Extensive papulonodular eruptions; destructive arthropathy • Systemic lesions (cardiac, bone marrow, etc.) • Possibly associated with solid organ malignancies, positive tuberculin skin test, autoimmune disease	• Circumscribed, non-encapsulated dermal and synovial infiltrate of multinucleate histiocytes with eosinophilic "ground-glass" cytoplasm 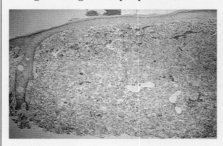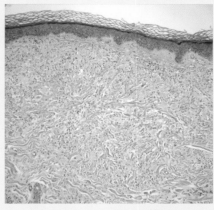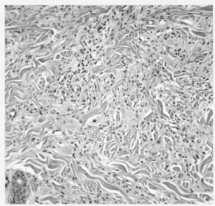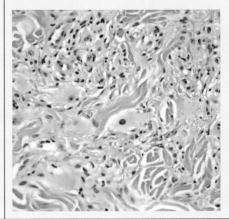

Name	Predilection and Clinical Key Features	Histopathology
Reticulohistio-cytoma [CD68, CD11b, HAM-56]	• "Solitary reticulohistiocytoma" • Similar to multicentric reticulohistiocytosis, but solitary and no arthritis or systemic lesions • Adults • Head and neck • Yellow–red nodule, which often resolves • May have mucous membrane lesions	• Similar to multicentric reticulohistiocytosis with histiocytes with "ground glass" cytoplasm
Familial histiocytic dermatoarthritis	• Child/adolescence • Face and limbs • Papulonodular eruption on face/limbs; symmetric destructive arthritis; ocular lesions	• Dermal mononuclear histiocytes with lymphocytes and plasma cells

Name	Predilection and Clinical Key Features	Histopathology
Necrobiotic xanthogranuloma (NXG) [CD68, Mac387]	<ul><li>Elderly (often in 60s)</li><li>Periorbital area, face, trunk, limbs</li></ul> 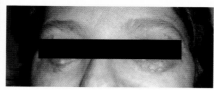 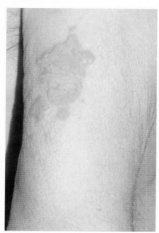 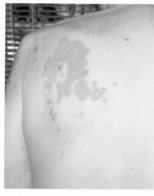 <ul><li>Multiple sharply demarcated, violaceous-to-red nodules/papules with a partly xanthomatous hue</li><li>Associated with paraproteinemia (IgG); ophthalmic complications (scleritis, keratitis); plasma cell dyscrasias</li></ul>	<ul><li>Zones of hyaline necrobiosis and granulomatous foci composed of histiocytes, foam cells, and lots of multinucleate giant cells with lots of nuclei</li><li>(Touton and foreign-body types); cholesterol clefts</li></ul> 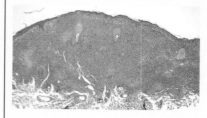 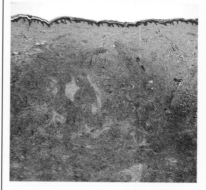 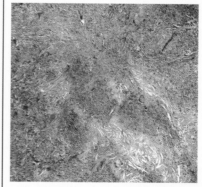 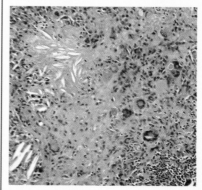 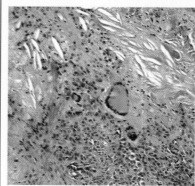

Name	Predilection and Clinical Key Features	Histopathology
Indeterminate cell histiocytosis [CD1a, S100, CD68]	• Self-limiting condition • All ages • Multiple red–brown to yellowish papules • Clinically, similar to generalized eruptive histiocytoma (See p. 738)	• Monomorphous infiltrate of mononuclear histiocytes intermingled with clusters of lymphocytes (but stain like both Langerhans and non-Langerhans cell histiocytosis) • Contains dentritic cells found in the dermis, which are similar to Langerhans cell that express S100 and CD1a; but this condition lacks Birbeck granules on EM and is positive for histiocytic markers such as CD68

Name	Predilection and Clinical Key Features	Histopathology
Rosai–Dorfman disease [S100; negative CD1a]	• "Sinus histiocytosis with massive lymphadenopathy" • Eyelids and malar region • First two decades • Cutaneous lesions vary; usually multiple nodules up to 4 cm or more; erythematous or xanthomatous papules; pustules, pigmented macules, plaques • Classic presentation: painless cervical lymphadenopathy, fever, anemia, elevated ESR and hypergammaglobulinemia (IgG)	• Dense dermal infiltrate of large histiocytes with abundant, eosinophilic cytoplasm and vesicular nuclei; possible septal and lobular panniculitis; emperipolesis (phagocytosis of inflammatory cells) • Emperipolesis = inflammatory cells inside macrophages (pictures above)

Name	Predilection and Clinical Key Features	Histopathology
Reactive histiocytosis	• Associated with cutaneous infection (histoplasmosis, toxoplasmosis, brucellosis, TB, leprosy, rubella, EBV)	

Xanthomatous infiltrates

Lipid metabolism	**Hyperlipoproteinemias**

• Triglyceride (TG) core = high in chylomicrons and VLDL
• Cholesterol ester core = high in LDL and HDL
• Lipoprotein lipase (liver) = mediates hydrolysis of VLDL with ApoC-II
• Apoprotein B-100 (VLDL, IDL, LDL) = major protein of LDL
• Apoprotein C-II (Chylo, VLDL, IDL, HDL) = activates lipoprotein lipase
• Apoprotein E (remnants, VLDL, IDL, HDL) = binds to LDL receptor
• HMG Co A reductase (liver) = rate-limiting cholesterol synthesis enzyme
	(Autosomal dominant except type I and III are recessive)
	• Type I (familial) = lipoprotein lipase deficiency:
	  • elevated chylomicrons, TG; but normal cholesterol
	  • no increased risk for coronary artery disease
	• Type II (hypercholesterolemia) = LDL receptor defect:
	  • increased LDL and cholesterol
	• Type III (dysbetalipoproteinemia) = apoprotein E defect (poor clearance):
	  • increased cholesterol and TG
	• Type IV (hypertriglyceridemia) = elevated VLD, TG; glucose intolerance
	• Type V = elevated chylomicrons, VLDL, and TG

| **Eruptive xanthoma** [CD68+] | • Seen in type I, IV, and V hyperlipoproteinemias
• Buttocks, thighs, extensor surfaces
• Multiple, small red–yellow papules (crops); erythematous halo; spontaneously resolve (weeks)
• Associated with elevated plasma chylomicrons (i.e. diabetes, alcohol, exogenous estrogens) | • "Foamy cells" with an inflammatory infiltrate in the upper dermis; lipid deposits in form of lace-like eosinophilic material between collagen bundles ("leaks" out)

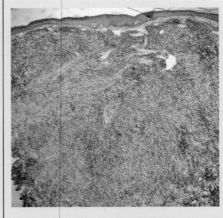
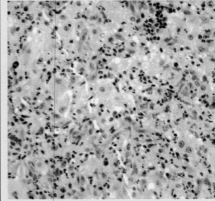 |

Name	Predilection and Clinical Key Features	Histopathology
Tuberous xanthoma	• Most characteristic of type III hyperlipoproteinemia (familial hyperlipoproteinemia); • Also seen with hepatic cholestasis, β-sitosterolemia • Elbows, knees, and buttocks • Yellowish nodules • Resolve with treatment of underlying hyperlipidemia • Elevated cholesterol and triglycerides	• Large aggregates of foam cells in dermis; fibroblasts; cholesterol clefts
Tendinous xanthoma	• Seen usually in type II hyperlipoproteinemias; may be due to cerebrotendinous xanthoma (CYP27A1 gene, metabolism of plant sterol); hepatic cholestasis • Extensor tendons of hands, feet, Achilles tendon • Firm to hard, flesh-colored nodule • Elevated LDL level (often due to LDL receptor defect)	• Tendinous xanthoma is similar to tuberous xanthomas (foam cells in dermis; fibroblasts; cholesterol clefts), except for tissue substrate

Name	Predilection and Clinical Key Features	Histopathology

Planar xanthoma	• Varies in location
	• May have normal lipid metabolism
	
	Variants of planar xanthoma:
	1. Xanthelasma:
	  • only 50% of patients have hyperlipidemia
	  • seen in type II and III
	  • eyelids, periorbital area
	  • yellow, soft macule or papule
	
	2. Intertriginous plane xanthoma:
	  • antecubital fossa, web spaces of fingers
	  • pathognomonic for type II (homozygous familial hypercholesterolemia)
	3. Xanthoma striatum palmaris:
	  • diagnostic for type III (dysbetalipoproteinemia)
	  • lesions present on palms and volar surface of fingers
	4. Diffuse plane xanthomas:
	  • adults
	  • trunk and neck
	  • macular, yellowish discoloration of the skin
	  • often associated with lymphoreticular neoplasms (i.e. multiple myeloma and adult T-cell lymphoma/leukemia)
		• Small aggregates of foam cells around vessels and hair follicles; no fibrosis or inflammatory cells)
		
		• Plane xanthoma (pictured above)
		
		• Xanthelasma (pictured above)

Name	Predilection and Clinical Key Features	Histopathology
Verruciform xanthoma [CD68, weakly positive for keratin and Factor XIIIa; negative S100]	• Normal lipid levels • Oral cavity, genitals • Solitary, asymptomatic, flat, pink–yellow plaques/warty lesions • May be seen in lymphedema, epidermolysis bullosa, GVHD, CHILD syndrome, etc.	• Verruca-like configuration; hyperkeratosis, focal parakeratosis and verrucous acanthosis; dermis filled with xanthoma cells • CD68 stain (below)
Papular xanthoma	• Any age • Face, trunk, mucous membranes • Multiple discrete yellow–red papules	• Infiltrate of foam cells in dermis, Touton giant cells; hemosiderin • Few to zero inflammatory cells (which differs from xanthoma disseminatum, eruptive xanthoma, and JXG)

Name	Predilection and Clinical Key Features	Histopathology
Langerhans cell infiltrates		

- Langerhans cells:
  - Bone marrow origin, type of dendritic cells that trap and process antigens for presenting to lymphocytes
  - Contain Birbeck granules ("tennis-racquet-shaped" organelles)
  - Stain with CD1a, S100, CD45, CD101, HLA-DR, and Lag (marker on Birbeck granule membranes)
  - High density areas of Langerhans cells = face, trunk; low density of Langerhans = palm/sole, anogenital, chronic UV, age

Name	Predilection and Clinical Key Features	Histopathology

Langerhans cell histiocytosis (LCH)
 	
[CD1a, HLA-DR, S100; negative CD68 and Mac387]
	• Children (age 1–3 years); boys.
	• Possible viral and immunologic etiology
	
	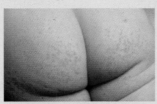
	
	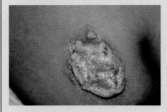
	
	• Crusted, scaly papules/vesicles or ulcerative lesion
	• Proliferation affects skin, bone, lung, liver, lymph nodes (may affect organ function)
	• Associated with increased risk of malignancy (especially solid tumors and leukemia)
	• Serum S100-B level to monitor disease progress
	
	Old subtypes not used anymore (see below):
	• Letterer–Siwe disease:
	  • prior age 2
	  • scalp, face, trunk, buttocks
	  • yellow–brown scaly papules or vesicles
	  • also see fever, anemia, lymphadenopathy, osteolytic lesions
	• Hand–Schüller–Christian disease:
	  • age 2–6
	  • triad = osteolytic bone lesions, diabetes insipidus (posterior pituitary infiltration), and exophthalmos
	• Eosinophilic granuloma:
	  • localized variant with bone lesions
	  • cutaneous noduloulcerative lesion in the mouth, genital, retroauricular regions
		• Large ovoid cells with indented or reniform ("coffee-bean") nucleus and abundant cytoplasm, often just below epidermis; various inflammatory cells; epidermotropism also seen (which differs from mastocytosis)
		• EM = Birbeck granules ("tennis racquet") within cell
		
		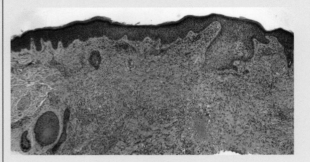
		
		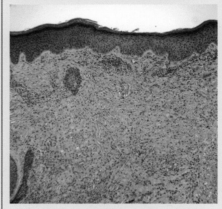
		
		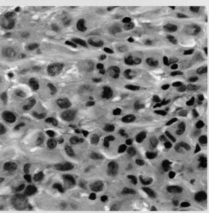

Name	Predilection and Clinical Key Features	Histopathology
Congenital self-healing reticulohistio-cytosis	• "Hashimoto–Pritzker disease" • Self-limited form of Langerhans cell histiocytosis • Present at birth (lasts weeks to 3 months) • Skin involvement only • Rapid healing of crusted papules/nodules; usually leave hyperpigmentation • R/O systemic involvement (liver, CBC, skeletal)	• Same histology as LCH

41 Cutaneous Lymphomatous and Leukemic Infiltrates

Differentiating Primary Cutaneous B-cell Lymphomas

(*Note:* lymphomas below are typically positive for CD20 and CD79a)

	Follicle Center Lymphoma	Marginal Zone B-cell Lymphoma	Diffuse Large B-cell Lymphoma, Leg Type	Diffuse Large B-Cell Lymphoma, Other
Positive antibody markers	CD10 and bcl-6 • Remember 10 letters in "follicular"	bcl-2	bcl-2	Depends on type (intravascular, plasmablastic, etc.)
Negative antibody markers	CD5, CD23	CD10, bcl-6, CD-5, CD23, cyclin D1 (bcl-1)	CD5, cyclin D1 (bcl-1)	bcl-2

Note:
- Cyclin D1 (bcl-1) positive in mantle cell lymphoma
- CD-5 and CD-23 positive in CLL/SLL: CD-5 is a normal T-cell marker, but is aberrantly expressed in mature B-cell lymphomas
    - Remember: there are 5 letters in "s-m-a-l-l" for CD-5 positive CLL/SLL

Tumor	Predilection and Clinical Key Features	Histopathology
Cutaneous T-cell and NK-cell lymphomas		

Mycosis fungoides (MF)	• 50% of all primary cutaneous lymphomas
	• Neoplasm of skin-homing T-cells
	• Typically, CD4 T-cells; exception is hypopigmented MF (CD8+)
	• Stains = positive CD3, CD4, CD45RO
	• Usually negative CD7 and CD30
	• Three clinical stages (see below):
	  1. Patch stage
	  2. Plaque stage
	  3. Tumor stage
	
	• *Note:* MF-like picture possible with drugs, such as captopril, carbamezepine, fluoxetine, phenytoin
	• Staging (and common treatments):
	  • Stage IA and IB = patch or plaque clinically:
	    • stage IA < 10% BSA
	    • stage IB > 10% BSA
	    • Possible Tx = topical steroid, PUVA
	  • Stage II = tumors and/or positive lymph nodes:
	    • Possible Tx = electron beam, PUVA, radiotherapy
	  • Stage III = erythrodermic:
	    • Possible Tx = plasmaphoresis, IFN-α
	  • Stage IV = nodal, visceral involvement:
	    • Possible Tx = CHOP chemotherapy, IL-12, denileukin	

Patch stage MF	• Hips, buttocks ("doubly-protected" areas from sunlight) • Eczematous ill-defined patches, often with a fine scale	• Epidermotropism of atypical lymphoctyes; often lichenoid or diffuse infiltrate • Pautrier microabscesses (intraepidermal nests of atypical cells) • "String of beads" along BMZ; clear halo around cells; uncommon microabscesses
Plaque stage MF	• Lower part trunk, thighs • Red to violaceous well-demarcated plaques, often with scale; often in annular or arciform arrangement	• 50% have Pautrier microabscesses • Prominent convoluted, indented nuclei

Tumor	Predilection and Clinical Key Features	Histopathology

Tumor stage MF	• Usually develops in pre-existing lesions
	
	• Violaceous to deep red lesions with a tense shiny surface (usually 1 cm or more in diameter)
	• May transform to CD30+ large cell lymphoma:
	  • occurs when >25% of cells are CD30+
	  • poor prognosis
		• Uncommon epidermotropism and Pautrier microabscesses; deep dermal and subcutaneous nodules of atypical cells

Tumor	Predilection and Clinical Key Features	Histopathology
Hypopigmented MF [CD3, CD4]	• Adults with darker skin type • Trunk and extremities • Hypopigmented scaly patches	• Similar to MF with exocytosis of lymphocytes, reduction in basal layer melanin and possible melanin incontinence • CD4 stain positive (above)
Folliculotropic MF [CD3, CD4; negative CD8]	• Variant of MF with neoplastic T-cell infiltrate; predominantly folliculocentric; epidermal involvement is absent/minimal • Adult males • Head and neck • Grouped folliculocentric papules; possible alopecia; pruritus common • Associated with lithium therapy • More resistant to therapies	• Follicular and perifollicular infiltrate of small to medium sized lymphocytes with or without follicular mucin; conspicuously cerebriform nuclei; possible mucin; does not involve the epidermis (or is minimal)

Tumor	Predilection and Clinical Key Features	Histopathology
Pagetoid reticulosis	• "Woringer–Kolopp disease" • Variant of MF • Adult males • Distal limbs • Large, solitary, slow-growing, erythematous, scaly or verrucous patch/plaque	• Epidermis is infiltrated by large atypical mononuclear cells with a pale eosinophilic cytoplasm, large nucleus, and prominent nucleolus; marked acanthosis with overlying hyperkeratosis and patchy parakeratosis

Tumor	Predilection and Clinical Key Features	Histopathology
Granulomatous slack skin	<ul><li>Elastolytic variant of MF (rare)</li><li>Axilla, groin</li><li>Drooping folds of skin (damaged elastic fibers)</li><li>One-third associated with Hodgkin's disease</li><li>Good prognosis</li></ul>	<ul><li>Granulomatous pattern with diffuse small T-cells (no epidermotropism); fragmented or absent elastic fibers [VVG stain]; psoriasiform hyperplasia; giant cells uniformly scattered in lymphocytic infiltrate</li></ul>
Sézary syndrome [CD3, CD4, CD45RO; negative CD8, CD30, often CD2, and CD7]	<ul><li>"Leukemic phase of MF"</li><li>Triad:<ol><li>Erythroderma</li><li>Lymphadenopathy</li><li>Circulating atypical mononuclear cells. Often keratoderma, intractable pruritus</li></ol></li></ul>	<ul><li>Lymph node (below)</li></ul> <ul><li>Sézary cells (below)</li></ul>

Tumor	Predilection and Clinical Key Features	Histopathology
Adult T-cell lymphoma/ leukemia (HTLV-1+) [CD3, CD4, CD25]	• Variant of peripheral T-cell lymphoma due to infection with human T-cell lymphotropic virus, type 1 (HTLV-1) • Japan and Caribbean • Skin lesions often the initial feature (50–70% cases) with erythematous patches, plaques; less common are erythroderma and vesiculobullous and purpuric eruptions • HTLV-1 transmitted sexually, via the blood, and by breastfeeding • Lifetime risk for lymphoma = 2–4%	• Similar to MF with epidermotropism and Pautrier microabscesses; but unlike MF, microabscesses may contain prominent apoptotic fragments; atypical lymphocytes, sometimes pleomorphic nuclei • *Note:* CD25+ differentiates ATLL from Sézary syndrome

Tumor	Predilection and Clinical Key Features	Histopathology

Anaplastic large cell lymphoma (ALCL)
 	
[CD30; negative CD15, unlike Hodgkin's]
	• Type of CD30+ T-cell lymphoproliferative disorder
	
	May be subdivided into:
	• Primary cutaneous:
	  • adult males
	  • most are ALK and EMA negative
	  • do not have a t(2:5) translocation
	• Primary systemic:
	  • males in 30s
	  • usually anaplastic lymphoma kinase [ALK+] and EMA positive
	  • have a t(2:5) translocation
	• Secondary types:
	  • arise in other lymphoproliferative disorders
		• "Hallmark cells" = large lymphoid cells with chromatin-poor, horseshoe-shaped or embryo-shaped nuclei, eosinophilic nucleoli, pale paranuclear hof, abundant cytoplasm; multinucleate cells (similar to Reed–Sternberg cells) may be seen

Tumor	Predilection and Clinical Key Features	Histopathology

Lymphomatoid papulosis (LyP)
[CD30, CD3, CD4]
	• Type of CD30+ disorder
	• Benign (90%)
	• Females in 30s–40s
	
	• Crops of papules or nodules that spontaneously regress
	• Associated with lymphoma, especially mycosis fungoides (40%), CD30+ T-cell lymphoma (30%), or Hodgkin's disease (25%)
		Variants:
		
		1. *Type A = most common variant of LyP:*
		  • Large CD30+ cells with at least one prominent nucleolus (may resemble Reed–Sternberg cells)
		  • "Bug-bite-like with large, atypical cells"
		  • Wedge-shaped, patchy and perivascular infiltrate of benign-appearing lymphocytes; extravasated RBCs in epidermis and dermis
		  • Epidermal necrosis; epidermotropism; possible vasculitis
		  • Associated with lymphoma
		
		2. *Type B (10% of patients):*
		  • Small atypical, cerebriform cells (rare CD30+ cells)
		  • Perivascular or band-like dermal infiltrate; epidermotropism common
		  • Associated with lymphoma (less than type A patients)
		
		3. *Type C (diffuse large cell):* sheets of large, anaplastic CD30+ cells; overlaps with primary cutaneous anaplastic large cell lymphoma

Tumor	Predilection and Clinical Key Features	Histopathology
Subcutaneous panniculitis-like T-cell lymphoma	• Aβ T-cell phenotype (CD8+ T-cells) • Legs • Single or multiple nodules • May be associated with systemic symptoms (fever, hemophagocytic syndrome) • See p. 357 also	• Lobular panniculitis-like histology; atypical lymphocytes rim adipocytes to form a lace-like pattern; phagocytic histiocytes ("bean-bag histiocytes") containing cell debris or RBCs
Extranodal NK-/T-cell lymphoma, nasal type [CD56, CD2]	• "Lethal midline granuloma" • Asia, South and central America • Nasal area • Associated with EBV • Nasal mass, often results in destruction of midline facial area; ulcerations	• Diffuse or angiocentric and periappendageal infiltrate; massive zonal necrosis, karyorrhexis

Tumor	Predilection and Clinical Key Features	Histopathology
B-cell lymphomas		
Primary cutaneous marginal zone B-cell lymphoma	• "Extranodal marginal zone lymphoma of MALT type" • Adult males • Arms and trunk • Red to purple, solitary, or multiple nodules	• "Top-heavy" or "bottom-heavy" infiltrate; epidermis spared; small lymphocytes with indented nuclei predominate; follicular centralized orientation; Dutcher bodies (PAS+ intranuclear inclusions) • Stain for bcl-2, CD20, CD79a (negative staining for CD5, CD10, CD23)
Primary cutaneous follicle center lymphoma	• "Follicular lymphoma" • Head and neck • Erythematous nodule; serum LDH level normal • *Note:* nodal lymphomas often show t(14,18) translocation, but not cutaneous follicular lymphomas (up to 40%)	• Normal epidermis; "bottom-heavy" infiltrate with varying size and shape; follicular architecture with small lymphocytes, histiocytes, and some eosinophils/plasma cells; germinal centers with poorly formed or absent mantle zones; can be graded 1–3 by centroblasts per high power field; also contain centrocytes (large, cleaved follicle center cells) • Stain for CD10 ("follicular" has 10 letters), bcl-6, CD20, MIB-1, CD79a (negative staining for CD5, CD23, bcl-2, and usually MUM1)

Tumor	Predilection and Clinical Key Features	Histopathology
Diffuse large B-cell lymphoma [bcl-2, CD20, CD79a; negative CD5, cyclin D1]	• Elderly women • Legs • Erythematous to red–brown nodules, rarely ulcerate • 5-year survival = approximately 50% • *Note:* primary cutaneous diffuse large B-cell lymphomas do not have t (14,18), but secondary cancer does contain the translocation	• Diffuse infiltrate; grenz zone • Contains large cells with nuclei twice the size of small lymphocytes and larger than macrophage nucleus

Tumor	Predilection and Clinical Key Features	Histopathology
Diffuse large B-cell lymphoma, leg type [bcl-2, MUM1]	<ul><li>Elderly</li><li>Legs</li><li>Rapidly growing erythematous tumor</li><li>5-year survival = 41% (poor prognosis)</li></ul>	<ul><li>Diffuse dermal infiltrate of large lymphocytes with features of centroblasts and immunoblasts; mitotic figures</li></ul>

Tumor	Predilection and Clinical Key Features	Histopathology
Diffuse large B-cell lymphoma, other		
Intravascular large B-cell lymphoma [CD20, CD79 inside vessels; negative CD3]	<ul><li>Rare form of systemic lymphoma</li><li>Characterized by an intravascular proliferation of large atypical lymphoid cells</li><li>Often present with multiple neurological defects; one-third have skin lesions (erythematous to blue plaques on extremities, trunk, face)</li><li>Likely due to tumor cells losing expression of CD29 (β1 integrin) and CD5 (ICAM-1) adhesion molecules, which are important in trafficking and transvascular migration</li></ul>	<ul><li>Blood vessels in dermis and subcutis partially or completely occluded with large atypical lymphoid cells; mitotic figures frequent; fibrin thrombi in vessels; upper dermis often spared</li></ul>

Tumor	Predilection and Clinical Key Features	Histopathology
Lymphomatoid granulomatosis (LG) [CD3, CD45RO, CD4]	• Variant of large B-cell lymphoma • Angiocentric T-cell-rich B-cell lymphoma • Middle age • Often involves lungs (death from respiratory failure) • 40–60% involve skin (especially trunk, lower extremities) • Often associated with Epstein–Barr virus • Common in immunodeficiency, such as HIV, post-organ transplant and Wiskott–Aldrich syndrome (X-linked; IgM deficiency, thrombocytopenia)	• Angiocentric polymorphous infiltrate in the dermis especially in perivascular, periappendageal, and perineural areas (sweat glands involved)
Precursor hematologic neoplasm		
Blastic plasmacytoid dendritic cell neoplasms [CD4, CD56]	• Adults (median age 67); males (2:1) • Localized or diffuse erythematous or bruise-like, red or purple patches, papules, nodules, or tumors • Skin involvement usually precedes a leukemic phase • Erythematous variant (pictures above)	• Infiltrate of uniform medium sized cells with little cytoplasm and nuclei with finely-dispersed cytoplasm and inconspicuous nucleoli; in the dermis and/or subcutis (resemble myeloblasts or lymphoblasts) • Epidermis is not involved and usually no necrosis, angio-invasion or inflammatory cells; "rimming" of adipocytes may be seen in subcutis if infiltrated • Initially defined by coexpression of CD4 and CD56, but can express CD123, TLC1, and BDCA-2

Tumor	Predilection and Clinical Key Features	Histopathology
Other T-/NK-cell lymphomas that may involve the skin		
Angioimmuno-blastic T-cell lymphoma (AITL) [CD2, CD3, CD45RO]	• Elderly • 50% of cases have rash • Non-specific generalized maculopapular rash or nodule	• Non-specific perivascular infiltrate of non-atypical lymphocytes with some vascular proliferation; proliferation of post-capillary venules often seen
Other B-cell lymphomas that may involve the skin		
Precursor B-lymphoblastic leukemia/ lymphoma [CD20, CD79a, CD99]	• Children to young adults • Head and neck • Erythematous or violaceous papule or nodules • LDH elevated	• Normal epidermis; "starry-sky" pattern; monomorphic, medium sized lymphoid cells with round or convoluted nuclei in dermis/subcutis and arranged in a "mosaic-stone" pattern

Tumor	Predilection and Clinical Key Features	Histopathology
Chronic lymphocytic leukemia/small lymphocytic lymphoma (B-CLL/SLL) [CD5+ ("small" has 5 letters), CD23+]	• Elderly • Localized or generalized erythematous papules or nodules • May transform to large cell lymphoma (Richter's syndrome), which is a poor prognosis	• Dermal infiltrate of monomorphous small lymphoctyes; possibly Dutcher bodies (pseudointranuclear inclusions), also in multiple myeloma
Mantle cell lymphoma [Cyclin D1+ (or bcl-1) is characteristic and CD20, CD5; negative CD23]	• Often skin disease secondary to nodal disease • Characteristic t(11:14) translocation	• Small to medium sized lymphoctyes with irregular or cleaved nuclei with dispersed chromatin and scant cytoplasm
Plasmacytoma	• See Chapter 40 for more information	
Other lymphomas		
Hodgkin's lymphoma [Reed–Sternberg cells are CD15, CD30+]	• Rarely involves skin • More commonly in lymph nodes, liver, spleen • Predicable nodal spread along consecutive areas, unlike non-Hodgkin's • Erythematous nodules or plaques • Non-specific manifestations (pruritus, herpes zoster, acquired ichthyosis)	• Normal epidermis with grenz zone; fibrosis; atypical Hodgkin's cells; Reed–Sternberg cells ("owl's eyes": binucleate cells that have prominent nucleoli with a halo)

Tumor	Predilection and Clinical Key Features	Histopathology
Cutaneous infiltrates of leukemias		
Leukemia cutis [CD43, CD45]	• Dissemination of leukemias to the skin • Associated with a poor prognosis • Solitary or multiple, violaceous or reddish-brown and hemorrhagic papules, nodules • In acute granulocytic leukemia, a granulocytic sarcoma or chloroma may form due to cutaneous involvement • A chloroma appears clinically as a green-colored tumor due to myeloperoxidase	• Perivascular and periappendageal infiltrate or confluent sheets of cells that involve the dermis and often the subcutis. Often basophilic cells with "Indian-file" pattern of cells (cohesive cells). Mitotic figures and apoptotic bodies often seen

Tumor	Predilection and Clinical Key Features	Histopathology
Lymphoid hyperplasias mimicking primary lymphoma		
Lymphoid hyperplasia simulating B-cell lymphoma	<ul><li>"Pseudolymphoma"</li><li>Females</li><li>Face (especially cheeks, earlobes), chest, upper extremities</li></ul><ul><li>Asymptomatic red–brown or violaceous papules; may be single, grouped, or widespread</li><li>Typically cause is unknown; possibly induced by arthropod bites, gold earrings, drugs (phenytoin, methotrexate), allergen injections, *Borrelia* infection (Europe)</li></ul>	<ul><li>Variably dense infiltrate; "top heavy" infiltrate > "bottom heavy"</li></ul><ul><li>Lymphoid centers with pale center area surrounded by dark area</li></ul>
Lymphomatoid drug reactions	<ul><li>Reaction that causes an atypical lymphoid infiltrate resembling mycosis fungoides</li><li>Regress after withdrawal of drug; but anticonvulsant reaction may persist >12 months</li><li>Associated with phenytoin sodium, carbamazepine, griseofulvin, atenolol, cyclosporine, ACE inhibitors, antihistamines</li></ul>	<ul><li>Band-like infiltrate resembling mycosis fungoides; contains atypical nuclei with cerebriform appearance; epidermotropism</li></ul>
Reactions resembling CD30+ lymphoproliferative disorders	<ul><li>Possible causes:<ul><li>Drugs (carbamazepine)</li><li>Viral infections (molluscum contagiosum, herpes simplex)</li><li>Arthropod bites</li></ul></li></ul>	

Tumor	Predilection and Clinical Key Features	Histopathology
Jessner's lymphocytic infiltrate	• Possible spectrum of lupus erythematosus or PMLE • Men • Face or neck • Asymptomatic, erythematous plaques • Average duration = 5 years	• Dense, superficial, and deep perivascular infiltrate of lymphocytes; small amount of mucin; epidermis normal without atrophy, basal vacuolar changes, or follicular plugs (unlike lupus) • DIF negative (unlike lupus)
Miscellaneous		
Extramedullary hematopoiesis [Immature myeloid cells are Leder stain +]	• Neonates that have multiple violaceous papulonodules ("blueberry muffin" baby) • Hematopoiesis occurs in: • Early embryos as a normal process • Neonates following intrauterine congenital infections (toxoplasmosis, rubella, CMV, Coxsackie virus) • Neonates with congenital hematological dyscrasias (hemolytic disease of newborn, "twin transfusion" syndrome) • Rarely, an adult complication of myelodysplastic and myeloproliferative disorders (CLL): most common association is myelofibrosis, particularly after a splenectomy	• Superficial and deep infiltrate with myeloid and erythroid components in various stages of maturation.

Index

A

Absidia spp., 463
acanthamebiasis, 491
Acanthamoeba spp., 491
acantholytic acanthoma, 212, 512
acantholytic dermatosis
  persistent, 214
  transient *see* Grover's disease
acantholytic dyskeratosis, 3, 211
  focal, 211
acantholytic solar keratosis, 104
acanthoma
  acantholytic, 212, 512
  clear cell, 62, 515
  epidermolytic, 211, 511
  large cell, 515
  pilar sheath, 572, 611
acanthosis, 5
  nigricans, 26, 387
acne conglobata, 307
acne fulminans, 300
acne inversa, 306
acne keloidalis, 305
acne necrotica, 301
acne necrotica miliaris, 301
acne vulgaris, 299
acquired brachial dyschromatosis, 227
acral angiofibroma, 618–19
acral erythema, 19
acral fibrokeratoma, 619
acral lentiginous melanoma, 556
acral persistent papular mucinosis, 268
Acremonium spp., 464
acro-osteolysis, 240
acroangiodermatitis, 710
acrochordon, 620
acrodermatitis chronica atrophicans, 249, 439
acrodermatitis enteropathica, 64, 374
acrogeria, 252
acrokeratoelastoidosis, 207, 262
acrokeratosis
  paraneoplastica, 86, 389
  verruciformis of Hopf, 4, 216
acromelanosis, 226
acrosyringeal nevus, 600
actinic cheilitis, 516
actinic folliculitis, 301
actinic granuloma of O'Brien, 156
actinic keratosis, 516
actinic lentigo, 29, 532
actinic prurigo, 401
actinic reticuloid, 402
actinic (solar) keratosis, 24
Actinomadura pelletieri, 459
Actinomyces israelii, 461
actinomycosis, 150, 461

acute febrile neutrophilic dermatosis *see* Sweet's
  syndrome
acute generalized exanthematous pustulosis, 68, 97
acute hemorrhagic edema of childhood, 171
acute intermittent porphyria, 378
acute superficial folliculitis, 301
Adams–Oliver syndrome, 246, 686
adenocarcinoma
  apocrine, 595
  ceruminous, 599
  digital papillary, 607
  Moll's glands, 599
adenoid cystic carcinoma, 597
adenoid squamous cell carcinoma, 522
adenolipoma, 652
adenoma
  apocrine, 591, 613, 614
  ceruminous, 599
  papillary eccrine, 601
  sebaceum, 618
  sebaceous, 584, 613
adenosquamous carcinoma, 523
adiposis dolorosa, 650
adnexal polyp of neonatal skin, 609
adult T-cell lymphoma/leukemia, 756
African trypanosomiasis, 491
AIDS
  necrotizing folliculitis, 301
  psoriasiform dermatitis, 54
ALA-dehydratase deficiency porphyria, 378
albinism
  oculocutaneous, 222
  partial, 221
Albright's hereditary osteodystrophy, 280
algal infections, 468
allergic contact dermatitis, 2, 67, 69, 74
alopecia
  androgenic, 319
  central centrifugal cicatricial, 321
  drug-induced, 320
  fibrosing in pattern distribution, 320
  lipedematous, 321
  postmenopausal frontal fibrosing, 320
  scarring, 320–1
    idiopathic, 320
    traction, 320
  temporal triangular, 319
  traumatic, 317
alopecia
  areata, 318
  musinosa, 275
  universalis congenita, 316
Alternaria spp., 456
Alternaria alternata, 458
alternariosis, 458
aluminum deposition, 293
amebae, 491

amebiasis, 491
amelanotic melanoma, 560
American trypanosomiasis, 491
amicrobial pustulosis associated with autoimmune
  disease, 98
amiodarone pigmentation, 294
amoxicillin reaction, 392
ampicillin reaction, 392
amyloid, 154
amyloid elastosis, 284
amyloidosis
  anosacral, 286
  auricular, 285
  biphasic, 285
  familial primary cutaneous, 286
  heredofamilial, 284
  macular, 285
  nodular, 286
  overall, 283
  poikilodermatous, 286
  primary systemic, 283
  secondary
    localized cutaneous, 286
    systemic, 283
anagen, 315
anagen effluvium, 320
anaplastic large cell lymphoma, 757
ancient nevus, 538
Ancylostoma braziliense, 499
androgenic alopecia, 319
anetoderma, 260
angioedema, 170
angioendotheliomatosis, reactive, 709
angiofibroma, 4, 715
  acral, 618–19
angiohistiocytoma, multinucleate cell, 708
angioimmunoblastic T-cell lymphoma, 765
angiokeratoma
  circumscriptum, 693
  corporis diffusum, 372, 693
  Fordyce variant, 693
  Mibelli variant, 693
  solitary/multiple, 693
angioleiomyoma, 659, 715
angiolipoma, 646, 651, 715
angiolymphoid hyperplasia with eosinophilia, 702
angioma
  cherry, 696
  tufted, 706
angiomatoid melanoma, 560
angiomatosis, bacillary, 430, 711
angiomyofibroblastoma, 715
  of vulva, 627
angiomyolipoma, 660
angiomyxolipoma, 652
angiomyxoma, 715
  superficial, 645